Integrated Electronic Health Records:

A Worktext for

Integrated Electronic Health Records:

A Worktext for

Third Edition

Lead Author: M. Beth Shanholtzer, MAEd, FAHIMA, RHIA

Director, HIM Program
Lord Fairfax Community College

Contributor: Amy L. Ensign, BHSA, CMA (AAMA), RMA (AMT)

Baker College

Contributor: Daniel J. Peterson, MBA, CMA (AAMA)

Herzing University

McGraw Hill Education

INTEGRATED ELECTRONIC HEALTH RECORDS: A WORKTEXT FOR GREENWAY
PRIME SUITE™, THIRD EDITION

Published by McGraw-Hill Education, 2 Penn Plaza, New York, NY 10121. Copyright © 2018 by
McGraw-Hill Education. All rights reserved. Printed in the United States of America. Previous
editions © 2015 and 2012. No part of this publication may be reproduced or distributed in any form or by
any means, or stored in a database or retrieval system, without the prior written consent of McGraw-Hill
Education, including, but not limited to, in any network or other electronic storage or transmission, or
broadcast for distance learning.
Some ancillaries, including electronic and print components, may not be available to customers outside the
United States.
This book is printed on acid-free paper.

5 6 7 8 9 0 LMN 21 20 19

ISBN   978-1-260-04823-0
MHID   1-260-04823-3

Chief Product Officer, SVP Products & Markets: *G. Scott Virkler*
Vice President, General Manager, Products & Markets: *Mike Ryan*
Vice President, Content Design & Delivery: *Betsy Whalen*
Managing Director: *Thomas Timp*
Executive Brand Manager: *William Lawrensen*
Director, Product Development: *Rose Koos*
Senior Product Developer: *Michelle L. Flomenhoft*
Digital Product Analyst: *Katherine Ward*
Executive Marketing Manager: *Roxan Kinsey*
Director, Content Design & Delivery: *Linda Avenarius*
Program Manager: *Angela FitzPatrick*
Content Project Managers: *Jessica Portz, Emily Windelborn, and Karen Jozefowicz*
Buyer: *Susan K. Culbertson*
Design: *Tara McDermott*
Cover Image: *©enjoynz/GettyImages*
Content Licensing Specialists: *Melissa Homer and Melisa Seegmiller*
Compositor: *SPi Global*
Printer: *LSC Communications*

The Internet addresses listed in the text were accurate at the time of publication. The inclusion of a website does
not indicate an endorsement by the authors or McGraw-Hill Education, and McGraw-Hill Education does not
guarantee the accuracy of the information presented at these sites.

mheducation.com/highered

brief contents

contents

preface

EHR Matters

Welcome to the third edition of *Integrated Electronic Health Records: An Online Course and Worktext for Greenway Prime Suite*™!

Healthcare is experiencing increased use of electronic health records in the United States, which is creating even more opportunities for people who want to work in the health professions. From front office staff to nurses, doctors, health information professionals, coders, and every worker in between, understanding how health information is transferred and how that information can improve the quality of healthcare is a valuable skill. Those working in healthcare settings will be impacted by electronic health records as they complete their daily tasks.

Developed as a comprehensive learning resource, this hands-on course for Integrated Electronic Health Records is offered through McGraw-Hill's *Connect. Connect* uses the latest technology and learning techniques to better connect professors to their students, and students to the information and customized resources they need to master a subject.

Integrated Electronic Health Records: A Worktext for Greenway Prime Suite complements the online *Connect* course and is written by an author with an extensive health information management/health information technology background: M. Beth Shanholtzer, MAEd, FAHIMA, RHIA. New contributors Amy Ensign and Daniel J. Peterson share their combined 40+ years of experience as clinical and administrative medical assistants and educators in the field.

Both the worktext and the online course include coverage of Greenway Prime Suite, an ONC-ATCB-certified, fully integrated, online electronic health records, practice management, and interoperable physician-based solution. The book is not meant to be an extensive user manual for Prime Suite; rather, it covers the key topics for electronic health records, with Prime Suite as the vehicle to demonstrate those topics. Attention is paid to providing the "why" behind each task so that the reader can accumulate transferable skills. The coverage is focused on using an EHR program in a doctor's office, while providing additional information on how tasks might also be completed in a hospital setting.

Electronic health records impact a variety of programs in the health professions; thus, this content will be relevant to health information management, health information technology, medical insurance, billing & coding, and medical assisting programs.

New to the Third Edition

In this third edition of *IEHR*, ICD-10-CM is the coding system used in exercises. New key terms have been added to several of the chapters. Each chapter ends with a key feature, Applying Your Skills, to give yet another opportunity for students to use what they have learned in each chapter. Additional Prime Suite exercises have been added as well, bringing the total to 70 exercises.

While content updates have been made to all of the chapters, here are the highlights:

Chapter 2

Additional roles and titles have been added in keeping with the expanding roles of health information and other allied health professionals. The end-of-chapter assessments have been expanded to capture these new roles and titles.

Chapter 4

The Applying Your Skills exercises previously found at the end of this chapter have been moved to Chapter 11, as part of a group of exercises that allow students to process a patient in the EHR from the time a single appointment is made until the claim for that encounter is paid.

Chapter 5

In the third edition, the use of scribes for documentation has been expanded upon.

Chapter 6

The third edition focuses on exercises based on ICD-10-CM, with a brief history of ICD-9-CM. Code linkage as part of the billing process, patient payments such as co-pays and coinsurances, adjudication, and the medical billing and documentation cycle are also discussed in greater detail.

Chapter 7

The third edition includes updates to HIPAA and security, and a lesson in information governance has been added to Chapter 7.

Chapter 9

The third edition discusses the current use of Stage 2 of Meaningful Use, along with the upcoming transition to Stage 3. A new figure depicting an example of a Meaningful Use dashboard has been added.

Chapter 10

The third edition includes a brief history of the initial adoption of electronic health records. It also discusses ancillary technologies, such as patient portals and personal health records, in greater detail.

Chapter 11

Chapter 11 is new to the third edition. Throughout this text, students learn their EHR skills by completing guided exercises using step-by-step directions. This chapter, however, provides them with the exciting opportunity to use those skills in a "real-world" application by following a scenario that takes them through the entire medical documentation and billing process. Using source documents and references to previous chapters, students must use their critical thinking skills to accomplish the tasks in this scenario.

The exercises in this chapter's scenario are consistent with previous exercises in that they are performed in a simulated environment, which facilitates instant feedback to the students and easier grading for instructors. Modules can also be assigned individually, making this chapter highly customizable.

McGraw-Hill Connect®
Learn Without Limits

Connect is a teaching and learning platform that is proven to deliver better results for students and instructors.

Connect empowers students by continually adapting to deliver precisely what they need, when they need it, and how they need it, so your class time is more engaging and effective.

> 73% of instructors who use **Connect** require it; instructor satisfaction **increases** by 28% when **Connect** is required.

Connect's Impact on Retention Rates, Pass Rates, and Average Exam Scores

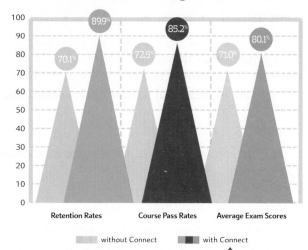

	Retention Rates	Course Pass Rates	Average Exam Scores
without Connect	70.1%	72.5%	71.0%
with Connect	89.9%	85.2%	80.1%

without Connect   with Connect

> Using **Connect** improves retention rates by **19.8%**, passing rates by **12.7%**, and exam scores by **9.1%**.

Analytics

Connect Insight®

Connect Insight is Connect's new one-of-a-kind visual analytics dashboard—now available for both instructors and students—that provides at-a-glance information regarding student performance, which is immediately actionable. By presenting assignment, assessment, and topical performance results together with a time metric that is easily visible for aggregate or individual results, Connect Insight gives the user the ability to take a just-in-time approach to teaching and learning, which was never before available. Connect Insight presents data that empowers students and helps instructors improve class performance in a way that is efficient and effective.

Impact on Final Course Grade Distribution

	without Connect		with Connect
A	22.9%		31.0%
B	27.4%		34.3%
C	22.9%		18.7%
D	11.5%		6.1%
F	15.4%		9.9%

> Students can view their results for any **Connect** course.

Mobile

Connect's new, intuitive mobile interface gives students and instructors flexible and convenient, anytime–anywhere access to all components of the Connect platform.

Adaptive

THE **ADAPTIVE** **READING EXPERIENCE**
DESIGNED TO TRANSFORM THE WAY STUDENTS READ

More students earn **A's** and **B's** when they use McGraw-Hill Education **Adaptive** products.

SmartBook®

Proven to help students improve grades and study more efficiently, SmartBook contains the same content within the print book, but actively tailors that content to the needs of the individual. SmartBook's adaptive technology provides precise, personalized instruction on what the student should do next, guiding the student to master and remember key concepts, targeting gaps in knowledge and offering customized feedback, and driving the student toward comprehension and retention of the subject matter. Available on tablets, SmartBook puts learning at the student's fingertips—anywhere, anytime.

Over **8 billion questions** have been answered, making McGraw-Hill Education products more intelligent, reliable, and precise.

STUDENTS WANT

Mc Graw Hill Education **SMARTBOOK**®

95% of students reported **SmartBook** to be a more effective way of reading material.

100% of students want to use the Practice Quiz feature available within **SmartBook** to help them study.

100% of students reported having reliable access to off-campus wifi.

90% of students say they would purchase **SmartBook** over print alone.

95% of students reported that **SmartBook** would impact their study skills in a positive way.

Mc Graw Hill Education

*Findings based on 2015 focus group results administered by McGraw-Hill Education

www.mheducation.com

A one-stop spot to present, deliver, and assess digital assets available from McGraw-Hill: McGraw-Hill Connect Integrated EHR

Seventy Hands-on Simulated Prime Suite Exercises are available through *Connect:*

- Prime Suite Exercises appear in Chapters 3–9 and 11. The exercises in Chapters 3–9 are correlated to Learning Outcomes, while the exercises in Chapter 11 include references back to earlier chapters.
- Prime Suite Exercises include the following modes (with the instructor deciding which modes to assign to the students):
  - *Demo Mode—watch a demonstration of the exercise (includes optional audio of the steps).*
  - *Practice Mode—try the exercise yourself with guidance (includes optional audio of the steps).*
  - *Test Mode—complete the exercise on your own.*
- Students receive a score from *Connect* after completing each mode. They receive 100% for completing all steps in Demo Mode and again in Practice Mode. They receive a percentage based on how many steps they execute correctly in Test Mode.
- For each Prime Suite Exercise, the same data is used for all of the modes in order to reinforce the skill being taught in that exercise.
- Each Prime Suite Exercise is labeled with
  - *HIM (Health Information Management)*
  - *PM (Practice Management)*
  - *EHR (Electronic Health Records)*
  - *Or some combination of the above three*

Much more information on how to complete the exercises in *Connect* can be found in the Library tab in *Connect* (instructor access only).

Instructor Resources

You can rely on the following materials to help you and your students work through the material in the book; all are available in the Instructor Resources under the Library tab in *Connect* (available only to instructors who are logged in to *Connect*).

Supplement	Features
Instructor's Manual (organized by Learning Outcomes)	Each chapter has • Lesson Plans and Teaching Tips • Outline of PowerPoint Presentations • Answer Keys for Check Your Understanding Questions and End-of-Chapter Questions
PowerPoint Presentations (organized by Learning Outcomes)	• Key Terms • Key Concepts • Created using MHE Accessible Template

Supplement	Features
Electronic Test Bank	- Computerized and *Connect* - Word Version - Questions are tagged with learning outcomes, level of difficulty, level of Bloom's taxonomy, feedback, ABHES, CAAHEP, and CAHIIM competencies.
Tools to Plan Course	- Transition Guide, by chapter, from Shanholtzer, 2e, to Shanholtzer, 3e - Correlations by learning outcomes to ABHES, CAAHEP, CAHIIM, and NHA - Sample Syllabi and Lesson Plans - Certificate of Completion - Asset Map—a recap of the key Instructor Resources, tied to the Learning Outcomes, as well as information on the content available through *Connect*
Tips for Prime Suite Exercises	- Multiple documents to help you and your students implement the Prime Suite Exercises in your course through *Connect*

Want to learn more about this product? Attend one of our online webinars. To learn more about them, please contact your McGraw-Hill learning technology representative. To find your McGraw-Hill representative, go to www.mheducation.com and click "Contact," then "Contact a Sales Rep."

Need help? Contact the McGraw-Hill Education Customer Experience Group (CXG). Visit the CXG website at www.mhhe.com/support. Browse our frequently asked questions (FAQs) and product documentation and/or contact a CXG representative.

Walkthrough of Integrated EHR Connect

EHR Matters . . . Be Prepared!

Complete 70 simulated Prime Suite Exercises, organized into the following modes (the instructor will determine which modes are assigned to the students):

DEMO: Watch a demonstration of the exercise. Note the Step Window on the right of the screen, which includes a Printer icon that allows you to print the steps when clicked. Audio is available with this mode.

PRACTICE: Try the same exercise yourself with guidance. The Step Window and audio are also available with this mode.

TEST: Complete the same exercise on your own, with a point given for each correct step.

FOR INSTRUCTORS

LIBRARY TAB: This includes access to the SmartBook eBook and the Instructor Resources.

about the Author and Contributors

M. Beth Shanholtzer, MAEd, FAHIMA, RHIA
Courtesy of the author

M. Beth Shanholtzer, MAEd, FAHIMA, RHIA has been in the health information management field for 37 years. Her experience has included HIM department management positions within hospitals in New Jersey, Pennsylvania, West Virginia, and Maryland. She has been in academics for nearly 23 years and is currently the program director for an HIM associate degree program, a medical billing and coding certificate program, and a medical administrative assistant certificate program at Lord Fairfax Community College in Middletown, Virginia. She previously held positions as program director and instructor of associate degree programs at Kaplan University.

She is active in AHIMA as chairperson and member of the Faculty Development Workgroup of the Council for Excellence in Education. On the state level, Beth has served as president, education chair, and legislative chair of the West Virginia Health Information Management Association.

Beth lives in Martinsburg, West Virginia, with her husband; they have three children.

Amy Ensign, BHSA, CMA (AAMA), RMA (AMT)
Courtesy of the author

Amy Ensign, BHSA, CMA (AAMA), RMA (AMT), has been in the medical field for over 20 years, working clinically, administratively, and in higher education. Beginning her career as a medical assistant with one of Michigan's major healthcare organizations, she moved into a leadership role working with senior management and supervising medical assistants. During this time, she began teaching as an adjunct instructor for Baker College and eight years ago moved into her current position as medical assistant and medical administrative specialist program director position for Baker College of Clinton Township. She is also active in the AAMA as treasurer of Michigan's Macomb Chapter. Amy lives in Grosse Pointe Woods, Michigan, with her husband and two children.

Daniel Peterson, MBA, CMA (AAMA)
Courtesy of the author

Daniel J. Peterson, MBA, CMA (AAMA), has been in the medical field on both the clinical and the business sides for over 20 years, starting his career as a medical assistant and then moving into management roles in clinics and hospitals. He has been in higher education for over 10 years. His experience has included medical assisting program chair at Corinthian Colleges and Minnesota School of Business, as well as health information management program chair at Minnesota School of Business. Dan is currently the business office supervisor at a large hospital in Minnesota. Dan lives in Blaine, Minnesota, with his wife; they have four children.

acknowledgments

Suggestions have been received from faculty and students throughout the country. This vital feedback is important for product development. Each person who has offered comments and suggestions has our thanks. The efforts of many people are needed to develop and improve a product. Among these people are the reviewers and consultants who point out areas of concern, cite areas of strength, and make recommendations for change. In this regard, the following instructors provided feedback that was enormously helpful.

Textbook Reviewers

Multiple instructors reviewed the book prior to publication, providing valuable feedback that directly impacted the book.

Laura Abel, BS, RHIT
ECPI University-Online Campus

Tammy L Burnette, PhD

Deborah Honstad, MA, RHIA
San Juan College

Patricia Jones, MBA, CPC, CMAA , CBCS
Ultimate Medical Academy

Fonzette Smith Leavell, MBA, M Ed
Ultimate Medical Academy

Donna Pritchard, RHIT LPN
Ozarks Technical Community College

Lisa Riggs, CPC, CPC-I
Ultimate Medical Academy-Online

Carla H. Ruffins, MS, RHIA, CHTS-PW
San Jacinto College

Patricia A. Saccone, MA, RHIA, CCS-P
Waubonsee Community College

Amber Schappaugh, MA, RMA (AMT)
Midstate College

Special thanks to the instructors who helped with the development of *Connect*, SmartBook, and the Prime Suite Exercises. These include:

Elaine Elder, ScD
Colorado Technical University

Savanna Garrity, CPC, MPA
Madisonville Community College

Leslie Gordon, MS, RHIA, FAHIMA
University of Alaska Southeast

Wendy M. Harrigan, CPC, CPMA
Ultimate Medical Academy

Lynnette Hessling, RHIA, MSHI, CHTS-PW, CHTS-TR
Ultimate Medical Academy

Susan Holler, MSEd, CPC, CMRS
Bryant & Stratton College

Deborah Honstad, MA, RHIA
San Juan College

Laura J. Michelsen, MJ, MS, RHIA, CHPS, CHDA

Corina Miranda, CMPC-I, CPC
American Academy of Professional Coders, Education Officer

Rolando Russell, MBA, RHIA, CPC, CPAR
Ultimate Medical Academy

Patricia A. Saccone, MA, RHIA, CCS-P
Waubonsee Community College

Patricia L. Tyhurst, CPC-I, COC, CPC

Jennifer Walters, BS, CMA
Delaware Technical Community College

Acknowledgments from the Author and Contributors

From Beth Shanholtzer: This text is dedicated to my family, friends, colleagues, and students who encourage and enlighten me every day. A special thanks goes to the McGraw-Hill Health Professions team for the opportunity to share my years of practical and academic experience through this text.

From Amy Ensign: I would like to say a special thank you to the McGraw-Hill Health Professions Team, namely Michelle Flomenhoft, Bill Lawrensen, and all of the folks who work behind the scenes to make the magic happen.

I would also like to thank a very special friend, Liz Hoffman, and Baker College for providing me with the opportunity many years ago to blend my medical background with academia. It has been a wonderful experience to reach out to the medical community and touch the lives of patients exponentially through my students. I am grateful!

A final thank you to my family, Jason, Ryan, and Brandon, who have been patient and supportive champions of every endeavor I undertake. You are the foundation of all of my successes!

From Dan Peterson: I want to thank the McGraw-Hill Health Professions Team, especially Michelle Flomenhoft and William Lawrensen, who gave me this opportunity and have been a continual source of support and encouragement.

I also need to thank my family who have supported me and have been so excited that dad is working on a "college book." To my wonderful wife Kristin, who has always been by my side with love and support throughout any situation we have been in. You are my best friend.

From All: Much appreciation goes to the McGraw-Hill staff for bringing this product to life: Bill Lawrensen, Executive Brand Manager for Health Professions; Roxan Kinsey, Executive Marketing Manager for Health Professions; Katie Ward, Digital Product Analyst for Health Professions; Michelle Flomenhoft, Senior Product Developer for Health Professions; Jessica Portz and Emily Windelborn, Content Project Managers; Sue Culbertson, Buyer; Tara McDermott, Designer; and Melissa Homer and Melisa Seegmiller, Content Licensing Specialists. Additional thanks go to Karen Jozefowicz for the support on the digital end, as well as to Melinda Bilecki, and Alyssa Heiber who lent their copyediting and reviewing skills to the project.

We would also like to thank our partners at Greenway Health™ for their continued support of this project, especially Angie Rhoads and Mike Kitchens.

An Overview of

Prime Suite's Practice Management and Electronic Health Record Software

At the end of this chapter, the student should be able to

1.1 Describe practice management applications.

1.2 List the advantages and disadvantages of an electronic health record.

1.3 Describe EHR applications.

1.4 Chart the flow of information from registration through processing of the claim.

1.5 Use the Help feature in Prime Suite.

Application

Care provider

Clearinghouse

Current Procedural Terminology (CPT)

Demographic (identifying) data

Electronic claims submission

Electronic health record (EHR)

Electronic medical record (EMR)

Encounter form (Superbill or routing slip)

International Classification of Diseases, 10th revision, Clinical Modification/Procedure Coding System (ICD-10-CM/PCS)

Interoperability

Master Patient (Person) Index

Patient List

Point of care

Practice management (PM)

Routing Slip (encounter form or Superbill)

Speech recognition technology

Superbill (encounter form or routing slip)

What You Need to Know and Why You Need to Know It

The purpose of this worktext is to introduce students to software used to gather, track, and store the clinical and administrative information of patients seen in the medical facility. This information is used for coordinating patient care; for filing claims for reimbursement; for reporting practice information to insurance carriers as well as government and nongovernment agencies; and for gathering statistics about the types of patients treated at the facility. We will be using Greenway Health's Prime Suite practice management (PM) and electronic health record (EHR) software throughout the text. This worktext is not meant to teach all the functionality of Prime Suite; instead, it is meant to demonstrate the most common electronic functions carried out in a medical office, hospital, or other healthcare facility.

This first chapter is an introduction and overview. The concepts in this chapter will be further explained throughout the text.

1.1 Practice Management Applications

Practice management Software used in physicians' offices to gather data on every patient and perform administrative functions from the time an appointment is made through the time the bill for each visit is paid.

Electronic health record (EHR) Comprehensive record of all health records for a patient, which is able to be shared electronically with other health providers as necessary.

Electronic medical record (EMR) The legal patient record that is created within any healthcare facility (hospital, nursing home, ambulatory surgery facility, physician's office, etc.). The EMR is the data source for the electronic health record (EHR).

for your information **fyi**

A healthcare facility is a hospital, a physician's practice, a dental practice, an outpatient diagnostic center, outpatient rehabilitation, outpatient psychological services, hospice, home healthcare, long-term care, or an ambulatory surgery center.

Typically, software (computer programs that carry out functions or operations) used in a medical office for administrative functions is known as **practice management (PM)** software. Filing an insurance claim for a patient is an example of an administrative function. Through the use of PM software, data are gathered on every patient from the time an appointment is made through the time the bill for each visit is paid. **Electronic health (medical) record (EHR/EMR)** software includes the clinical documentation of patient care. The patient's chief complaint, record of vital signs, results of physical examination, and past medical history are all examples of clinical data.

Greenway Health's Prime Suite is both a PM and an EHR solution using a single database. The use of this single database to document the administrative and clinical aspects of patient care allows the provider to concentrate on the care of the patient, improve the quality of the documentation collected, and share that documentation with other healthcare providers as appropriate, with the result of better coordination of the patient's overall care.

We will first look at the applications typically found in practice management software, including Prime Suite. *Practice management* is a term used in physicians' practices. In other healthcare facilities, including hospitals, these functions will also be computerized but are referred to as registration, admission, discharge, transfer (R-ADT); billing systems; or something similar.

The main applications include

- Entering each patient seen into a master list
- Scheduling appointments
- Assigning ICD-10-CM/PCS and CPT codes
- Completing a billing claim form for each visit
- Sending the insurance claims to insurance carriers

More details on each of these applications follow.

Entering Each Patient Seen into a Master List

Each patient seen, whether in a physician's office or a hospital, is only entered once into what is known as the **Patient List** or **Master Patient (Person) Index** (listings of all patients seen in an office or hospital). These will be further discussed in a future chapter. This is done during the registration process. The first time a patient is registered, the patient is entered into the Master Patient Index/Patient List; on subsequent visits, the Master Patient Index/Patient List is searched for that patient, and any changes in demographic information, such as change in address, phone number, or a change in insurance coverage is/are made. The current encounter appears once the registration is complete as well.

It is during the registration process that consent forms to treat as well as to bill insurance are typically signed.

Scheduling Appointments

To maintain efficiency in an office, it is important that appointment times are entered accurately. Think of it this way—if a patient were told to come to the office for an appointment at a particular date and time, but the appointment book showed another date and time for that patient to be seen, the end result would be disorganization for the office as well as unhappy patients and staff. Computerizing this function allows sufficient time to be allotted to each patient based on the reason for his or her visit, and it allows for more efficient scheduling of the provider's time.

Assigning ICD-10-CM/PCS Diagnosis and CPT Procedure Codes

You may have noticed during a visit to your own physician's office that you are given a piece of paper when you leave the examining room. This is referred to as an **encounter form, a Superbill, or a routing slip**. There are many numbers, known as codes, on this paper. Every diagnosis made by a care provider is written in narrative form in a patient's health record and then carried over to the Superbill. These narrative diagnoses are converted into alphanumeric form with a coding system known as **International Classification of Diseases, 10th revision, Clinical Modification Procedure Coding System (ICD-10-CM/PCS)**. The same occurs for each procedure performed, but the coding system used is **Current Procedural Terminology (CPT)**. The Superbill and coding functions will be covered in detail in the chapter on insurance and billing functions of this text. Most likely, you will have a separate course or courses in billing and coding as well.

Completing a Billing Claim Form for Each Visit

In order to submit bills to health insurance carriers, a claim form must be generated for each visit. This is done by compiling the patient's identifying data, his or her insurance data, and the ICD-10-CM/PCS and CPT codes into claim forms such as the CMS-837P (electronic), CMS-1500 (paper), which are used by physicians' practices and other outpatient settings, or the UB-04, which is used to bill hospital, rehabilitation, end-stage renal facility, and other long term care-type settings.

Master Patient Index (MPI)/ Patient List A permanent listing of all patients who have received care in a hospital (inpatient or outpatient). In physicians' offices often referred to as a Master Patient List or Patient List. May also be known as a Master Person List or Master Person Index.

Encounter form A document (paper or electronic) that is used in medical offices to capture the diagnoses and services or procedures performed and from which the CMS-1500 billing form is completed. Also known as a routing slip or Superbill.

International Classification of Diseases, 10th revision, Clinical Modification/Procedure Coding System (ICD-10-CM/PCS) The classification system used to convert narrative diagnoses and procedures into numeric codes. Effective October 1, 2015, replaced ICD-9-CM.

Current Procedural Terminology (CPT) Coding system used to convert narrative procedures and services into numeric form. CPT is used to code procedures and services in a physician's office; in a hospital setting, it is used for outpatient coding (emergency room, outpatient diagnostic testing, or ambulatory surgery, for example).

Sending the Insurance Claims to Insurance Carriers

Once the claim form is generated, it is submitted to the insurance carrier for payment. Some hard-copy claim forms are still mailed to the insurance carrier, but the majority of forms are sent by **electronic claims submission**. Filing a claim electronically means that the information is sent by wire to a **clearinghouse** or directly to the insurance carrier. Filing claims electronically reduces billing errors and processing time, which results in faster payment. A clearinghouse is a service that processes data into a standardized billing format and checks for inconsistencies or other errors in the data.

The patient's **demographic (identifying) data** are collected as part of the administrative (non-clinical) information, as well as information needed for the business processes that take place in a healthcare facility—for instance, gathering insurance information, completing a claim form, and submitting a claim.

Administrative data include insurance and financial data, authorization to bill the insurance company, correspondence related to billing matters, and the like. Demographic data identify the patient—name, address, phone numbers, sex, race, and so on. The demographic data are specific administrative data that help differentiate one patient from another with the same name.

Electronic claims submission
Submitting insurance claims via wire to a clearinghouse or directly to the insurance carrier.

Clearinghouse A service that processes data into a standardized billing format and checks for inconsistencies or other errors in the data.

Demographic (identifying) data
Data that identify the patient. Consist of name, date of birth, sex, race, and Social Security number (may vary by facility policy).

Check Your Understanding

1. Is Prime Suite a practice management tool or an electronic health record? Support your answer.
2. List the types of data that insurance companies need to be provided with on a billing claim form.

1.2 Why Adopt Electronic Health Record Applications?

The widespread acceptance of an electronic health record has been slow compared to other industries such as banking or retail. Healthcare administrators and care providers have long been leery of electronic health records. Security concerns, the lengthy implementation process, and the high cost of implementing an EHR headline the reasons for a culture of uncertainty and a "let's wait and see" attitude. The perception has been that paper records are more secure—not as susceptible to loss, theft, or tampering, since there is a tangible object that can be seen or carried from place to place by a human being. In reality, paper records are potentially more susceptible to loss or tampering than an electronic record. A paper record cannot be "followed," whereas every entry, change, or view of an electronic record can be tracked and reported. With proper backup procedures, EHRs cannot be lost or misfiled, which is not the case with paper records. Of course, if a patient's name is misspelled or if a patient used a different name on a previous registration, then location will be difficult, but there are other ways to search for the record such as by date of birth, which is not possible with a paper record. Security will be discussed in more detail in the chapter on privacy and security.

The initial purchase and implementation costs of an EMR/EHR are high—much higher than the cost of file folders and filing equipment in a paper system. The research and development of an electronic system by service providers (software companies), the allocation of human resources for planning and training, and the cost of hardware and additional software all contribute to these costs. There is an ongoing cost of maintaining any system, paper or electronic. The return on investment of an electronic system is in enhanced patient safety and improved quality of care, less duplication of effort, a more efficiently run office, instant access to patient health records, and the data needed for reporting purposes. Though for a time the paper system will still be maintained, gradually the costs of filing supplies, the physical space needed for paper records, and long-term storage (archiving) will lessen once the electronic system is in place.

For care providers, there is a high learning curve, and they must be willing to devote time to the new system before it is second nature to them. Though care providers are often resistant to putting in that investment of time, in the end they will find their time is used more for patient care than for "charting." The productivity of healthcare professionals such as nurses, laboratory technicians, and medical assistants will be negatively impacted in the beginning until they, too, learn the electronic system.

As for administrative staff, learning an EHR system is more time consuming and has a higher learning curve than the manual processes associated with paper records. After all, filing, whether alphabetic or numeric, is more intuitive than searching a computer database or knowing which screen a particular piece of data resides on; and again, a piece of paper or a folder full of papers is tangible, whereas an electronic system is not.

Sharing information has also been a sticking point. Though patients have had access to their records for many years, they were not well informed about how to gain that access, and many did not know that they could even request an amendment to their health records. Healthcare providers have been fearful of releasing patients' health records to others, including other healthcare providers, because there is a sense of loss of control over the information and lack of confidentiality.

This sharing of health information with other healthcare providers or entities is possible because of **interoperability**. It means that many different functions can take place and information can be shared between computer systems, or within applications of the same computer system, which is not possible with a manual or paper record system. For instance, in her physician's practice, Alicia Matthews' medical information is readily accessible and just a couple of clicks away, regardless of whether a pharmacy needs a list of her allergies before refilling a prescription or the practice's billing staff needs her policy number. Also, let's say Alicia is a patient of Dr. Ingram. She has been seen for repeated bouts of strep throat. Dr. Ingram has referred her to Dr. Johnson, an otorhinolaryngologist (ear, nose, and throat specialist). Her appointment with Dr. Johnson is set up for July 2. When she arrives for her appointment, Dr. Johnson already has her records from Dr. Ingram, and rather than having to take all of Alicia's information over again, the doctor can spend the time examining Alicia and determining a plan of care. Because the computer systems at the two offices are interoperable, the information can be shared seamlessly.

In recent years, this "wait and see" culture has been subsiding. As research shows that there has been a decrease in medical errors and an increase in timeliness of diagnosis and treatment due in large part to timely

Interoperability Many different functions can take place and information can be shared between computer systems, or within applications of the same computer system, which is not possible with a manual or paper record system.

TABLE 1.1   Comparison of Paper to Electronic Health Records

Paper Health Records	Electronic Health Records
Security concerns include theft and tampering with documentation.	Security concerns include loss of data and computer hackers.
Individual records are easily lost or misfiled.	Misfiling is not an issue as long as the patient's name is spelled correctly.
Startup costs are relatively inexpensive.	Startup costs are relatively high.
Operating costs are relatively inexpensive, as the system does not change drastically from year to year.	Operating costs are dependent on level of support from software vendor, maintenance costs, and cost of upgrades.
Records take up a great deal of space.	They do not take up physical space other than the desktop computers.
Archiving costs are high.	Archiving costs are for disk or server space.
Training staff is a relatively short and inexpensive process.	Staff and physician training is time consuming.
Physicians perceive that writing or dictating is easier than typing into a computer.	Once learned, documentation is easily done by point and click or voice recognition systems.
Documentation by care providers tends to be less detailed.	Documentation by care providers tends to be more detailed.
Sharing health information with other care providers or healthcare facilities is a time-consuming process and may delay diagnosis or treatment.	Sharing health information with other care providers or healthcare facilities is done in a timely manner and may assist in timely diagnosis and treatment.

access to information—for instance, a patient's allergy to penicillin or the fact that a patient has already had her gallbladder removed—care providers and administrators are more open-minded and are pushing for totally paperless systems within their facilities. Increasingly, healthcare providers are accepting that an informed patient is a more compliant patient and that patients should have a say in their medical care.

Ensuring regulatory compliance is also made easier and more efficient through use of an electronic health record. Report-writing capabilities available in electronic systems allow for fast, reliable data submission and retrieval.

Table 1.1 shows a comparison of issues encountered in paper record-keeping versus electronic record-keeping (Table 1.1).

From a more global perspective, the use of electronic medical records will allow for the collection of incredible amounts of clinical data for use in medical research and epidemiology, which will have a profound effect on healthcare worldwide.

Check Your Understanding

1. Is a paper-based system of records more secure than an electronic one? Explain your answer.
2. Why are startup costs significantly higher with EHRs versus paper-based records?

Now, let's take a look at the electronic record using Prime Suite.

It is through the EHR functionality that clinical information is collected and includes the patient's medical history, the patient's current condition(s), the treatment rendered, the results of treatment, the prognosis, the plan of care, the diagnosis, and any instructions given by the provider.

Prime Suite's EHR **applications** (functionality) include

- Clinical documentation of a patient's visit (the progress note) by the **care provider**
- The prescription of medications and their electronic submission to the patient's pharmacy of choice through use of the ePrescribing solution
- Exchange of clinical information between medical providers or other entities with a need to know, through the Greenway Exchange solution
- The ability to access clinical trials, evidence-based medicine, and pharmaceutical research to improve patient care, as well as access to clinical and financial benchmarking services to enhance financial management by using the Prime Research solution
- Mobile EHR applications available on personal digital assistants (PDAs) or smartphones to allow providers instant access anytime and anywhere through Prime Mobile.
- **Point of care** dictation of progress notes by the provider through Prime Speech, which is a form of **speech (voice) recognition technology**. Speech recognition technology allows documentation to occur on the computer screen as the care provider dictates notes. *Point of care* refers to the dictation that occurs at the very time the patient is being seen.

Application Software that has a special purpose, such as word processing or spreadsheet, or for a particular industry such as practice management or electronic health record software.

Care provider Term used to refer to a physician, physician's assistant, dentist, psychologist, nurse practitioner, or midwife.

Point of care Documentation, dictation, ordering of tests and procedures that occur at the same time the patient is being seen.

Speech recognition technology Software that recognizes the words being said by the person dictating, and converts the speech to text. Speech recognition technology "learns" the dictator's voice as corrections are made by an editor, while voice recognition does not.

Check Your Understanding

1. What does Prime Suite's Greenway Exchange function do?
2. What is Prime Speech?
3. Dr. Harrison's office uses Prime Suite as its practice management (PM) and electronic health record (EHR) solution. For each of the following, which application within Prime Suite would be used? Would it be PM, EHR, Prime Speech, Greenway Exchange, or Scheduling? Select the *best* answer. (An application may be used more than once or not at all.)
    a. Elaine Verados is a patient of Dr. Harrison, and he has referred her to Dr. Smithton, an otorhinolaryngologist, for an opinion on treating a persistent problem with her right ear. Dr. Harrison documents the patient's history and request for consultation, which is electronically submitted to Dr. Smithton's office.
    b. Dr. Harrison dictates the letter requesting Dr. Smithton to give her opinion of Elaine Verados' condition using _____.
    c. Carl Pike calls the office of Dr. Harrison because he wishes to establish care at that office. Dr. Harrison is taking new patients, so a mutually agreed-upon time is set up for Carl to have a physical exam by Dr. Harrison. The application used to do this is _____.
    d. Dr. Harrison documents Carl Pike's known drug allergies. This is done in the _____.
    e. Dr. Harrison dictates the results of Carl Pike's physical examination, and his words appear on the computer screen as he is speaking. This application is _____.
    f. A listing of all patients ever seen in Dr. Harrison's office is found in which solution?

If you think about your past experiences visiting a physician's office, you will recognize many of these steps and how similar they are to your experience. Of course, not every step is exactly the same in every office, but the basic premise is the same.

In step one (Figure 1.1) an appointment is made. Of course, if you were going to an urgent care center or an emergency room, this step is not necessary. Once the appointment is made, you go to the office on the day and time of the appointment and you are "checked in." This is known as registration— some of your administrative data may have been taken over the phone, but the data may be verified and more may be collected when you appear for the appointment. Also, if new authorization forms or other administrative forms need to be signed, that is done at this point.

After you are checked in, you wait to be seen by the care providers (Figure 1.2). First, you are called back to the exam room by a healthcare professional (Figure 1.3); your height, weight, and vital signs (temperature, pulse, blood pressure) are taken; and you are asked questions about why you are being seen today and your medical history. Once those are complete, the care provider steps in for the actual exam (Figure 1.4).

Once the care provider has completed the exam, assessed your condition, and given you a plan of care, including instructions, the business functions begin (Figure 1.5 and Figure 1.6). These include the check-out and billing procedures. Some of these procedures are repeated or continue for several weeks or months until the claim is paid and the patient's account reflects a zero balance.

In cases where the care provider has ordered diagnostic procedures such as x-rays or laboratory tests, the clinical documentation steps are repeated (Figure 1.7).

for your information **fyi**

The term *care provider* will be used to refer to any physician, physician's assistant, dentist, psychologist, nurse practitioner, or midwife.

for your information **fyi**

The medical assistant, nurse, receptionist, health information technician, medical biller/coder, and office administrative personnel will be referred to as *healthcare professionals* throughout the text.

Appointment Scheduling

New Patient Calls the Office

Patient Search/ Add New Patient

Scheduling Dashboard/ Wizard/ Quick Search

Make Appointment for Patient

Referral Management (Alt:R)

Link to Patient Information/ Update Insurance for Automated Eligibilty Verification

Figure 1.1 **Appointment Scheduling Flowchart**

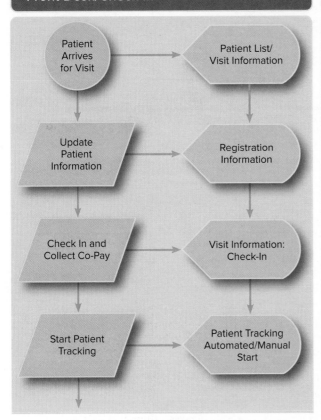

Figure 1.2 Front Desk Check-In Flowchart

Figure 1.3 Nursing/Clinical Support Flowchart

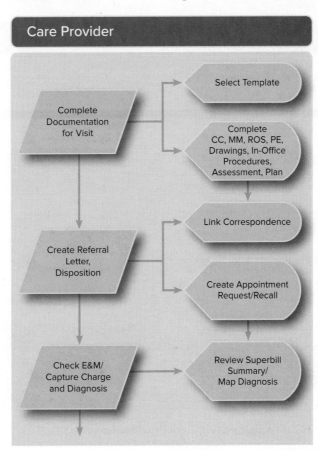

Figure 1.4 Care Provider Flowchart

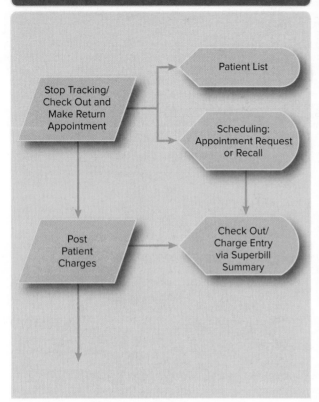

Figure 1.5   Check-Out Desk Flowchart

Figure 1.6   Business Office/Billing Flowchart

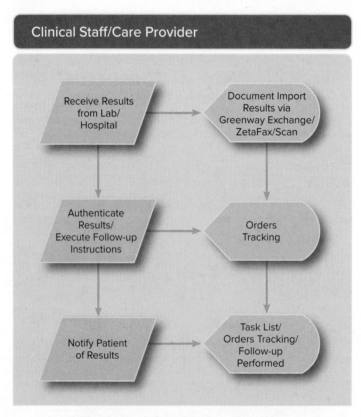

Figure 1.7   Clinical Staff/Care Provider Flowchart

1. Put the following steps in the flow of information into the correct order: front desk checks in the patient; business office/billing processes charges; patient is processed at check-out desk; appointment scheduling personnel make patient's appointment; nursing/clinical support sees patient; clinical staff/care provider examines patient.

2. Under what circumstances would clinical documentation steps need to be repeated?

1.5 Use of the Help Feature

The use of Help text or of a Help function is standard in most software applications. You have no doubt used it from time to time when preparing word processing or spreadsheet applications. Prime Suite is no different.

Prime Suite Help text can be accessed through any screen, as you see in Figure 1.8.

By clicking on Help, the care provider or healthcare professional will gain access to the entire user's guide (Figure 1.9). The guide can be searched by topic, or by using the index or glossary. For instance, if you want to know more about vocabulary reconciliation, clicking on index allows you to access a keyword search, where the system begins to predict what you are

Figure 1.8   Accessing Help Screen from Desktop

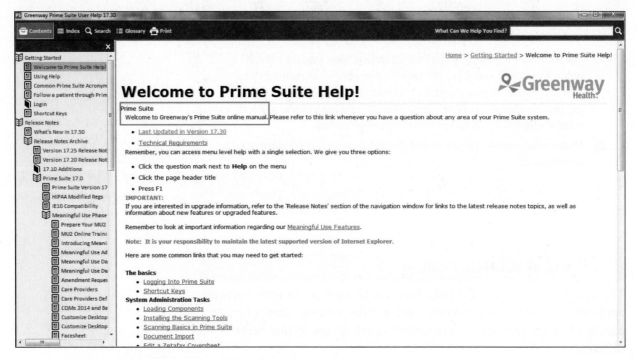

Figure 1.9   Prime Suite Online Manual (User's Guide)

searching for based on the first few characters typed or by an entire word typed in the search field (Figure 1.9).

The important thing about Help is that it is there for just that—to help you learn Prime Suite, to assist you when you are unsure of the steps you need to complete, and to keep you up to date with changes or new functionality added to the software.

Check Your Understanding

1. How do you access the Help feature in Prime Suite?
2. How many ways are there to locate information?
3. Using the Help feature, describe how to add a new allergy to a patient's chart.

APPLYING YOUR SKILLS

This worktext covers electronic health records and, to some extent, practice management functionality through the use of Greenway Health's Prime Suite software. Many other software systems are also available; searching out other software and becoming aware of what is available are things a health-care professional (and provider) should do periodically. Take some time now to do an Internet search of PM software and EHR software. Write a brief summary of three or four vendors of each software package.

chapter 1 **summary**

LEARNING OUTCOME	CONCEPTS FOR REVIEW

1.1 Describe practice management applications.	– What is practice management?
	– Practice management applications
	  • Master Patient Index/Patient List
	  • Schedule appointments
	  • Assign ICD-10-CM/PCS and CPT codes
	  • Complete billing claim form
	  • Send insurance claims to carriers

1.2 List the advantages and disadvantages of an electronic health record.	– Disadvantages
	  • Increased security functions
	  • High cost of implementation
	  • Training requirements
	– Advantages
	  • Possibly more secure than paper records
	  • High return on investment
	  • All information in one place
	  • Interoperability
	  • Assures regulatory compliance
	  • Exchange of information with those who have a need to know

1.3 Describe EHR applications.	– Clinical documentation – Electronic prescribing – Exchange of clinical information – Research evidence-based medicine, pharmaceutical research, clinical and financial benchmarking studies – Speech recognition

1.4 Chart the flow of information from registration through processing of the claim.	– Appointment scheduling
	– Front desk check-in
	  • Verify demographic information
	  • Sign authorization/administrative forms, if necessary
	– Patient taken to examining room
	  • Height, weight, vital signs taken
	  • Patient states the reason for today's visit (chief complaint)

(continued)

	– Care provider meets with the patient
	   • Provider verifies reason for visit; updates history
	   • Provider examines patient
	   • Provider makes referrals, if necessary
	   • Prescriptions electronically sent to pharmacy, if necessary
	   • Provider completes the chart, which then starts the coding and claims process
	   • Provider completes the visit and provides patient with a Superbill, routing slip, or encounter form
	– Patient stops at the check-out desk
	   • Superbill/routing slip/encounter form given to staff member at the check-out desk
	   • Patient pays co-pay, if not paid during check-in process
	   • Patient leaves the office
	– Business office/billing
	   • Insurance claim form is completed electronically
	   • Insurance claim is submitted electronically
	   • Insurance payment (or notice of denial) is received
	   • Payment is entered in the system
	   • Patient's account is updated
	   • Statement is sent, if necessary
	– Follow-up
	   • Results of diagnostic tests received, if applicable
	   • Record is updated with results
	   • Provider reviews results
	   • Patient is contacted, if necessary

1.5 Use the Help feature in Prime Suite.	– Use of Help from menu bar – Other means of accessing Help feature – User's guide

chapter **review**

MATCHING QUESTIONS

Match the terms on the left with the definitions on the right.

_____ 1. **[LO 1.2]** interoperability

_____ 2. **[LO 1.3]** application

_____ 3. **[LO 1.3]** care provider

_____ 4. **[LO 1.1]** clearinghouse

_____ 5. **[LO 1.1]** electronic claims submission

_____ 6. **[LO 1.1]** encounter form

_____ 7. **[LO 1.3]** point of care

_____ 8. **[LO 1.1]** practice management software

_____ 9. **[LO 1.3]** speech recognition

_____ 10. **[LO 1.1]** demographics

a. form generated at the completion of an office visit, a portion of which details the patient's diagnosis, the procedures and services performed, and the charge for each procedure/service

b. filing of a healthcare claim using a computer rather than paper

c. technology that digitally transcribes spoken words

d. specialized computer software that performs administrative and billing procedures in medical offices

e. documented patient information such as age, sex, and race

f. procedures that take place at the time of care, rather than at a remote location or at a point in time after care is complete

g. person, usually a physician, who performs health-care services requiring specialized education and training

h. software with a unique purpose, such as word processing, or used for a specific industry

i. allows syncing of multiple, unrelated functions or systems

j. service that assists in claims processing by standardizing billing and performing error checks

MULTIPLE-CHOICE QUESTIONS

Select the letter that best completes the statement or answers the question:

1. **[LO 1.1]** EHR/EMR software is more comprehensive than practice management software because it
   a. is computerized.
   b. contains more menu options.
   c. includes clinical documentation.
   d. submits insurance claims.

Enhance your learning by completing these exercises and more at http://**connect.mheducation.com**!

2. **[LO 1.3]** Prime Suite
   a. allows for ePrescribing.
   b. has mobile applications.
   c. assists in information exchange.
   d. all of these

3. **[LO 1.1]** A patient is entered into the Patient List
   a. once.
   b. twice.
   c. after a procedure.
   d. each time he or she is seen.

4. **[LO 1.2]** When transitioning from a paper to an electronic health record, healthcare facilities can expect the costs associated with health records to _____.
   a. increase
   b. decrease
   c. stay the same
   d. disappear

5. **[LO 1.4]** The patient's demographic information, for instance their address or phone number, is typically updated at what point in the information cycle?
   a. patient history
   b. physical exam
   c. registration (check-in)
   d. check-out

6. **[LO 1.3]** Clinical documentation of a patient's visit is known as the
   a. Superbill.
   b. progress note.
   c. medical claim.
   d. point of care.

7. **[LO 1.1]** An encounter form is also known as a/an
   a. EHR.
   b. history.
   c. claim form.
   d. Superbill.

8. **[LO 1.1]** The _____ is a form used to bill patient claims in physicians' offices.
   a. CMS-1500
   b. ICD-10
   c. CPT
   d. UB-04

9. **[LO 1.2]** One factor that might contribute to slow acceptance of EHRs is
   a. security fears.
   b. laziness.
   c. fear of change.
   d. space concerns.

10. **[LO 1.5]** Prime Suite's user guide is accessed through the _____ feature.
    a. help
    b. information
    c. lookup
    d. query

11. **[LO 1.3]** Which of the following illustrates clinical information collected through an EHR?
    a. insurance policy
    b. plan of care
    c. research effects
    d. regulatory guidelines

12. **[LO 1.2]** _____ is not easily attained when using a manual record system.
    a. Communication
    b. Data capture
    c. Interoperability
    d. Maintenance

SHORT-ANSWER QUESTIONS

1. **[LO 1.4]** List the steps included in patient flow of information.

2. **[LO 1.2]** Outline at least three advantages to electronic health records as discussed in the text.

3. **[LO 1.1]** What functions are performed in practice management software?

4. **[LO 1.3]** What feature of Prime Suite allows practitioners to access clinical trials and other research?

5. **[LO 1.5]** If you needed to use Prime Suite's help feature to look up how to register a patient, how would you do that?

6. **[LO 1.4]** What is the first step in the patient flow of information?

7. **[LO 1.1]** Why is a claim form completed for every patient visit?

8. **[LO 1.3]** Mobile EHR applications are currently available on what mobile devices?

9. **[LO 1.2]** Define interoperability and give an example of how it might be used in the healthcare field.

10. **[LO 1.1]** What is electronic claims submission? Why is this the preferred method of claims submission?

11. **[LO 1.1]** List at least three main applications found in a typical practice management program.

12. **[LO 1.4]** What is the final step in the front desk/check-in process?

Enhance your learning by completing these exercises and more at http://**connect.mheducation.com**!

APPLYING YOUR KNOWLEDGE

1. **[LO 1.2]** Your medical office is preparing to transition from a paper-based office to an electronic one; you are really excited about this change. One day you receive an email from one of your colleagues, Sari Murray, negatively discussing the change and wondering why things cannot stay how they are now. Your colleague is looking to you and asking your opinion on the upcoming transition. Write an email back to Sari, discussing your thoughts on the change to electronic records.

2. **[LOs 1.1, 1.2, 1.3, 1.5]** The physician partners in your practice have asked you to write up a justification for purchasing a PM/EHR software package such as Greenway Health. Write a thorough justification for their review.

3. **[LO 1.4]** Denise Cruz arrives at your office for her annual check-up appointment with Dr. Smith. Discuss what will happen with Denise as she moves through each step of patient flow.

4. **[LOs 1.2, 1.3]** A patient is seen in a hospital emergency department after experiencing constant, severe abdominal pain for the past three hours. After numerous tests, no cause for the abdominal pain can be determined. Discuss how EHRs might help diagnose this patient.

5. **[LOs 1.1, 1.2, 1.3]** Compare and contrast a typical day in a paper-based office with a day at an office that uses practice management software.

6. **[LOs 1.1, 1.2, 1.3, 1.4, 1.5]** The medical office you work in recently transitioned into an electronic office and is implementing practice management software. You are excited about this change and are learning all you can about the new technology. However, some of your coworkers are having trouble grasping the basics and are now saying they don't want to use the software at all. What steps could you take to assist your struggling coworkers?

chapter references

Content related to Greenway Health™, Greenway Prime Suite™, or other related products retrieved from http://www.greenwayhealth.com (or earlier iterations of the website) from 2011–2016.

Health Data Structure, Collection, and Standards

Learning Outcomes

At the end of this chapter, the student should be able to

2.1 Describe the roles of six healthcare professionals who maintain or use practice management and electronic health record applications.

2.2 Explain the difference between data and information.

2.3 Define information governance and the HIM professional's role in it.

2.4 Identify computer-based health information media.

2.5 Relate how screen-based data collection tools are used in healthcare.

2.6 Demonstrate how individual data elements are collected.

2.7 Describe electronic health record applications.

2.8 Identify laws, regulations, and standards that govern electronic health information.

2.9 Distinguish between practice management software and hospital health information software.

Key Terms

American Recovery and Reinvestment Act of 2009 (ARRA)
Certification Commission for Health Information Technology (CCHIT)
Clinical decision support (CDS)
Data
Health and Medicine Division (HMD)
Health information exchange (HIE)
Health Information Technology for Economic and Clinical Health (HITECH) Act
Health Insurance Portability and Accountability Act (HIPAA)
Healthcare administrator
Healthcare systems administrator
Information
Information Governance

Institute of Medicine (IOM)
Meaningful Use (MU)
Merit-based Incentive Payment System (MIPS)
National Academies of Sciences, Engineering, and Medicine (the National Academies)
Nationwide Health Information Network (NwHIN)
National Provider Identifier (NPI)
Office of the National Coordinator for Health Information Technology (ONC)
Personal health record (PHR)
Picture Archiving and Communication System (PACS)
Protected health information (PHI)
Regional extension center (REC)
Regional Health Information Organization (RHIO)
Structured data
Unstructured data

What You Need to Know and Why You Need to Know It

As a healthcare professional you will be one of many who will be selecting, maintaining, and using electronic health record and management software. Knowing who within the organization is using the software and how they are using it is important to selecting a system that meets the needs of the organization. The collection of data must be done efficiently while meeting the documentation requirements of licensing and accrediting agencies, as well as insurance carriers (including Medicare), and conforming to the legal definition of an electronic health record. We will begin this chapter by reviewing the professionals involved and the positions they hold within the organization. Then, the concepts of data structure, collection, and standards will be introduced in preparation for a more detailed level of instruction in the remaining chapters of the text. We will also cover how data are collected; the tools used to collect the data; how data are transformed into information; and the regulations and standards that dictate the collection, maintenance, use, and storage of health information in an electronic form.

Health information management spans a wide range of functions and processes within a healthcare organization. Just about every decision is based on statistics that are largely collected from the health records of a facility. The data that are captured will result in information used by care providers to make decisions regarding patient care and to justify reimbursement. In addition, various levels of administrators will use information in risk management activities, budgeting, strategic planning, quality assessment, and financial reporting. Report writing will be discussed in greater detail in the chapter covering decision and compliance support.

Table 2.1 depicts many of the medical professions within healthcare, the education or certifications they may hold, and the responsibilities they may have as they pertain to the collection and use of data. This is not an exhaustive list, as there are myriad other positions such as therapists, laboratory technicians, and radiology technicians, just to name a few. Those listed are the positions held by individuals who are more likely to be involved in selecting, implementing, maintaining, and using the electronic systems in a healthcare facility.

During the process of selecting the system, it is imperative that people with knowledge of health information standards, structure, and content be involved. The health information professional fulfills this role, particularly in hospitals. In addition, administrative staff who are responsible for the effective operation of the entire organization, including facility- or enterprise-wide information systems, are key to the process as well. That is not to say that individual department managers (laboratory, nursing, radiology, etc.) do not have a say—but the administrators responsible for those departments may be the key players in the early stages of system selection.

In large practices, there may be an office manager or other administrative staff member with a health information background or credentials who will oversee the process. In smaller offices, the services of a consultant may be used, or the EHR vendor may have the health information expertise to oversee the process.

TABLE 2.1   **Medical Professions within Healthcare**

Profession	Certifications	Description/Positions Held
Health information and informatics	• Registered Health Information Administrator (RHIA®) • Registered Health Information Technician (RHIT®) • Certified Health Data Analyst (CHDA®) • Certified in Healthcare Privacy and Security (CHPS®) • Certified Professional in Health Information and Management Systems (CPHIMS)	• Work in any healthcare setting, but most often in acute care or specialty hospitals • Work in healthcare-related professions such as consultants, software trainers and installers, and employees of government agencies, and staff of insurance companies and law offices • Associate's, bachelor's, and master's degrees available • Many healthcare facilities, particularly hospitals, require certification Positions held in the following areas: • Health information department management • Information technology and systems management • Project management • Software analysis • Implementation support • Information system design • EHR implementation and management • Data analysis • Documentation management • Privacy/security assurance • Release of healthcare information oversight • Risk management • Compliance management • Utilization management • Quality assessment/assurance • Cancer registry management • Medical staff coordination
Health information specialty areas (AHIMA Certified Healthcare Technology Specialist [CHTS] credentials)	Require completion of nondegree educational programs that prepare students for competency in • Assessing workflows • Selecting hardware and software • Working with vendors • Installing and testing systems • Diagnosing IT problems • Training practice staff on systems	• The most recent health information/informatics roles • May work in any healthcare facility, inpatient or outpatient • Each competency exam is specific to a particular role that plays a part in meaningful use of the electronic health record (EHR) • Registration /Scheduling staff within healthcare facilities, particularly hospitals
Coding professionals	• Certified Coding Associate (CCA®) • Certified Coding Specialist (CCS®) • Certified Coding Specialist-Physician-based (CCS-P®) • Certified Professional Coder (CPC®) • Certified Outpatient Coder (COC®) • Certified Inpatient Coder (CIC®) • Certified Interventional Radiology Cardiovascular Coder (CIRCC®) • Specialty coding designations	• Work in all healthcare settings • Work in healthcare-related settings such as consulting firms, software vendors, insurance companies • Certificate or associate's degree Positions held in the following areas: • Medical coder • Reimbursement specialist • Insurance biller • Chargemaster specialist • Insurance claims specialist

(continued)

Profession	Certifications	Description/Positions Held
Medical assistants	• Certified Medical Assistant (CMA) • Registered Medical Assistant (RMA)	• Typically employed in physician's office or other outpatient setting • Requires associate's degree or certificate • Perform clinical duties such as prepping patients, taking vital signs, taking medical histories, assisting physician during exams, explaining minor procedures and giving instructions based on physician's orders, and collecting specimens • Perform administrative duties such as answering phone, making appointments, registering patients, maintaining health records, handling correspondence, filing health insurance claims, scheduling outpatient services, arranging referrals, and managing the office in general • May hold positions as office managers or business managers within a medical practice
Healthcare administrators	• Certified Health Care Facility Manager (CHFM) • Fellow of the American College of Healthcare Executives (FACHE) • American College of Medical Practice Executives (ACMPE) certification • Certified Practice Manager (CPM) • Certified Medical Practice Compliance Specialist (CMPCS) • Certified Physician Practice Manager (CPPM®)	• Work in all healthcare organizations • Bachelor's or master's degree typically required • Plan, organize, coordinate, and direct facility or department operations Positions held with the following titles: • Hospital administrator • Chief information officer/manager • Project manager • Department manager • Office manager • Office administrator • Compliance officer
Care providers	• Physicians—Doctor of Medicine (MD), Doctor of Osteopathy (DO) • Physicians' Assistants (PA, PA-C) • Certified Nurse Practitioners (CNP) • Certified Registered Nurse Midwives (CRNM)	• Work in any healthcare setting • Requires advanced education, licensure, and possibly certification • The only medical professionals who can diagnose a patient, order diagnostic testing and therapeutic (including medications) measures
Nursing	• Registered Nurse (RN) • Licensed Practical Nurse (LPN)	• Provide direct care to patients • May also hold non–direct care positions in utilization management, risk management, quality assessment, and general management within a healthcare facility • Nursing informatics • Requires associate's or bachelor's degree at a minimum; management positions and informatics positions may require a master's degree

2.1 The Professionals Who Maintain and Use Health Information

In the inpatient setting, the **healthcare administrator** may be a chief executive officer (CEO), chief operating officer (COO), chief financial officer (CFO), or chief information officer (CIO). These individuals typically have a bachelor's or master's degree (preferred) in healthcare administration and are responsible for overseeing several departments (or the entire organization, in the case of the CEO). Their degree is most likely in healthcare administration, healthcare management, or health systems administration. These individuals concentrate on the big picture—the operation of the organization as a whole. **Healthcare systems administrators** are concerned with how all automated systems, including the electronic health record, affect individual departments. For example, will all the information needs of the board of directors and administration for adequate, easily obtainable decision support data be met by the current (or proposed) electronic health record system? Will the clinicians have fast, easily accessible, accurate clinical information? Is the system secure and does it meet all standards and regulations? The healthcare systems administrator may be known as the chief information officer and will typically have a great deal of knowledge and experience related to the technical aspects of automated systems.

In a hospital setting, the director of the health information department and the chief information officer work closely. Each plays a key role in the selection of the product. Health information professionals have basic clinical knowledge, technical knowledge of automated systems, and expertise in record-keeping practices, putting them in a position to lead automation of health information efforts. Depending on the level and content of his or her education, a health information management professional may hold the position of chief information officer. Traditionally, the data have been the health information manager's main concern, and the actual use of the technology has been the chief information officer's domain. The staff of the health information department will need to enter, maintain, and retrieve data from electronic health records and may be certified by the American Health Information Management Association (AHIMA). Various certifications are listed in Table 2.1, as well as other certifications for health information professionals. The most recent development in health information careers and competencies is the recognition of competency exams in specialty areas, which are also explained in Table 2.1.

In a medical office or other outpatient setting, healthcare administrators may have the same titles as those used in the inpatient setting, or they may be called office manager, office administrator, business manager, and the like. These individuals are keenly aware that electronic systems can greatly enhance the efficiency of an office or can just as easily be a negative force that causes inefficiencies; therefore, they are at the forefront of selecting and maintaining electronic systems that meet the needs of the practice and its practitioners. Certification of professionals in the outpatient setting is just as important as in the inpatient setting.

Healthcare professionals such as medical assistants, nurses, medical coders and billers, and other administrative professionals will be using the software in a medical practice and will want it to be "user friendly," since they will be required to enter and retrieve data quickly yet accurately. The office administrator (manager) will be gathering information from the practice management and EHR systems to ensure claims are filed and paid accurately and in a timely manner, to ensure the requirements of managed care organizations are met, and to ensure compliance with **Meaningful Use (MU)** and **Merit-based Incentive Payment System (MIPS)** requirements. At the time of this writing, the repeal of MU as it was originally passed, and the subsequent adoption of MIPS, is an ongoing process.

The American Health Information Management Association (AHIMA), the American Association of Medical Assistants (AAMA), the American Medical Technologists (AMT), the Healthcare Information and Management and Systems Society (HIMSS), and the Physician Office Management Association of America (POMAA) are all professional associations offering certifying exams; providing members with up-to-date, relevant information about their respective fields; and offering continuing education opportunities, networking opportunities, publications, and career assistance. Each has an extensive website accessible by a search of the name.

Check Your Understanding

1. What roles might be held by a healthcare administrator?
2. What is the difference between a medical assistant and an office administrator?

2.2 Data versus Information

Throughout this worktext you will see the terms **data** and **information**. They are often used interchangeably, but they are not entirely the same. Look up each term in a dictionary, and you will see within the definitions that the terms are almost interchangeable, or synonymous. Think of it this way, though: Data are single facts, such as *the patient is 60 years old,* or *the patient is female,* or *the patient is African American.* Single facts come together to form information. For example, the fact that Elena Jones is allergic to penicillin is a piece of data. But add to that piece of data the fact that she breaks out in hives, has difficulty breathing, and required an emergency room visit for her last allergic reaction, and we have information about Elena and her allergy to penicillin. It is vital that each piece of data is accurate, valid, and timely to ensure that the information resulting from the data is also accurate, valid, timely, and in a usable format to ensure quality medical care.

Data may be **unstructured** or **structured**. Unstructured data are written in narrative form, such as in a sentence. Structured data are in a specified format such as numeric, alphabetic, or alphanumeric, and is of a specified length and format. Examples of unstructured data are a transcribed report based on a physician's dictation, a written progress note, voice files, and scanned images of original documents. In this unstructured format, it is difficult, if not impossible, to track or trend statistics or to share information with healthcare agencies, public health agencies, or insurance carriers. Structured data—such as standard templates that are used to collect the elements of a dictated report or progress note, bar codes to identify types of reports or individual files, or numeric codes that equate to a written diagnosis or procedure—allow computers to process the data into usable information.

Data A single, raw fact such as a patient's name, height, or weight. Often used interchangeably with information, though they are not synonymous terms.

Information Raw facts that, when viewed as a whole, have meaning. Example: a report of all patients treated in the emergency department of Memorial Medical Center with a primary diagnosis of streptococcal pharyngitis (strep throat), sorted by patients' age.

Structured data Data that fit a particular model or format, which can be tracked and may be part of a database. Examples include ICD-10-CM/PCS codes, CPT codes, a patient's temperature, or a patient's age.

Unstructured data Data in the form of words or audio files that cannot be tracked. Examples include emails, written narratives, and audio files from speech recognition technology.

Check Your Understanding

1. Define data.
2. Differentiate between structured and unstructured data. Give an example of each.

2.3   Information Governance

Information governance As defined by AHIMA, information governance is "the enterprise-wide framework for managing information throughout its life-cycle and supporting the organization's strategy, operations, regulatory, legal, risk and environmental requirements."

Information governance is not a new concept; however, since the electronic collection, maintenance, and storage of health information are relatively new to healthcare, so is the concept of **information governance**. The acceptable protocol and structure for electronically preserving health information is at the core of information governance.

The American Health Information Management Association (AHIMA) defines information governance as "an organization-wide framework for managing information throughout its lifecycle and for supporting the organization's strategy, operations, regulatory, legal, risk and environmental requirements" (AHIMA information governance glossary retrieved at http://www.ahima.org/topics/infogovernance/ig-glossary).

In Section 2.2, you learned that data come together to form information. The data gathered are used for myriad reasons throughout healthcare: to diagnose a patient's condition; for financial reasons; to show compliance with various rules, regulations, and standards; for quality assessment activities and risk management; to defend the legal interests of the facility, healthcare practitioners, and providers; and to carry out administrative responsibilities at all levels.

One of the principal responsibilities of HIM professionals is the capture, handling, and storage of data. Not only does data have to be captured and stored, it must be accurate, timely, credible, and secure—all attributes of information governance, and thus logical responsibilities for the HIM professional. There are rules surrounding the capture and storage of the data (which becomes information). The rules come from licensing agencies, accrediting agencies, private insurers, government agencies, and internal bylaws or policies. HIM professionals analyze health records to ensure these rules are met, and the health record is the source document to ensure that the rules are being followed. HIM professionals ensure required content is present in health records; for instance, the surgery schedule for the day may be reviewed by a member of the medical transcription staff to ensure that all scheduled surgical patients have had a history and physical examination dictated, transcribed, and posted to the patients' health records prior to their posted surgery start time. After discharge, records are analyzed to ensure that all entries are authenticated (signed), that records of all patients who have undergone surgery include a dictated operative report, and that all inpatient records include a discharge summary by the patient's attending physician. This is known as quantitative analysis.

HIM professionals may review health records qualitatively as well—for instance, the medical history of a 60-year-old patient being seen with a chief complaint of a persistent cough should reflect whether that patient has been a smoker, the patient's current and past occupations, and whether there is a family history of lung cancer. And finally, HIM professionals code diagnoses and procedures that will allow the collection of data, which will be used not only for reimbursement purposes but also for public health initiatives—to collect statistics on mortality and morbidity locally, nationally, and globally—and for decision making in healthcare facilities to allocate resources for purchases of equipment, staffing, and expansion (or decrease) of services.

In a physician's practice, quantitative and qualitative reviews of documentation should be done on an ongoing basis, though the review may be done by a medical administrative assistant rather than a health information professional. Often, coding is done as a function of the billing software, and that is even more reason for frequent reviews of coding quality by a coding professional.

Check Your Understanding

1. Why would information governance be important in a field such as health information?

2. Dr. Smith saw Carol Brady in the emergency department of Memorial Hospital on January 5. She dictated the results of the physical exam performed on the patient on January 7. Should that be of concern to the individual responsible for information governance at Memorial Hospital? Why or why not?

2.4 Computer-Based Health Information Media

Prior to there being an electronic health record system, clinicians relied on one medium to collect and access information about patients, that is, paper. Many pieces of paper make up a health record, and records of patients are often several inches thick. Paper records are contained in a folder that is filed numerically by a medical record number or alphabetically by the patient's last name. Paper is still in use to some degree, and there are still providers who do not want to give up paper records, but electronic media are gaining acceptance in the healthcare community, and by 2017 the electronic health record will be a requirement rather than a choice, thanks to the **Health Information Technology for Economic and Clinical Health (HITECH) Act**, which will be covered more thoroughly later in this chapter. In addition, many health insurance plans are making electronic **personal health records (PHRs)** available to their subscribers and have been doing so for the past few years. Some patients keep their own PHR in a folder, in paper form, or in computerized form—for instance, in a spreadsheet. When a patient maintains his or her own PHR, it often contains the patient's health history, immunization status, current and past medications, allergies, and instructions given by a care provider, as well as patient education materials. The PHR—whether kept by the patient on paper, in a spreadsheet, or on the patient's insurer's software—does not replace the legal health record kept by the patient's care provider or hospital.

In addition to being the repository for all of the clinical data about individual patients, electronic health records provide physicians with **clinical decision support (CDS)** software as well, which is used to access current information about a disease or condition. This technology alerts the care provider to possible medication interactions, gives treatment options based on results of clinical trials or research, and alerts the provider that a

Health Information Technology for Economic and Clinical Health (HITECH) Act A portion of the American Recovery and Reinvestment Act (ARRA) that is meant to increase the use of an electronic health record by hospitals and physicians through a monetary incentive program.

Personal health record (PHR) A record, kept by the patient, that contains a person's health history, immunization status, current and past medications, allergies, and instructions given by a care provider; it often includes patient education materials as well.

Clinical decision support (CDS) Allows access to current treatment options for a disease, through electronic or remote methods. Alerts the care provider to possible medication interactions, gives treatment options based on results of clinical trials or research, and alerts the provider that a patient may have a particular diagnosis based on the data found in the patient's electronic record.

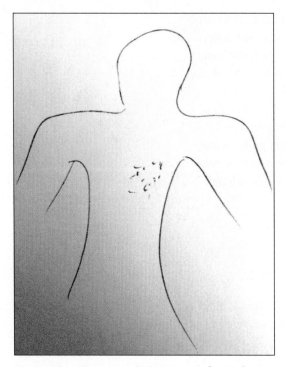

Figure 2.1 **Drawing of Placement of a Rash on a Patient's Back as It Would Have Appeared in a Paper Health Record** Source: Beth Shanholtzer

patient may have a particular diagnosis based on the data found in his or her electronic record. Not so long ago, physicians were opposed to this technology, thinking it was "cookbook medicine"; this is no longer the case, since great advances in the diagnosis and treatment of illnesses occur so quickly, making it very difficult or impossible to keep up with the most recent studies, findings, and recommended treatments. Thus, decision support applications within an EHR software package help to keep physicians up to date as well as improve the quality of patient care.

Physicians can use computerized models within the EHR to show where a patient's rash is located, for example, rather than a crudely drawn picture of a patient's back (Figures 2.1 and 2.2).

The use of videos or DVDs is not new technology, although they are now used more often to educate patients about the procedure they are about to undergo than are handouts or educational booklets. The care provider may choose to show patients a video while they are in the office, or provide a link to a video for patients to view from their home computer. Using this type of media ensures that the information used to educate patients is consistent. Other types of presentation software, such as graphs or anatomy images, such as the one seen in Figure 2.2, are also used to educate patients or to capture a more succinct representation of the patient's problem.

Most EHRs now provide educational materials, which can be specific to a particular patient's conditions, including treatment options and medications. The educational materials may be printed out for the patient or provided through a secure portal the patient accesses from home.

Physicians and administrators may want to visually present findings of a study or to consult with another physician and show a patient's disease progression. This can be done through the use of software that has been available for years—presentation software such as Microsoft PowerPoint® or OpenOffice Impress. Spreadsheets are often useful in making a point as well. EHR software provides the ability to visually chart changes in a patient's

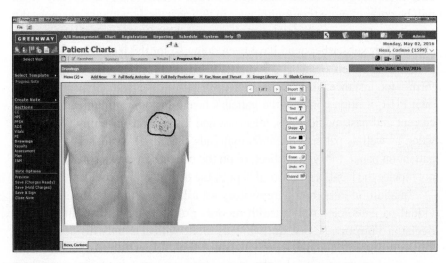

Figure 2.2 **Computer-Generated Drawing of Placement of a Rash on a Patient's Back**

vital signs, for example, and show trends or statistical changes. Patient care and treatment are greatly enhanced with the ability to track vital signs over time, thus alerting the care provider to changes in a patient's condition.

Let's look at a particular scenario. Patti Wolfe has been seeing Dr. Raszkowski for the past five years. She has been faithful about having a yearly physical exam. For the past four years, her blood pressure has increased on each visit. In 2013, her blood pressure was 130/80; in 2014, it was 135/82; in 2015, it was 130/83; and in 2016, it was 140/88. Seeing this steady climb, Dr. Raszkowski explained the situation to Mrs. Wolfe and started her on a treatment regimen. Without this quick visual of her blood pressures, the physician may not have picked up the subtle changes, and her high blood pressure might have gone untreated.

Speech recognition technology is a medium that has been available for many years and has steadily gained in popularity. This software translates what a provider is saying and types those words into text. Whereas physicians used to dictate into a microphone and a medical transcriptionist typed the words using word processing software, through the use of speech recognition software the physician still dictates, but the software captures his or her words, then converts speech into text. The software is not 100 percent accurate, however, and in the world of medicine, it needs to be. Thus, a human being must still review the final document for accuracy and make all necessary corrections. With speech recognition, the medical transcriptionist's role has changed from transcriber to editor. As the corrections are made, the software "learns" the dictator's voice so that future dictations do not reflect those same errors. Let's look at an example: Dr. Curtis dictates the sentence "There is no further medical history of note," but the speech recognition software translates that sentence as "There is no murmur history of note." The word *further* may have been heard as "murmur" because of a particular inflection in the physician's voice The next time the same physician dictates the word *further,* the software will understand the physician's tone and voice inflection and transcribe the word correctly.

A **Picture Archiving and Communication System (PACS)** allows providers to view images such as x-rays, scans, and ultrasounds. Originally used as a means to store x-ray film, PACS makes it possible for providers to remotely view x-ray film to aid in clinical decision support. The improved image quality using PACS as well as the ability to add alerts or reminders based on the findings noted in PACS greatly improve patient care. Figure 2.3 illustrates a typical PACS used to view radiologic images.

Picture Archiving and Communication System (PACS) Computerized system for enhanced viewing and sharing of images such as x-rays, scans, ultrasounds, and mammograms.

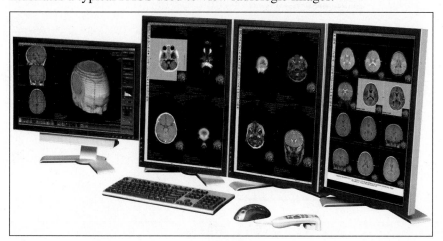

Figure 2.3   DR Systems, Inc., PACS © DR Systems, Inc.

Check Your Understanding

1. In the past, physicians marked the location of a patient's pain by drawing on a picture of a body. With the advantage of EHRs, what are they now able to do?
2. What does PACS stand for?
3. What does PACS allow providers to do?

2.5 Screen-Based Data Collection Tools

Those who are entering (also known as capturing) data typically do so on a computer screen. It may be done on a desktop computer, a laptop, a notebook computer, or a personal digital assistant (PDA). On all of these devices, data are entered and then retrieved using a computer screen. Think of the screen as the replacement for paper. Advantages include the portability of the hand-held devices used to enter the data, the ability to have multiple monitors showing different images at the same time, and the ability to customize a screen based on user preference. With paper records, there is typically an order in which the individual papers are filed within the folder, but not all care providers prefer the same order. Take a look at the two screens showing a patient's history in Figures 2.4 and 2.5—you see that the same information is collected but that the information is in different places on the screen.

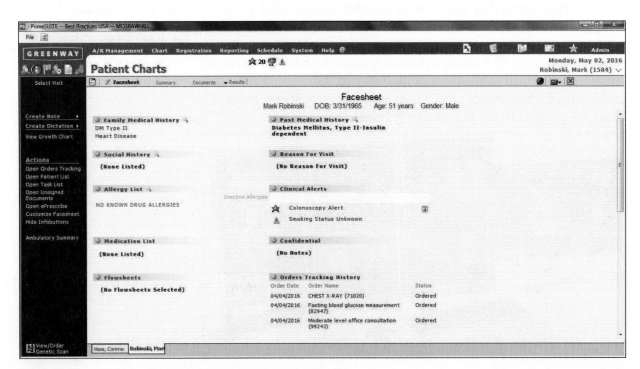

Figure 2.4 Facesheet Format Preferred by One Care Provider

Figure 2.5 Facesheet Format Preferred by a Different Care Provider

Check Your Understanding

1. What types of computers are used for data capture?
2. What are some advantages of screen-based data collection tools?

2.6 Collecting Data Elements

So, we have this data, but how did we get it in the first place? It all starts when the patient makes an appointment with a physician's office or goes to the hospital for an emergency department, outpatient diagnostic, outpatient therapy, or outpatient surgery encounter or an inpatient admission. We collect identifying information verbally from the patient (or representative), or we ask the patient to complete a form (or a combination of both). See Figure 2.6 for an example of a patient registration form.

The patient's past medical, surgical, social, and family histories are collected and entered into the EHR as well. Figure 2.7 illustrates documentation in Prime Suite; each of the areas, when clicked on, includes more detailed information about the patient. Medication allergies, current medications, and immunization history are typically captured as part of the past medical history. The history is taken from a history form and/or the patient is asked questions in order to capture those data elements in the EHR. Remember, attention to detail is essential when documenting in the EHR.

The care provider then documents the history of present illness (HPI) and performs and documents a physical exam. He or she views all of this information to make an assessment of the patient (diagnoses the patient's conditions) and then determines a treatment plan (also called a plan of care).

Greensburg Medical Center
REGISTRATION FORM
(Please Print)

Today's date:	Care Provider:

PATIENT INFORMATION

Patient's last name:	First:	Middle:	❑ Mr. ❑ Miss ❑ Mrs. ❑ Ms.	Marital status (circle one) Single / Mar / Div / Sep / Wid

Is this your legal name? ❑ Yes ❑ No	If not, what is your legal name?	(Former name):	Birth date:	Age:	Sex: ❑ M ❑ F

Street address:	Social Security no.:	Home phone no.:

P. O. Box:	City:	State:	ZIP Code:

Occupation:	Employer:	Employer phone no.:

E-mail address:	Cell phone:

Race:	Ethnicity:	Primary language:	Religion:

Other family members seen here:

INSURANCE INFORMATION
(Presentation of Insurance Card is required at time of each visit)

Person responsible for bill:	Birth date: / /	Address (if different) :	Home phone no.: ( )

Is this person a patient here?   ❑ Yes   ❑ No

Occupation:	Employer:	Employer address:	Employer phone no.: ( )

Is this patient covered by insurance?   ❑ Yes   ❑ No

Please indicate primary insurance	❑ McGraw-Hill Healthmark Insurance	❑ BlueCross/Shield	❑ [Insurance]	❑ [Insurance]	❑ [Insurance]
❑ [Insurance]	❑ Workers' Compensation	❑ Medicare	❑ Medicaid *(Please provide card)*	❑ Other	

Subscriber's name:	Subscriber's S.S.no.:	Birth date: / /	Group no.:	Policy no.:	Co-payment: $

Patient's relationship to subscriber:	❑ Self	❑ Spouse	❑ Child	❑ Other	Effective Date:

Name of secondary insurance (if applicable) :	Subscriber's name:	Group no.:	Policy no.:

Patient's relationship to subscriber:	❑ Self	❑ Spouse	❑ Child	❑ Other

IN CASE OF EMERGENCY

Name of local friend or relative (not living at same address) :	Relationship to patient:	Home phone no.: ( )	Work phone no.: ( )

The above information is true to the best of my knowledge. I authorize my insurance benefits be paid directly to the physician. I understand that I am financially responsible for any balance. I also authorize [Name of Practice] or insurance company to release any information required to process my claims.

Patient/Guardian signature	*Date*

Figure 2.6   Patient Registration Form

In addition, the patient's previous health records are often used as a source of data. This information may be sent to the facility in a paper format, which is later scanned into the patient's health record, or the information can be retrieved electronically, eventually becoming part of the patient's record.

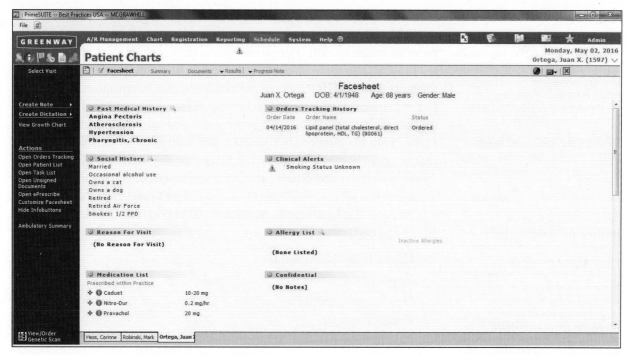

Figure 2.7   Prime Suite Documentation of Patient's Past Medical History

---

Check Your Understanding

1. Besides a patient's medical, social, surgical, and family histories, what other data are entered into his or her EHR?

2. Can a patient's previous health records be used as a source of data? Explain your answer.

3. Name two ways that identifying information is collected from a patient.

2.7   Electronic Health (Medical) Records (EHRs) (EMRs)

A health record that is in electronic form is referred to as an electronic health record (EHR) and sometimes an electronic medical record (EMR). The Office of the National Coordinator for Health Information Technology (ONC), however, differentiates between the two, based on a white paper by Garets and Davis. According to Garets and Davis, the EMR is the legal patient record that is created within any healthcare facility (hospital, nursing home, ambulatory surgery facility, physician's practice, etc.). The information in that EMR relates solely to that episode of care, and the EMR is the data source for the EHR. The individual records feed into the EHR so that healthcare providers, patients, employers, and insurance carriers can access a patient's health records as appropriate and in accordance with **Health Insurance Portability and Accountability Act (HIPAA)** regulations. Only those who have a need to know should access the information found in a patient's record.

Let's look at an example. Alison Holt is seen in the emergency room of Memorial Hospital on July 15, 2015. An EMR is compiled for that visit. She also has an EMR for an inpatient stay in Memorial Hospital from October 5 to October 10, 2014. There are additional EMRs for Alison Holt that pertain

for your information

The Garets and Davis paper can be found at http://www .providersedge.com/ehdocs/ ehr_articles/Electronic_Patient_ Records-EMRs_and_EHRs.pdf.

Health Insurance Portability and Accountability Act (HIPAA)
Passed in 1996, this act includes regulations that afford people who leave their employment the ability to keep their insurance or obtain new health insurance even if they have a pre-existing medical condition. Also sets standards for storing, maintaining, and sharing electronic health information while ensuring its privacy and security.

for your information

To avoid any confusion caused by use of the acronyms EMR and EHR, throughout this worktext we will use the term *electronic health record (EHR)*.

to various physician office visits and outpatient diagnostic testing. Then, in April 2016, Ms. Holt sees a pulmonary specialist, who needs to review her previous health records. Her providers and the hospitals she has been admitted to are able to share information through a **Regional Health Information Organization (RHIO)**, which includes healthcare organizations in her area that exchange patient information in order to improve care. This **health information exchange (HIE)** results in the quick and easy sharing of her medical history with the pulmonary specialist. Her individual records thus becomes part of an EHR. In effect, an EHR allows for the exchange of information among caregivers and others (insurance, employers, etc.) who have a need to know, but in a secure environment and according to certain standards.

In 2003, the **Institute of Medicine (IOM)** defined the functions of an EHR. The eight core functions are

- Health information and data
- Result management
- Order management
- Decision support
- Electronic communication and connectivity
- Patient support
- Administrative processes and reporting
- Reporting and population health

We will no doubt continue to use the terms *EMR* and *EHR* interchangeably, but it is important to remember that in order for the benefits of the EMR to be realized, an EHR must exist. Without the EMR, the EHR, by definition, would not exist.

Of note, as of March 15, 2016, the Institute of Medicine was renamed. It is now the Health and Medicine Division (HMD) of the **National Academies of Sciences, Engineering, and Medicine (the National Academies)**. The HMD is continuing the work of the IOM but is broadening its focus on a broader range of health-related issues.

Check Your Understanding

1. The legal patient record created for one episode of care is known as the _____.

2. Who is allowed to access the information contained in a patient's record?

2.8 Laws, Regulations, and Standards

Health Insurance Portability and Accountability Act (HIPAA)

As a healthcare professional, you will get used to the fact that there are many outside influences that affect how and why we do our jobs. We will start our journey through the agencies, regulations, and laws that govern the keeping and exchange of health information with HIPAA, although many laws and standards came before it. HIPAA stands for Health Insurance Portability and Accountability Act. HIPAA was passed on August 21, 1996, with a multifaceted purpose. It included regulations that afforded people who left their employment the ability to keep their insurance or obtain new health insurance, even if they had a pre-existing medical condition. It also set standards for several aspects of storing, maintaining, and sharing electronic health information while ensuring the privacy and security of health information.

Several rules are addressed in HIPAA, including the Privacy Rule, with an effective compliance date of April 14, 2003. Its intent was to ensure the privacy of health information and the use of **protected health information (PHI)**, which is information that identifies the patient. The Office of Civil Rights enforces compliance with the Privacy Rule. All healthcare facilities and providers are required to comply with HIPAA. The specifics of the Privacy Rule will be covered in more detail in the Privacy, Security, Confidentiality, and Legal Issues chapter; however, it is important to know that electronic data collection, maintenance, use, and storage are all governed by standards, and many of these come from HIPAA. Health records are legal documents and must be compliant with state and federal regulations, as well as with standards set forth by accrediting agencies and insurance carriers.

In February 2003, the Security Rules were published. The deadline for facilities to implement the Security Rules was April 20, 2005. These security standards require healthcare organizations to implement safeguards (administrative, physical, and technological) that ensure health information is protected, that it is kept private, and that it is retrievable in the event that the integrity of the electronic system is compromised.

The Electronic Healthcare Transactions, Code Sets, and National Identifiers Rules require that medical providers who submit claims electronically be compliant with regulations requiring standardization of electronic collection and exchange of health information. Hospitals, physicians' offices, and clearinghouses (entities that process medical claims prior to payment) are required not only to submit claims (and diagnosis and procedure codes) electronically but also to receive information, such as remittance advices, from insurance companies electronically. Compliance was required by October 23, 2003. On January 1, 2012, HIPAA version 5010 of the Code Set Rule went into effect and is part of the electronic transaction standards of HIPAA. This is an upgrade from version 4010, which had been in use since 2000. Like any other software, it had become outdated and was in need of upgrading. The driving force behind the effective date, though, was the impending ICD-10-CM/PCS change. In order to accept and transmit codes that are alphanumeric and that vary in length, new software was necessary; 4010 could not accommodate the new coding structure. In addition, version 5010 includes improved instructions for the use of the **National Provider Identifier (NPI)** number, which is a unique identifier that must be used on insurance claims to identify the care provider and/or group practice that rendered care to the patient. The NPI implementation was the last of the original HIPAA regulations to take effect.

Health Information Technology for Economic and Clinical Health Act (HITECH)

The Health Information Technology for Economic and Clinical Health (HITECH) Act is part of the **American Recovery and Reinvestment Act of 2009 (ARRA)**, which was signed into law by President Obama on February 17, 2009. The HITECH portion of ARRA is meant to increase the use of

Protected health information (PHI) Any piece of information that identifies a patient, including a patient's name, date of birth, address, email, telephone number, employer, relatives' names, Social Security number, medical record number, account numbers tied to the patient, fingerprints, photographs, and characteristics about the patient that would automatically disclose his or her identity. PHI also includes any clinical information about an identified patient.

National Provider Identifier (NPI) A unique, 10-digit identifier, issued by the Centers for Medicare and Medicaid Services (CMS), that must be used on insurance claims to identify the care provider and/or group practice that rendered care to the patient.

American Recovery and Reinvestment Act (ARRA) Signed into law by President Obama on February 17, 2009; this economic "stimulus plan" includes provisions for the Health Information Technology for Economic and Clinical Health (HITECH) Act.

an EHR by hospitals and physicians. The incentive program, made possible through HITECH, includes $18 billion in funding for this purpose. Physicians and hospitals that show meaningful use of the information collected through use of an EHR will benefit from HITECH. The incentives can be used for implementation of new EHR systems or for upgrades to those that are already in place. Later in this text, we will demonstrate the meaningful use of data. There are three stages of Meaningful Use; the first is the collection and use of data, the second is the secure exchange of information, and the third is the use of patient data to improve patient outcomes. Figure 2.8 depicts the HITECH interim final rule from the Health and Human Services (HHS) website.

Office of the National Coordinator (ONC)

Office of the National Coordinator for Health Information Technology (ONC) The principal federal entity charged with coordination, implementation, and use of health information technology and the electronic exchange of health information.

From ARRA also came the **Office of the National Coordinator for Health Information Technology (ONC)**. The ONC was created in 2004 through a presidential order but was later mandated by legislation (HITECH). According to the ONC website, "ONC is the principal Federal entity charged with coordination of nationwide efforts to implement and use the most advanced health information technology and the electronic exchange of health information."

National Health Information Network (NHIN)

National Health Information Network (NHIN) A set of standards, services, and policies that enable the secure exchange of health information over the Internet.

The ultimate goal of using EHR technology is to improve patient care—sharing information to improve diagnosis, treatment, and prognosis—while doing so in an economically efficient manner. In order to share health information electronically, though, standards must be set, and policies must be adhered to. According to the ONC website, the **National Health Information Network (NHIN)** is "a set of standards, services, and policies that enable the secure

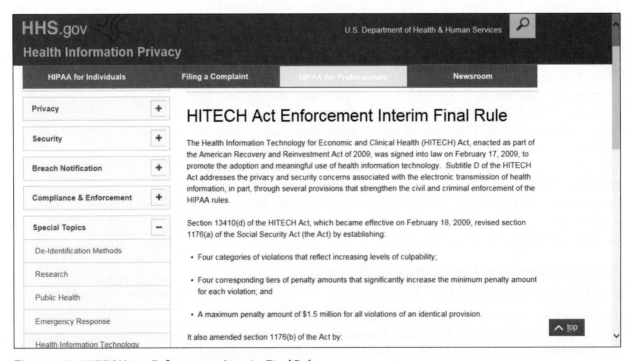

Figure 2.8   HITECH Act Enforcement Interim Final Rule

Source: www.hhs.gov

exchange of health information over the Internet" (National Health Information Network: Overview).

Current activities of the NHIN include

Nationwide Health Information Network (NwHIN)—"a set of standards, services, and policies that enable the secure exchange of health information over the Internet" (HealthIT.gov)

National eHealth Collaborative (NeHC)—created through a grant from the ONC, a public-private partnership that enables secure and interoperable nationwide health information exchange to advance health and improve healthcare. "The broad mission of NeHC is threefold: consumer engagement in eHealth, health IT education, and HIE" (National eHealth Collaborative).

Direct Project—a project aimed at developing standards and services that will enable secure exchange of information on a local level among trusted providers to support stage 1 of the Meaningful Use incentives, which went into effect on January 1, 2011

CONNECT—free, open source software that supports health information exchange

Since the first edition of this text was written, there has been progress in healthcare reform in the United States. New reimbursement models are on the horizon, and with them comes more of an emphasis on competitiveness in providing healthcare, as well as more of a shared risk/shared reward system (Berry). Data is required in order to measure healthcare quality, and the resulting quality measures are necessary to roll out these new models of reimbursement; therefore, the exchange of health information also becomes a necessity.

A downside to this, at least from the perspective of providers of healthcare, is a decrease in revenue from the standpoint that sharing health information will result in a reduction of duplicate testing and unnecessary tests or procedures.

Certification Commission for Health Information Technology (CCHIT) and Other Certifying Agencies

In the first several years of HITECH, to ensure that health information was shared securely, and that the shared information was used for its intended purpose, the **Certification Commission for Health Information Technology (CCHIT)** was founded to develop certifying criteria for the functionality, interoperability, and security of EHRs. A nongovernmental, nonprofit organization, CCHIT began certifying EHR systems in 2004 and ended operations in November 2014. Since then, certification of EHR systems is the responsibility of the Office of the National Coordinator for Health Information Technology (ONC).

Certification Commission for Health Information Technology (CCHIT) A nonprofit, nongovernmental agency whose purpose was to certify electronic health records for functionality, interoperability, and security.

The Healthcare Information and Management Systems Society (HIMSS), a nonprofit organization that focuses on the use of information technology (IT) and management systems needed to improve healthcare, provides important information regarding the EHR on its website, found at http://www.himss.org/ASP/topics_ehr.asp.

The Medicare and Medicaid EHR Incentive Programs require the use of certified EHR technology; a listing of certified EHR technologies can be found at http://onc-chpl.force.com/ehrcert. When you access this list, you will see that there are other EHR certifying agencies, which will be discussed in a later chapter.

Regional Extension Centers

Regional extension center (REC)
An organization that assists healthcare providers with the selection and implementation of electronic health record systems.

As part of HITECH, extension centers are funded by the federal government. The purpose of the extension centers is to lend technical assistance and guidance regarding best practices in the selection, implementation, and maintenance of an EHR that will satisfy the Meaningful Use requirements. Each **regional extension center**, or **REC** (pronounced R-E-C), is responsible for a geographic region in the United States and is a nonprofit entity. Accomplishments of each REC can be found at https://www.healthit.gov/providers-professionals/rec-highlights

Thus, you can see that many entities exist to ensure that health information is shared so that safe, effective, quality medical care is provided, yet in a manner that allows for the security and privacy of that information exchange.

Check Your Understanding ✔

1. The original agency/organization responsible for developing the criteria for and then certifying EHR systems was _____.
2. Name the four subcategories of HIPAA.
3. What does PHI stand for?
4. The organization currently responsible for certifying EHR systems is _____.
5. What office ensures compliance with the Privacy Rule?
6. Explain the necessity behind upgrading to HIPAA 5010.

2.9   Similarities and Differences between a Physician's Office and Hospital Information Systems

Regardless of the healthcare setting—inpatient or outpatient—every patient seen must have a health record that describes his or her history of present illness, past medical and surgical history, record of physical exam, record of treatment rendered, results of diagnostic tests, plan of care, and diagnoses. In a physician's office setting, the patient schedules an appointment, which is part of the registration process. In a hospital setting, a patient may arrive without an appointment for an emergency department visit or to have outpatient lab work done, for example. In either case, appointments are typically unnecessary or impossible. In other instances, such as for a CT scan, which requires a significant amount of time and specially trained staff, an appointment is necessary. And, in a hospital setting, a patient may be scheduled for an elective surgery such as cholecystectomy (removal of the gallbladder), which would also be a scheduled (planned) visit.

The steps taken to capture the fact that a patient was seen, no matter what the setting, are most easily (and accurately) done using computerization. In a physician's office, this is done using practice management (PM) software. In a hospital, these captured records are called the Master Patient (Person) Index (MPI), and the MPI is part of the R-ADT (Registration, Admission,

Discharge, Transfer) functions of the hospital's automated information system. Each patient is entered only once into the MPI, although there may be several visits (encounters) for each patient as a subset of the main entry. This allows the documentation of each individual visit to be filed in one place within the MPI.

Increasingly in the past decade, single hospitals and physician practices have been purchased by large hospital systems. The single hospitals/offices then become part of an "enterprise." In some cases, the individual institutions or offices maintain their own records and operate autonomously. In others, the MPI is shared (an enterprise-wide MPI) and more than likely will result in duplicate patient records and an increase in incorrect data. Obviously, correct data in the MPI is always a priority, but when an enterprise-wide MPI is used, it becomes even more imperative to have staff that continually monitor for and clean up any inaccurate, duplicate, erroneous, or unreliable data. It also becomes more important for registration staff to do a thorough check of the MPI before adding a patient as new or before selecting an existing patient.

Practice management software is used to handle office administrative functions such as listing all patients who have been seen in that practice; capturing insurance and demographic information; entering charges and diagnosis and procedure codes; filing, maintaining, and following up on medical claims and collections (billing procedures); running statistical reports about the practice; and scheduling patients' appointments.

The capture of the identifying information and clinical documentation discussed earlier in this chapter is part of the electronic health record in both hospitals and physicians' offices.

The various functions performed all have different names in different settings, but their goals are the same: registration of the patient and then compilation of a health record for every encounter the patient has in that facility or office.

Table 2.2 compares common jargon used in a hospital to that used in a physician's office. For instance, a "SOAP" note stands for Subjective (the patient's complaint in his/her own words), Objective (a description of what

TABLE 2.2	Comparison of Outpatient to Inpatient Setting	
Action	**Physician's Office or Other Outpatient Setting**	**Hospital**
Patient seeks care	Schedule patient or make an appointment	Register or admit a patient
Health record compiled	Documentation in a SOAP note format, narrative progress note or "chart"	End product is a health (medical) record
Listing of all patients seen by the facility	Once the patient is registered one time, he or she appears in the Patient List	Once the patient is registered one time, he or she appears in the Master Patient (Person) Index (MPI)
Patient has outpatient care	Each is called an encounter or visit	Each is called an encounter
Patient stays overnight	n/a	Patient is an admission or inpatient
Patient is finished with the encounter	Patient checks out	Patient is discharged

the care provider observes or measurable findings), Assessment (the diagnosis), and Plan (the treatment) and is a format used to document progress notes in any setting, but it is most often used in outpatient settings such as physicians' offices. SOAP notes would be equivalent to what are referred to as progress notes in inpatient settings.

The objective of an EHR is to capture timely, accurate, usable health information to ensure quality medical care; provide for coordination of care; support the medical necessity for diagnostic testing; protect the legal interests of the patient, provider, and hospital; collect data used in statistical reporting; and file insurance claims.

In order to select, implement, maintain, and use practice management software or the electronic health record, a team of professionals is typically assembled to investigate several software options. Those on the team should include individuals who understand not only how to use the software but also what to look for when selecting software that will meet the stiff regulations that govern the keeping of health information. It is vital that this health information be maintained in a way that is private, confidential, and secure yet readily available when needed. In addition, the information must be accurate, reliable, and valid. Over the past several years, the federal government has affirmed that there is an urgent need for an electronic health record that will provide for more efficient, effective, and safe healthcare for Americans.

Check Your Understanding

1. The SOAP note format of writing progress notes is generally used in a/an _____ setting.
2. Could a patient ever have outpatient care in a hospital setting? If so, what is an episode of outpatient care called?
3. What term refers to a hospital's historical list of patients?

APPLYING YOUR SKILLS

You have learned much about how healthcare is structured in the United States and the professionals who manage various aspects of healthcare, and you have been introduced to the organizations that govern the electronic systems used in healthcare facilities. To tie all of this together, you will set out on a virtual scavenger hunt. Use the Internet to answer the following questions about your region of the country.

1. Find the website for a hospital near you. Who is the CEO?
2. By searching the Web or reading a newspaper or magazine article, find information related to healthcare, such as current cancer rate, death rate for a particular region, or proven treatment for a particular disease. What makes this information rather than data?
3. Using the Internet, find the regional extension center for your state.
4. Using the Internet, find the health information exchange for your state.
5. Find three hospitals or physician practices within a 100-mile radius of your home. For each, is the hospital or practice stand-alone or part of an enterprise system?

chapter 2 **summary**

LEARNING OUTCOME	CONCEPTS FOR REVIEW

2.1 Describe the role of six healthcare professionals who maintain or use practice management and electronic health record applications.	– Healthcare professionals, their educational background, their certifications, and how they use health information:
	  • Chief information officer
	  • Health information professionals
	  • Chief financial officer
	  • Healthcare adminstrators/managers/office administrators
	  • Care providers
	  • Nurses, medical assistants

2.2 Explain the difference between data and information.	– Often used interchangeably – Data are single facts. – Single facts come together to form information. – Structured vs. unstructured data
2.3 Define information governance and the HIM professional's role in it.	– Define information governance. – List the uses of healthcare data. – List the attributes of data.

2.4 Identify computer-based health information media.	– Role of the Health Information Technology for Economic and Clinical Health (HITECH) Act in the adoption of an electronic health record
	– Define personal health record (PHR).
	– Electronic health record includes
	  • Decision support technology
	  • Computerized models and images
	  • Presentation aids
	  • Voice recognition technology
	  • Picture Archiving and Communication System (PACS)

2.5 Relate how screen-based data collection tools are used in healthcare.	– Hardware used to collect health information:
	  • Desktop computers
	  • Laptop computers
	  • Notebook computers
	  • iPad
	  • iPhone
	  • Personal digital assistant (PDA)
	– Advantages include portability and customization.

(continued)

LEARNING OUTCOME	CONCEPTS FOR REVIEW
2.6 Demonstrate how individual data elements are collected.	– Data collected through use of forms or in person – Registration forms used as method of collecting patient identifying and demographic information – Patient history form used as method of collecting past medical, surgical, family, and social histories; allergies; medication history
2.7 Describe electronic health record applications.	– Differentiate between electronic medical record (EMR) and electronic health record (EHR). – Role of the Office of the National Coordinator for Health Information Technology (ONC) – Differentiate between Regional Health Information Organization (RHIO) and health information exchange (HIE). – List the functions of the EHR as detailed by the Institute of Medicine (IOM)/ Health and Medicine Division of the National Academies (HMD).
2.8 Identify laws, regulations, and standards that govern electronic health information.	– Identify the Privacy, Security, Transactions, and Code Set Rules of HIPAA. – Define protected health information (PHI). – Define National Provider Identifier (NPI) number. – Describe the Health Information Technology for Economic and Clinical Health (HITECH) Act and its role in requiring electronic health records. – Define Meaningful Use of data collected through use of an EHR. – Describe the purpose of the Office of the National Coordinator for Health Information Technology (ONC). – Explain the National Health Information Network (NHIN). – Explain the Certification Commission for Health Information Technology (CCHIT). – Relate the purpose of regional extension centers (RECs).
2.9 Distinguish between practice management software and hospital health information software.	– Describe the functions of practice management software. – Differentiate between R-ADT systems and EHR systems within a hospital setting. – Discuss the use of a Master Patient (Person) Index and Patient List. – Articulate the purpose of an EHR.

chapter review

MATCHING QUESTIONS

Match the terms on the left with the definitions on the right.

_____ 1. **[LO 2.2]** data

_____ 2. **[LO 2.7]** health information exchange

_____ 3. **[LO 2.2]** unstructured data

_____ 4. **[LO 2.1]** healthcare systems administrator

_____ 5. **[LO 2.1]** Meaningful Use

_____ 6. **[LO 2.4]** clinical decision support

_____ 7. **[LO 2.9]** Master Patient Index

_____ 8. **[LO 2.8]** protected health information

_____ 9. **[LO 2.8]** Office of the National Coordinator (ONC)

_____ 10. **[LO 2.7]** Institute of Medicine (IOM)

_____ 11. **[LO 2.3]** information governance

a. any piece of identifying or clinical information about a patient

b. organization that is responsible for certifying electronic health records for viability

c. staff member whose responsibilities include management of a facility's IT functions

d. use of health information in an effective and efficient manner to improve patient care

e. single facts often used interchangeably with information

f. The original entity to define the functions of an EHR; now known as the Health and Medicine Division of the National Academies

g. method of accessing current treatment options for a disease, through electronic or remote methods

h. haring of health information among various entities, using standardized and secure processes

i. record of the names of all patients seen in a hospital setting

j. details that cannot be tracked, such as emails and voice recognition technology audio files

k. organization-wide framework for managing information throughout its lifecycle and for supporting the organization's strategy, operations, regulatory, legal, risk, and environmental requirements.

MULTIPLE-CHOICE QUESTIONS

Select the letter that best completes the statement or answers the question:

1. **[LO 2.7]** The acronym HIE stands for
   a. health information exchange.
   b. hospital information exchange.
   c. health information electronically.
   d. hospital institutional exchange.

2. **[LO 2.5]** An advantage of using screen-based data collection tools is that the layout of the information can be
   a. printed.
   b. deleted.
   c. shredded.
   d. customized.

3. **[LO 2.7]** The _____ defined the eight core functions of an EHR.
   a. National Institutes of Health
   b. American Recovery and Reinvestment Act
   c. Institute of Medicine
   d. HITECH Act

4. **[LO 2.8]** Which of the following is a goal of HIPAA?
   a. establish standards for keeping health information
   b. ensure that patients receive timely treatment
   c. allow a person's insurance to transfer from one job to another
   d. guide how Picture Archiving and Communication Systems are used

5. **[LOs 2.6, 2.9]** In a physician's office, patient data collection begins when
   a. the patient exam begins.
   b. the patient calls to make an appointment.
   c. the medical assistant takes the patient's vital signs.
   d. the patient signs in at the front desk.

6. **[LO 2.4]** An advantage of EHRs is that patients are now able to _____ about procedures they are undergoing.
   a. negotiate charges with insurance representatives
   b. see diagrams
   c. ask questions
   d. view patient education videos

7. **[LO 2.2]** "Jim Smith had a heart attack when he was 53" is an example of
   a. data.
   b. information.
   c. support.
   d. technology.

8. **[LO 2.9]** When patients are finished with their encounter at a hospital, they
   a. are admitted.
   b. check out.
   c. complete a SOAP note.
   d. are discharged.

9. **[LO 2.8]** If a hospital uses information gathered through its EHRs to justify the purchase of state-the-art equipment to improve patient care, it is
   a. violating the Privacy Rule.
   b. engaging in Meaningful Use.
   c. abusing protected health information.
   d. following CCHIT.

SHORT-ANSWER QUESTIONS

1. **[LO 2.1]** List the six healthcare professionals involved in EHR use and explain the role of each.

2. **[LO 2.8]** Explain the evolution of CCHIT.

3. **[LO 2.1]** Explain the differences among a healthcare administrator, a healthcare manager, and a health systems administrator.

4. **[LO 2.9]** List the six objectives of an EHR.

5. **[LO 2.8]** HIPAA is an acronym for _____.

6. **[LO 2.7]** Contrast an EHR with an EMR.

7. **[LO 2.2]** Explain the difference between data and information and give an example of each.

8. **[LO 2.4]** Why were so many physicians opposed to clinical decision support in the past?

9. **[LO 2.5]** List and explain the four types of histories entered into a patient's electronic record.

10. **[LO 2.5]** Name two advantages of using screen-based data collection tools.

11. **[LO 2.1]** If someone has the letters "RHIA" after his or her name, what does that mean?

12. **[LO 2.9]** What does the R-ADT acronym mean in a hospital setting? Explain its purpose.

13. **[LO 2.8]** Explain the purpose of a regional extension center (REC).

14. **[LO 2.4]** Discuss at least one way that voice recognition technology can be used in a medical setting.

15. **[LO 2.3]** In a physician's practice, which staff position is likely to be responsible for functions of information governance?

APPLYING YOUR KNOWLEDGE

1. **[LOs 2.4, 2.5, 2.7, 2.8]** Discuss any potential drawbacks to the full-scale use of EHRs and explain what precautions or regulations have been put in place to deal with each drawback.

2. **[LO 2.8]** Incentives are a significant part of the HITECH Act. Discuss the advantages and potential disadvantages associated with using incentives as a tool for implementing EHRs.

3. **[LOs 2.2, 2.6]** In the following case study, determine what would be considered data and what would be considered information: New patient Alice Jones is a 32-year-old female who presents with chest pains. She tells you that, in the past, she has been diagnosed with rosacea and is allergic to latex. In addition, she has had surgery for a broken arm. She does not smoke, is a social drinker, and has no family history of heart problems.

4. **[LO 2.9]** A physician's office and a hospital employ different terminology and process flow when maintaining records and monitoring patient flow. Why is there no set protocol that is used by all healthcare settings?

5. **[LO 2.4]** Describe a scenario where presentation software might be used in a physician's practice.

 Enhance your learning by completing these exercises and more at http://**connect.mheducation.com**!

6. **[LO 2.9]** Think about the six main objectives of an EHR. Which of the six do you feel would be most useful for care providers? For patients? For office managers? Explain your answers.

7. **[LO 2.8]** Visit the HIPAA Fast Facts website located in the FYI box in Section 2.8. Summarize the information found on the website and write a brief scenario that illustrates how the information could be put into practice at a physician's office or a hospital.

8. **[LO 2.1]** Choose one of the professional associations listed in Section 2.1. Locate the association's website and create an outline for a sample presentation you might give to your office staff that highlights the important aspects of that association's influence on health information management.

9. **[LO 2.3]** One of the physicians in your practice thinks it is a waste of time to review the quality of documentation of the health records in this three-physician practice. You are the office manager. Explain to the physicians why the quality, thoroughness, and timeliness of documentation are so important.

chapter references

Berry, Kate. (2013, March). HIE Quality Check. *Journal of AHIMA, 84*(3): 28–32.

Certification Commission for Health Information Technology. (2013). *About the Certification Commission for Health Information Technology.* Retrieved from http://www.cchit.org/about.

Department of Health and Human Services, Centers for Medicare and Medicaid Services. (2016). *Administrative Simplification Overview.* Retrieved from https://www.cms.gov/Regulations-and-Guidance/Administrative-Simplification/HIPAA-ACA/.

Department of Health and Human Services, Centers for Medicare and Medicaid Services. Medicare Learning Network. (2014). *The National Provider Identifier (NPI): What You Need to Know.* Retrieved from http://www.cms.gov/MLNProducts/downloads/NPIBooklet.pdf.

Garets, D., and Davis, M. (2005, October). Electronic Patient Records: EMRs and EHRs. *Healthcare Informatics.* Retrieved from http://www.providersedge.com/ehdocs/ehr_articles/Electronic_Patient_Records-EMRs_and_EHRs.pdf.

Health Care Administrator. (2004). Retrieved from Health Careers Center website: http://www.mshealthcareers.com/careers/healthcareadmin.htm.

HealthIT.gov. Interoperability Portfolio: Nationwide Health Information Network. (2013). Retrieved from http://www.healthit.gov/policy-researchers-implementers/nationwide-health-information-network-nwhin.

National Academies of Sciences, Engineering, and Medicine. Health and Medicine Division. About Our Division and Website. Retrieved at http://www.nationalacademies.org/hmd/

National Academies: Health and Medicine Division (HMD). (2013). *Key Capabilities of an Electronic Health Record System.* Retrieved from http://nationalacademies.org/hmd/reports/2003/key-capabilities-of-an-electronic-health-record-system.aspx.

Newby, Cynthia. (2009). *HIPAA for Allied Health Careers.* New York: McGraw-Hill Companies.

SmartData Collective. (2014). *A Quick Guide to Structured and Unstructured Data.* Retrieved from http://www.smartdatacollective.com/michelenemschoff/206391/quick-guide-structured-and-unstructured-data.

U.S. Department of Health and Human Services, Office of the National Coordinator for Health Information Technology. (2011). *National Health Information Network: Overview.* Retrieved from http://www.healthit.gov/policy-researchers-implementers/nationwide-health-information-network-nwhin

U.S. Department of Health and Human Services, Office of the National Coordinator for Health Information Technology. Retrieved from http://www.healthit.gov/newsroom/about-onc.

U.S. Department of Health and Human Services, Office of the National Coordinator for Health Information Technology. *HITECH and Funding Opportunities.* Retrieved from http://www.healthit.gov/policy-researchers-implementers/hitech-programs-advisory-committees.

Content of the Health Record— Administrative Data

At the end of this chapter, the student should be able to

3.1 Identify administrative data elements.

3.2 Explain the administrative uses of data.

3.3 Explain the use of EHR data in an Accountable Care Organization (ACO).

3.4 Explain the use of the Master Patient (Person) Index (MPI).

3.5 Apply procedures to register a new patient in Prime Suite.

3.6 Apply procedures to schedule a patient's appointment in Prime Suite.

3.7 Apply procedures to edit demographic information in Prime Suite.

3.8 Follow the steps performed upon patient check-in.

3.9 Apply procedures to capture insurance information in Prime Suite.

3.10 Locate the Help feature in Prime Suite.

Key **Terms**

Accountable Care Organization (ACO)
Administrative data
Chief complaint
Clinical Documentation Architecture (CDA)
CMS-1500
Continuity of Care Document (CCD)
Data dictionary
Default value
Demographic (identifying) data

Health Level Seven (HL7)
Interoperability
Library
Medical record number
Medicare Access and CHIP Reauthorization Act
National Provider Identifier (NPI)
Merit-based Incentive Payment System (MIPS)
Quality Reporting Document Architecture (QRDA)
UB-04

What You Need to Know and Why You Need to Know It

In previous chapters we talked about the importance of each patient's having only one record in the EHR of that facility. Remember, though, that one record may have many individual encounters attached to it, one for each visit to a healthcare facility as a patient. In this chapter we will discuss the administrative data, including demographic (identifying) data that are collected about each patient, thus forming the master record or Master Patient Index for each patient.

3.1 Administrative Data Elements

Administrative data is nonclinical data and does not include data relative to the diagnosis, prognosis, treatment, or plan of care. **Demographic data** is a subset of administrative data and includes data collected to identify a particular patient. It includes the patient's full name, date of birth, race, ethnicity, gender, marital status, address, and phone number. The Social Security number used to be an additional identifier that was widely used. Because of identity theft concerns, that practice is now not as common, or some practices request only the last four digits of the patient's Social Security number. Additional information that is typically collected includes employed/student status, employer name and address, next of kin, and insurance policy name, policy number, and group number. In addition to identifying patients, many administrative data elements are required to complete insurance claim forms such as the **CMS-1500** and the **UB-04**, as required by HIPAA. The CMS-1500 form is used to bill outpatient encounters, and the UB-04 is used to bill hospital admissions/encounters. Examples of the CMS-1500 and the UB-04 are available in the Appendix.

Identifying information for inpatients and outpatients, as included in the core health data elements recommended by the National Center for Vital and Health Statistics in 1996, should include the data elements listed here:

- Patient's full name
- Previous name (maiden name or previous married name)
- Personal/unique identifier—this is also referred to as medical record number or chart number
- Account (billing) number
- Date of birth
- Gender
- Race
- Ethnicity
- Residence (address)
- Marital status
- Current or most recent occupation (employer)
- Type of encounter (inpatient, emergency room visit, physician's office visit, ambulatory surgery, outpatient diagnostic visit, etc.)
- Admission date (inpatient) or date of encounter (outpatient)
- Discharge date (inpatient)

Administrative data Identifying information, insurance-related information, authorizations, and business correspondence found in a patient's health record.

Demographic (identifying) data Data that identify the patient. Consists of name, date of birth, sex, race, and Social Security number (may vary by facility policy).

CMS-1500 The form used by physicians' offices to submit insurance claims.

UB-04 The form used to submit insurance claims for hospital patients.

- Facility identification (unique identifier of the medical office, hospital, outpatient surgery center, etc.)
- Type of facility/place of encounter (hospital, physician's office, surgi-center, etc.)
- Healthcare practitioner identification number (outpatient)
- Provider location or address of encounter (outpatient)
- Attending physician identification (inpatient)
- Patient's expected sources of payment (Medicare, Medicaid, insurance, self-pay, etc.)
- Whether injury is related to employment or accident
- Total billed charges

Health Level Seven (HL7) A set of standards that makes sharing of data between or among healthcare entities possible.

These data elements are also included in the **Health Level Seven (HL7)** standards. HL7 allows different software packages to interface with one another, that is, it allows them to share data. Many different companies develop healthcare applications and systems, and by writing the software according to HL7 standards, the applications "talk to each other"; if they did not, the data would have to be entered separately in each application. Hospitals and medical practices may have different vendors for different systems. For instance, there may be one service provider for the laboratory system, one for the pharmacy system, one for tracking incomplete records, and so on. Through use of HL7 standards, if a piece of data is changed in one application system, say the patient's telephone number, the change will be reflected in each system. This is a very important requirement, because without this standard language, **interoperability** (sharing data through a single database) would not be possible.

Interoperability Many different functions can take place and information can be shared between computer systems, or within applications of the same computer system, which is not possible with a manual or paper record system.

HL7 has been the most widely used and recognized standard in the healthcare industry. HL7 now recognizes new, more specific standards, which include **Clinical Documentation Architecture (CDA)** and **Quality Reporting Document Architecture (QRDA)**. The CDA is used for an important piece of the Meaningful Use legislation in preparing a **Continuity of Care Document (CCD)**, and the QRDA is important for quality reporting purposes as well as for sharing information between providers or facilities. The Continuity of Care Documents tie directly to one of the major goals of an electronic health record—that is, improving patient care and patient outcomes through information. The ability to electronically share important clinical data among caregivers, even those from different or even competitive healthcare facilities, is a step toward improving overall quality of care. Service providers (EHR and PM software vendors) are finding it more beneficial to work together to form new partnerships, resulting in collaborative relationships, than to concentrate on selling their product(s) alone.

Clinical Documentation Architecture (CDA) Developed by HL7, a document markup standard that specifies the structure and semantics of clinical documents such as discharge summary, operative report, etc.

Quality Reporting Document Architecture (QRDA) Based on HL7's approved Clinical Documentation Architecture (CDA), QRDA is a data standard used for reporting quality measure data and that is EHR compatible across different health IT systems.

Commonwell Health Alliance is an example of how health information technology vendors are working together to collaborate toward the ultimate goal of true interoperability of healthcare electronic systems. According to Commonwell's website, "The Alliance intends to be an independent, not-for-profit trade association that will support and promote the seamless interoperability of and access to patient data across the healthcare system."

Continuity of Care Document (CCD) A document exchange standard used to share patient summary information, such as in the case of a patient being referred from one healthcare provider to another.

Meaningful Use will be covered in more detail in the chapter on decision and compliance support in this worktext. A detailed explanation about the protocols themselves for HL7 is not necessary in this text, but they will be covered in a more advanced information technology course.

One of the data elements listed above is previous name (maiden name or previous married name). Collecting this data element allows for cross-referencing of files. If a woman was previously seen at a facility under her maiden name, but is being seen for the first time using her married name, she should be listed only one time in the master list of patients.

In an outpatient setting, the data elements listed previously are collected on a patient registration form, which is completed at the time care is established with that facility or office. The information should be verified with the patient each time he or she is seen to ensure that there has been no change in information, and that there have been no additions or deletions to the information. Examples include changes in address, telephone number, marital status, or expected source of payment. In a hospital setting, the information may be required prior to a patient's undergoing an elective admission, or it may be collected face-to-face in the registration department when the patient presents for care.

Equally important when collecting sufficient identifying information is that each data element is consistently defined by the facility. Use of a **data dictionary**, as seen in Figure 3.1, will ensure that each member of the registration staff has defined the data element correctly, and that only valid entries are made in a particular data element.

Data dictionary A document that specifies the format of each data field as well as a detailed explanation or definition for that field, which allows for consistency of data collection.

Let's look at a few examples. First, consider the possible data dictionary choices for marital status. The typical choices are single, married, separated, widowed, divorced, and unknown. If that is the definition of marital status in your facility, then those are the *only* choices available in the practice management system. Data dictionaries should be very specific. An example is the definition of "separated." Some facilities may consider a patient to be separated only if she presents a legal document stating such, and if she cannot do that, she is considered married for data collection purposes, even though she considers herself to be separated in the legal sense. Another example is the patient's full name. In the facility's data dictionary, the full name may be defined as the patient's last name, first name, middle name. Or it may be defined as the last name, first name, middle initial. Thus, when a patient is registered, the name should be collected exactly as defined in that facility's data dictionary. Failure to follow the data dictionary definitions will result in unreliable data.

For consistency of wording and to save time, many fields in Prime Suite have a **library** of possibilities from which to choose. These are called drop-down menus. Examples of libraries are employers, common medications, religions, ethnicities, medical conditions, and elements of a physical exam. Clinical templates are also found in libraries (Figure 3.2).

Library In computer software, a listing or choice of entities, for instance, employers, insurance plans, ICD-10-CM codes, or CPT codes.

Field Name	Data Type	Field Length	Description
Last name	Alphabetic	18	Patient's legal surname
First name	Alphabetic	10	Patient's first name
Middle name	Alphabetic	10	Patient's middle name
DOB	Numeric	08	Date of birth as it appears on birth certificate
Phone number	Numeric	10	Preferred phone number including area code

Figure 3.1 Excerpt from a Data Dictionary

Figure 3.2 Library of Clinical Templates Found in Prime Suite

3.2 Administrative Uses of Data

In addition to identifying a particular patient, administrative data are also used to satisfy HIPAA data requirements, which in turn are used to file electronic health claims for reimbursement. The CMS-1500 form is used to submit claims electronically for outpatient encounters, and the UB-04 is used to submit hospital claims. There are five major sections or levels on the claim form (refer to the CMS-1500 and UB-04 forms found in the Appendix).

1. Provider information

The name, address, **National Provider Identifier (NPI)** number, and telephone number of the provider

2. Subscriber and patient information

This section includes information about the policyholder (subscriber) of the insurance and the patient identifying information. These may be one and the same, if the patient is the policyholder (the primary insured). Following is a partial list of information collected but it is not limited to

- Policyholder's (subscriber's) name
- Group or insurance plan name
- Identification (policy) number
- Patient's relationship to the policyholder

3. Payer information

- Group or insurance plan name
- Plan identification
- Address
- Assignment of benefits authorization (allows payment to be made directly to the provider)
- Release of information authorization (allows clinical information to be released to the insurance company)
- Referral number (if patient was referred by another provider)
- Prior authorization number (obtained when insurance plan requires procedures to be approved for payment in advance)

4. Claim details—a partial list of data includes

- Individual account number or identification for that particular encounter

National Provider Identifier (NPI) A unique, 10-digit identifier, issued by the Centers for Medicare and Medicaid Services (CMS), that must be used on insurance claims to identify the care provider and/or group practice that rendered care to the patient.

- Total charges submitted
- Place of service code
- Provider signature
- Details about the onset of the illness/accident
- Date(s) of service
- Amount collected from the patient
- Unique identifier (medical record number or chart number)
- International Classification of Diseases, 10th revision, Clinical Modification (ICD-10-CM) diagnosis codes. ICD-10-CM is a classification system that converts diagnoses into alphanumeric form. It is published by the World Health Organization (WHO) and is the required code set for documenting diagnoses on all patients in any care setting. For example, the ICD-10-CM code for a patient with type II diabetes mellitus with diabetic nephropathy is E11.21.
- Whether the encounter was due to an auto or other accident or was a work-related injury

5. Services
- Procedures performed as indicated by Current Procedural Terminology (CPT) codes. CPT codes convert written procedures and services into numeric form. This code set is published by the American Medical Association (AMA) and is the required code set for submitting procedures and services for outpatients. An example of a CPT code is 82247, which is the code for a total bilirubin test. For hospital inpatients, ICD-10-PCS codes are assigned to convert procedures into coded form. For example, the ICD-10-PCS code for a left heart catheterization is 4A023N7. ICD-10-PCS is only used in the United States, as opposed to ICD-10-CM, which is used internationally.
- Date(s) of service

Information collected in each of these major sections may overlap. For instance, the place of service code or the dates of service code would be collected only once but satisfies the claim details as well as the services section requirements.

Administrative data, as well as clinical data, which describe the patient's diagnosis and procedures, may also be used to satisfy reporting requirements. For instance, capturing the race and ethnicity of all patients and then completing a report requested by the state department of health regarding race and ethnicity distribution is an example of the administrative use of data and an example of the meaningful use of data. Other administrative data elements that are required to satisfy Meaningful Use requirements are the patient's preferred language, gender, and date of birth. An example of a clinical data element that is collected from within the provider's documentation or in the health history is the patient's smoking status (if the patient is 13 years of age or older). A report that includes the total number of patients living in a particular ZIP code with a diagnosis of COPD (chronic obstructive pulmonary disease) is an example of a report that uses both administrative and clinical data. Another is the total number of patients between the ages of 13 and 50 years of age who are smokers and have a diagnosis of asthma. Either of these reports may be used by public health agencies or in educational materials used in a smoking cessation class.

The Patient Protection and Affordable Care Act (ACA) is part of the health-care reform legislation passed in 2010. Included in that piece of legislation is the formation of the **Accountable Care Organization (ACO)**. An Accountable Care Organization is a healthcare model whereby a group of physicians, hospitals, and/or other healthcare providers (e.g., home health agencies) form a partnership that provides high-quality, coordinated care to a population of patients. The payment for the care is based on quality measures, as opposed to the traditional fee-for-service model. Data are necessary to report the results of each quality measure (Washington).

ACO models include the Centers for Medicare and Medicaid Services (CMS) models and various commercial payer models.

The ACO models are reliant on the data gathered from individual providers' EHR systems. The exchange of health information that we discussed earlier is critical to the success of ACOs, since the point is coordination of care and the reduction of redundant or unnecessary treatments or diagnostics. Though this may result in a decrease in revenue for providers, it is essential if healthcare costs are to be contained. Health information professionals and practice managers play a major role in the ACO model, since quality data in the form of diagnosis and procedure codes, patient identification, and so on is essential in ensuring accurate, quality measurement and data integrity. ACOs will remain important as healthcare organizations prepare for the Medicare Access and CHIP Reauthorization Act of 2015 (MACRA).

Medicare Access and CHIP Reauthorization Act of 2015 (MACRA)

The **Medicare Access and CHIP Reauthorization Act**, or MACRA is known as the "Doc Fix Act." It ends the Sustainable Growth Rate formula that had been used to determine payments to providers for healthcare services billed to Medicare beneficiaries. MACRA provides a framework that rewards care providers who give better (not necessarily more) care to Medicare beneficiaries and combines existing quality reporting systems into one new system. The new payment program is called the **Merit-based Incentive Payment System or MIPS**. Eligible professionals (physicians) will be measured on quality, resource use, clinical practice improvement, and meaningful use of certified EHR technology. (Centers for Medicare and Medicaid Services)

The Master Patient (Person) Index, or MPI, contains the identifying or administrative data on each patient. The acronym MPI is used more in the hospital setting than in the outpatient setting, although the objective is the same: one file of all the patients seen in the facility, with each patient listed in the index only *once*. In a medical practice, this may be referred to as the Patient List or Master Patient List. Each patient then has a second level of information that reflects individual visits to the facility. For instance, James Philips has been a patient at Memorial Hospital. He was admitted as an inpatient in January 2010 for appendicitis. He was then seen in the emergency department of the hospital in June 2010 for a fracture of his right radius. In September he underwent outpatient blood work ordered by his primary care physician. In this instance,

---

Accountable Care Organization (ACO) A reimbursement model where hospitals, physicians, and other healthcare providers form partnerships whereby all are accountable for the quality of care, efficiency of medical services (to contain costs), and patient satisfaction; a pay-for-performance model of healthcare reimbursement.

Medicare Access and CHIP Reauthorization Act (MACRA) Ends the Sustainable Growth Rate formula that had been used to determine payments to providers for healthcare services billed to Medicare beneficiaries. Also known as the Doc Fix Act.

Merit-based Incentive Payment System (MIPS) A new Medicare provider payment program based on quality of care, resource use, clinical practice improvement, and meaningful use of certified EHR technology.

for your information [fyi]

Examples of Medicare Shared Services Accountable Care Organizations include Adena Healthcare Collaborative, LLC; Bassett Accountable Care Partners, LLC; Bluegrass Clinical Partners, LLC; and Carroll ACO, LLC. An Internet search of any of these will give you a better understanding of an Accountable Care Organization and its structure.

James will have one entry in the MPI, but he will have three individual encounters attached to his record (one inpatient, two outpatient encounters).

The MPI must be kept permanently, since it is the master list of all patients seen at a particular facility. In the hospital setting, records are filed by **medical record number**, which is a unique number assigned to each patient. The medical record number for each patient is linked to the patient's name in the MPI. Thus, if the MPI is destroyed or unavailable for some reason, it would be difficult, if not impossible, to locate the patient's health record in a paper record system. Though physicians' offices typically file alphabetically by the patient's last name, best practice still dictates that a master index (list) of all patients be kept.

In some facilities and offices, the MPI is still kept manually. With the move toward an electronic record, an electronic MPI is more the norm. Figure 3.3 is an example of a manual MPI card. Figure 3.4 is an example of the equivalent of an MPI entry in Prime Suite (for a different patient). Notice that in the electronic version, much more demographic information is collected and stored in this patient's master file than for the patient with the manual MPI card.

Medical record number A unique number assigned to each patient seen by a facility or office.

MEMORIAL HOSPITAL 7652 HORIZON WAY ANYWHERE, TX 44555			
Last Name, First Name, Middle Name Philips, James Bernard		**DOB** 07/31/1990	Gender Male Race Caucasian **Medical Record Number** 07-45-85
Home Address 1234 Oriole Way, Anywhere, TX 44555			**Telephone Number** 555-555-3333
Previous Name n/a			**Social Security Number** 123-45-6780
ADM/ENCOUNTER DATE	**DISCHARGE DATE**	**TYPE OF SERVICE**	**PROVIDER**
1/15/2014	1/28/2014	IP	Howard Hinkins, MD
6/22/2014	6/22/2014	ED	Sylvia Crowell, MD
9/30/2014	9/30/2014	OP	Lloyd Wright, Md

Figure 3.3   **Master Patient Index (MPI) Card**

Figure 3.4   **Example of Prime Suite Demographic Screen**

Before any information, administrative or clinical, is entered for a patient, he or she must be registered in the practice management software, which in turn populates basic information in the EHR as well. This function is carried out in every healthcare setting. It is important to have pertinent information about the patient available to the office staff. In Exercise 3.1, perform the steps necessary to view this information on the desktop.

EXERCISE   3.1

Go to http://connect.mheducation.com to complete this exercise.

The Patient Information Screen

Using a computer to store data about all patients allows us to retrieve that data more quickly and is more efficient than using manual systems. There is certain data the healthcare professional needs to access often. In order to efficiently access this common information, the Prime Suite Desktop can be modified by changing the Patient Information Settings.

The Patient Information Settings screenshot shown in Figure 3.5 is the screen used to change the information settings.

Figure 3.5   Patient Information Settings Screenshot in Prime Suite

In this exercise, you will select common data elements to display on the Desktop screen.

Follow these steps to complete this exercise:

1. Click the View Patient Info icon.
2. Click the Customize Patient Information icon.
3. Select Patient Picture.
4. Select Patient Name.
5. Select Patient ID.
6. Select Age.
7. Select Date of Birth.
8. Select Social Security Number (SSN).
9. Select Sex.
10. Select Primary Language.
11. Select Emergency Contact.
12. Select Address.
13. Select Home Phone.

14. Select Cell.
15. Select Email.
16. Select Preferred Communications.
17. Select Patient Balance.
18. Select Insurance Balance.
19. Select Total Balance.
20. Select Primary Insurance.
21. Select Primary Co-Pay.
22. Select Secondary Insurance.
23. Select Secondary Co-Pay.
24. Select Preferred Provider.
25. Select Primary Care Provider.
26. Select Next Appt. Info.
27. Select Preferred Pharmacy.
28. Select Pharmacy Fax.
29. Select Pharmacy Phone.
30. Select Pharmacy Address.
31. Click the Patient Info icon to close.

☑ **You have completed Exercise 3.1**

In a physician's office, the registration process is completed by the reception staff at the time the patient arrives for care. In the hospital setting, the process takes place when the patient presents for care and is done by registration staff, often called Patient Access. Some hospitals have a centralized registration department, meaning that regardless of the type of patient (inpatient or outpatient), all registration is done from a central location. Other hospitals have decentralized registration, meaning that there is an admissions department that registers inpatients, an emergency department registration area for emergency patients, and an outpatient registration area for diagnostic testing such as radiology, laboratory, physical therapy, and so on. It is important for the physician's office reception and scheduling staff to know what type of registration model is used by the local hospital(s), since communication with the registration staff is common. In Exercise 3.2 we will follow a patient through registration in a physician's office.

 connect Go to http://connect.mheducationl.com to complete this exercise.   **(PM)**   **EXERCISE**   **3.2**

Register a New Patient

In this exercise, we will be registering a new patient, Alfredo J. Garza. He has called Greensburg Medical Center, asking if any of the providers were taking new patients. The healthcare professional tells him that Dr. Ingram, a family practice physician, is taking new patients and asks if he would like to establish care with Dr. Ingram. Since Mr. Garza does want to do so, the following steps are completed to register him in the practice management and EHR system of Greensburg Medical Center.

(continued)

 Prime Suite Tip

Information must be entered in test mode exactly as it appears in the source documentation. For instance, the telephone number must be entered as 770-555-5555.

From the initial phone call, basic information such as full name, date of birth, address, and telephone number(s) is taken. He tells the healthcare professional that his name is Alfredo Jose Garza. He was born on 07/31/1945. His address is 117 Greenway Blvd, Carrollton, GA 30117, and his phone number is 770-555-5555.

The healthcare professional will mail Mr. Garza some paperwork to complete before he arrives for his appointment. Typically, the paperwork includes a form to collect administrative information, a past medical history form, and authorization forms. The administrative information includes information such as address, telephone number, next of kin, insurance information, ethnicity, and race. The insurance information is entered as soon as it is available so that verification of insurance can be done (more about insurance verification is in the financial management chapter).

For our purposes, we will assume that Mr. Garza completed the initial paperwork and brought it to the office before the day of his appointment with Dr. Ingram, as noted in Figure 3.6.

Follow these steps to complete the exercise on your own once you have watched the demonstration and tried the steps with helpful prompts. Use the registration form in Figure 3.6 to complete the following steps:

1. Click the Patient Information icon.
2. Click the *Last Name: field.
3. Type "Garza".
4. Click the *First Name: field.
5. Type "Alfredo".
6. Click the Middle Name field.
7. Type "Jose".
8. Click Search.
9. Click OK.
10. Click the Date Of Birth field.
11. Type "07/31/1945".
12. Click the Sex drop-down menu.
13. Click Male to select it.
14. Click the Home Phone field.
15. Type "770-555-5555".
16. Click the Work Phone field.
17. Type "770-555-6666".
18. Click Add New.
19. Click Yes.
20. Click Registration.
21. Click Information.
22. Click the *Race 1: drop-down menu.
23. Click Declined to select it.
24. Click the *Primary Language: field.
25. Type "Sp" in the Primary Language field and hit Enter.
26. Click "Spanish".
27. Click the Religion drop-down menu.
28. Click Catholic to select it.
29. Click the *Ethnicity: drop-down menu.
30. Click Hispanic or Latino to select it.
31. Click the Address *Line 1 field.

(continued)

Greensburg Medical Center
REGISTRATION FORM
(Please Print)

Today's date: March 17, 2016

Care Provider: Dr. Ingram

PATIENT INFORMATION

Patient's last name:	First:	Middle:	x Mr. ☐ Mrs.	☐ Miss ☐ Ms.	Marital status (circle one)
Garza	Alfredo	Jose			(Single) / Mar / Div / Sep / Wid

Is this your legal name?	If not, what is your legal name?	(Former name):	Birth date:	Age:	Sex:
☒ Yes ☐ No			07/31/1945	68	☒ M ☐ F

Street address:	Social Security no.:	Home phone no.:
117 Greenway Blvd.		770-555-5555

P. O. Box:	City:	State:	ZIP Code:
	Carrollton	GA	30117

Occupation:	Employer:	Employer phone no.:
Project Manager	Greenway	770-555-6666

E-mail address: ajgarza@greenwaymedical.com	Cell phone: 770-555-7777

Race: declined **Ethnicity:** Hispanic   **Primary language:** Spanish   **Religion:** Catholic

Other family members seen here:

INSURANCE INFORMATION

(Presentation of Insurance Card is required at time of each visit)

Person responsible for bill:	Birth date:	Address (if different):	Home phone no.:
Alfredo Garza	07/31/1945		

Is this person a patient here?   ☒ Yes   ☐ No

Occupation:	Employer:	Employer address:	Employer phone no.:

Is this patient covered by insurance?   ☒ Yes   ☐ No

Please indicate primary insurance	☒ McGraw-Hill Healthmark Insurance	☐ BlueCross/Shield	☐ [Insurance]	☐ [Insurance]	☐ [Insurance]
☐ [Insurance]	☐ Workers' Compensation	☐ Medicare	☐ Medicaid (Please provide card)	☐ Other	

Subscriber's name:	Subscriber's S.S. no.:	Birth date:	Group no.:	Policy no.:	Co-payment:
Alfredo Jose Garza		07/31/1945	6500	GAR5679009	$ 20.00

Patient's relationship to subscriber: ☒ Self   ☐ Spouse   ☐ Child   ☐ Other   Effective Date: 01/06/2013

Name of secondary insurance (if applicable):	Subscriber's name:	Group no.:	Policy no.:
None			

Patient's relationship to subscriber: ☐ Self   ☐ Spouse   ☐ Child   ☐ Other

IN CASE OF EMERGENCY

Name of local friend or relative (not living at same address):	Relationship to patient:	Home phone no.:	Work phone no.:

The above information is true to the best of my knowledge. I authorize my insurance benefits be paid directly to the physician. I understand that I am financially responsible for any balance. I also authorize [Name of Practice] or insurance company to release any information required to process my claims.

Patient/Guardian signature   _Date_

Figure 3.6 Alfredo Garza Registration Form

32. Type "117 Greenway Blvd".
33. Click the *Zip: field.
34. Type "30117".
35. Press "Tab".
36. Click the Cell field.
37. Type "770-555-7777".
38. Click the Email field.
39. Type "ajgarza@greenwaymedical.com".
40. Click the *Preferred Communications: drop-down menu.
41. Click Email to select it.
42. Click the Search Employer icon.
43. Type "Greenway".
44. Click Search.
45. Click Select.
46. Click the Status drop-down menu.
47. Click Full-time to select it.
48. Click the Occupation field.
49. Type "Project Manager".
50. Click Save.

☑ **You have completed Exercise 3.2**

3.6 Scheduling an Appointment

In Prime Suite, the "Appointment Scheduling" function is used to make the appointment with the provider who has been assigned to that patient. In Alfredo Garza's example, he was a new patient and was assigned to Dr. Ingram.

In an office setting, the healthcare professional will need to know the reason for the visit in order to allot enough time for it. For example, a follow-up visit for hypertension is going to take less time than a physical exam. The scheduler or healthcare professional will also ask for convenient days and times before beginning the search for the appointment. In a hospital setting, outpatient procedures such as CT scans or MRIs are scheduled in advance, and the process is similar.

Each care provider is set up in the PM system to show his or her typical schedule. For instance, Dr. Ingram may prefer to start the day at 9:00 a.m., break for lunch from noon to 1 p.m., and end his day at 5:30 p.m. Dr. Pueblas, on the other hand, may prefer to start seeing patients at 8 a.m., break from seeing patients between 11 and 11:30 a.m. to return phone calls and perform administrative tasks, see patients from 11:30 a.m. until 1:00 p.m., and then break for lunch from 1:00 p.m. until 2:00 p.m. Her last appointment of the day is scheduled for 4:30 p.m. In addition, some care providers prefer to do complete physical exams only in the morning. Many offices leave open appointment times for urgent visits. Patients who do not show up for an appointment, or who cancel at the last minute, can wreak havoc on a schedule!

Schedule an Appointment

Recall that we registered Mr. Garza in Exercise 3.2, so his name is located in Prime Suite's Master Patient List. The healthcare professional asked Mr. Garza which days of the week work best for him. He does not have a preference of day, but he would like to be seen soon, so the healthcare professional starts the search beginning with March 28th. Since Mr. Garza is establishing care with this office, the type of visit he will have is a Routine Office Visit (ROV). He will be having a complete exam. By selecting the correct type of visit, the amount of time allotted for that visit is automatically assigned by the system. In this case, it will be a 30-minute appointment. He then states that a morning visit on a Wednesday is best for him, so 9:30 on March 30th is selected by the healthcare professional. Mr. Garza also stated that he was having shortness of breath, so that will be entered as his **chief complaint**, which is the reason (in the patient's own words) that he has made the appointment.

Now we will perform the process of scheduling an appointment for Alfredo Garza.

Follow these steps to complete the exercise on your own once you have watched the demonstration and tried the steps with helpful prompts.

1. Click Search for Patient.
2. Type "Garza" in the *Last Name: field.
3. Click Search.
4. Click the line with the patient record for Alfredo Jose Garza.
5. Click Select.
6. Click Appointment Scheduling.
7. Click the plus sign by Providers.
8. Click the check box by Dr. Ingram's name.
9. Click the check box next to Greensburg Medical Center.
10. Click the *From Date: field.
11. Type "03/28/2016".
12. Click View Schedules (in the far right corner).
13. Click the Next Day blue arrow.
14. Click the Next Day blue arrow again.
15. Click the plus sign by Office Visits.
16. Drag the ROV - New Patient Exam icon to the 09:30 AM time slot.
17. Click the Chief Complaint: field.
18. Type "Shortness of breath".
19. Click the Save button.

 You have completed Exercise 3.3

Chief complaint The reason for which a patient has made an appointment (usually in his/her own words, for instance, "I have a sore throat.").

Prime Suite Tip **PS**

In Prime Suite, when the search function is used, the first patient who meets the criteria entered (in this case, the last name Garza) is highlighted. By clicking anywhere on the line of the patient you are actually looking for, then clicking Select, you will choose the correct person.

Prime Suite Tip **PS**

A plus sign (+) next to a menu designates that there are more submenus available for that item. To find them, click on the plus sign.

3.7 **Editing Demographic Data**

People move, their last names change, their emergency contact information changes—just about anything except their first name and date of birth can change. It is important that an office always have up-to-date information on a patient.

At the time of check-in, many offices print out the identification page and have the patient review it, either on a yearly basis or even every time a patient is seen. If changes need to be made, the patient communicates them to the office staff, and the information is edited appropriately. To save paper, some offices have a computer terminal where the patient can view the information on the screen, or the healthcare professional may just swivel the screen around for the patient to view and either verify that no changes are necessary or state what information does need to be changed.

EXERCISE 3.4 Go to http://connect.mheducation.com to complete this exercise.

Edit Demographic Information

In this exercise, Mr. Garza realizes that he has moved since initially completing the registration paperwork; he calls in to the office to give his new address. He tells the healthcare professional that his address is now 2024 Peachtree Parkway, Carrollton, GA 30117.

Follow these steps to complete the exercise on your own once you've watched the demonstration and tried the steps with helpful prompts.

1. Click the Patient Information icon.
2. Type "Garza" in the *Last Name field.
3. Click Search.
4. Click Jose.
5. Click Select.
6. Click Information.
7. Click the Address *Line 1: field.
8. Type "2024 Peachtree Parkway".
9. Press "Tab".
10. Click Save.

✓ **You have completed Exercise 3.4**

Default value A value that automatically appears in a field each time it appears on a screen (e.g., the current date in a date field, the local area code in a home phone number field).

Prime Suite Tip

Default values are used throughout Prime Suite. This means that the most common entry in a particular field is already placed in a field when the screen appears. If that information is correct, the healthcare professional simply tabs through the field. If the default information for that patient is not correct, then the drop-down menu of choices is searched for the appropriate information. Examples include the Visit Type and Service Location fields.

3.8 Checking In a Patient

One of the advantages of using PM software is the ability to track a patient's flow through the office. The flow starts when the patient checks in. As a patient, you are aware of this part of the process—it is when you either sign your name on a log sheet or verbally inform the healthcare professional that you have arrived. This process is used in a physician's office setting but would not necessarily have a use in the hospital environment, other than in the outpatient registration area.

The typical flow is the following:

Patient checks in at front desk > patient is seen by clinical support team (MA or nurse) > patient is seen by the care provider (physician or physician's assistant or nurse practitioner) > patient stops at the cashier or check-out desk > billing processes begin.

Check In a Patient Who Has Arrived

In the following exercise, Alfredo Garza has arrived and he has just signed the log, which alerts the healthcare professional to check him in for his appointment.

Follow these steps to complete the exercise on your own once you have watched the demonstration and tried the steps with helpful prompts.

1. Click Registration.
2. Click Visit Information Check-In.
3. Click Garza, Alfredo J.
4. Click Close.
5. Click the *Visit Type drop-down menu.
6. Click Routine Office Visit to select it.
7. Click the *Service Location drop-down menu.
8. Click Greenway Medical Clinic South to select it.
9. Click Check-In.

☑️ **You have completed Exercise 3.5**

3.9 Capturing Insurance Information

Although a medical practice or hospital is in business to care for patients, in the end, it is also just that—a business. In order to stay financially viable, there must be organized, effective policies and procedures in place to ensure cash flow and fiscal success.

You will learn about the intricacies of setting up fee schedules, billing insurance plans, and collection procedures in another course. In this exercise, though, you will learn about the information that must be collected for any patients who have a private or group insurance plan or who participate in a government health plan.

Figure 3.7 is a sample insurance card. This card should be presented each time a patient arrives for an encounter. Office staff may scan the front and back of the card as an image that will reside in Prime Suite, or they may photocopy the front and back of the card and keep it in the patient's chart.

The information must be entered in Prime Suite exactly as it appears on the insurance card. For instance, say Alfredo Jose Garza does not use his first name; instead, he uses A. Jose Garza. But his insurance card reads Alfredo Jose Garza. In Prime Suite, or any other PM software, he should be entered as Alfredo Jose Garza.

Any typographical errors within Prime Suite will result in a delayed or denied claim. That will slow payment, which is not good business practice for the office!

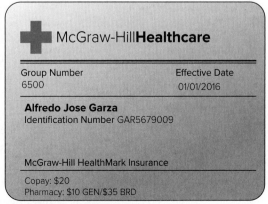

➕ McGraw-Hill**Healthcare**

Group Number	Effective Date
6500	01/01/2016

Alfredo Jose Garza
Identification Number GAR5679009

McGraw-Hill HealthMark Insurance

Copay: $20
Pharmacy: $10 GEN/$35 BRD

Figure 3.7 Sample Insurance Card

Capture Insurance Information of a Patient

In the exercise that follows, Mr. Garza has presented his insurance card to the healthcare professional and has completed the insurance information on his registration form (Figure 3.6). Mr. Garza has coverage through only one insurance company, so that is the primary insurance (the first insurance that is billed).

Follow these steps to complete the exercise on your own once you have watched the demonstration and tried the steps with helpful prompts.

1. Click the Priority drop-down menu.
2. Click Primary to select it.
3. Click "Click here to search for plan".
4. Click the Insurance Co: drop-down menu.
5. Click McGraw-Hill HealthMark to select it.
6. Click Search.
7. Click Select.
8. Press "Tab".
9. Press "Tab".
10. Type "Garza, Alfredo" in the Policy Holder field.
11. Press "Tab".
12. Type "GAR5679009" in the Policy Number field.
13. Press "Tab".
14. Type "6500" in the Group Number field.
15. Press "Tab".
16. Type "01/01/2016" in the Effective Date field.
17. Press "Tab".
18. Type "t" in the Expiration Date field.
19. Click Save.
20. Click the View/Edit Patient Flags icon.
21. Click Co-pay $20.
22. Click Save.

✓ **You have completed Exercise 3.6**

3.10 Utilizing the Help Feature

The "Help" feature is a staple of almost any computer software program. What is important is that you *use* the Help feature when you need to. For many of us, it is easier to ask someone how to perform a particular function than to search for the solution ourselves. The problem is, the person you are asking may give you the incorrect answer, or you may be in a position where you need an answer fast and there is no one around to ask. It shows initiative and will help you remember the steps more easily if you seek out the answer on your own. Consider this analogy—you remember how to get to a particular destination when you have driven there yourself rather than as a passenger, correct? The same applies here. You will remember and *understand* the process if you look up the steps on your own.

Use the Help Feature

In this scenario, you are fairly new to Greensburg Medical Center, but you have been employed there for several weeks and are comfortable using Prime Suite. You would like to learn more about appointments and, more specifically, appointment scheduling. You know how to schedule a basic office visit but you would like to know more, so you go to Prime Suite Help for more guidance.

Follow these steps to complete the exercise on your own once you have watched the demonstration and tried the steps with helpful prompts.

1. Click Help.
2. Click Prime Suite Help.
3. Click the "What Can We Help You Find?" field.
4. Type "Appointments".
5. Click the Search icon.
6. Click Appointment Scheduling.
7. Click the scroll bar.

☑ **You have completed Exercise 3.7**

Selecting the Help feature will connect you to the Prime Suite User's Manual. Features you may typically use are

- Getting Started and Navigating Prime Suite Help
- Prime Suite Topics
- Frequently Asked Questions (FAQ)
- Work Flow Solutions

Also readily available in Prime Suite Help is material that speaks to the newest upgrades in functionality, as well as a listing of what Greenway has determined to be the most frequently asked questions about topics (Figure 3.8).

Figure 3.8 Help Feature, Prime Suite User's Manual

APPLYING YOUR SKILLS

In this chapter we discussed how important accurate data is. Let's take a look at a situation that is not all that uncommon.

Cindy, at Dr. Clark's office, is in the midst of checking in a patient, Diana G. Pike, while also listening to her supervisor, Emily, giving her instructions about something unrelated. Mrs. Pike has filled out the new patient registration form and mentioned to Cindy that she is a new patient. Mrs. Pike has a seat, and Cindy is completing her registration. She types in the last name of Pike and sees that there is a Diana Pike in the system. Diana G. Pike has a date of birth of 9/18/1957 and lives at 367 Elmwood Drive, Carollton, GA. Diana Pike has a date of birth of 8/18/1957 and lives at 387 Elmhurst Drive, Carollton, GA. She assumes that someone inaccurately entered Diana Pike into the system, and she enters information about today's appointment under Diana Pike's record in the Master Patient Index.

Is there a problem? If so, what is it? How could it have been avoided? What impact could this have on other steps of the process?

chapter 3 **summary**

LEARNING OUTCOME	CONCEPTS FOR REVIEW
3.1 Identify administrative data elements.	– Demographic data are identifying data. – Administrative data include demographic data as well as additional nonclinical data. – A data dictionary is necessary to ensure consistency and reliability of data. – CMS-1500, UB-04, and HIPAA regulations dictate much of the administrative data captured.
3.2 Explain the administrative uses of data.	– Insurance purposes (file claims) – Satisfy regulatory requirements and Meaningful Use – Five sections of the claim form • Provider • Subscriber • Payer • Claim detail • Services
3.3 Explain the use of EHR data in an Accountable Care Organization (ACO).	– Patient Protection and Affordable Care Act (ACA) – Definition of an ACO • A new healthcare reimbursement model • Partnership between healthcare providers to provide high-quality, coordinated care – Reimbursement based on quality measures, not fee for service – Need data from EHR to report results of each quality measure – ACO model used by Medicare and some commercial insurance plans – Medicare Access and CHIP Reauthorization Act – (MACRA) • Merit-based Incentive Payment System (MIPS) – Health information professionals as well as office administrators must ensure quality data collection and reporting.
3.4 Explain the use of the Master Patient (Person) Index (MPI).	– Means of tracking that a patient was seen in a healthcare facility – Only one entry per patient • Each encounter has its own entry, filed under the patient's master entry. – Medical record (chart) number unique to each patient—links the patient to his/her health record – Can be manual or electronic – Kept permanently

LEARNING OUTCOME	CONCEPTS FOR REVIEW
3.5 Apply procedures to register a new patient in Prime Suite.	– Patient must have an entry in the Master Patient Index or Patient List before any other functions can occur (scheduling, patient's chart, etc.). – Registration process occurs in every healthcare setting. – Registration process ultimately results in the patient's being a part of the MPI. – In a physician's office setting, this is done by a healthcare professional. – In a hospital setting. this is done by the registration department.
3.6 Apply procedures to schedule a patient's appointment in Prime Suite.	– Before scheduling an appointment, a provider has to be assigned, if a new patient, or select the patient's usual provider. – Must know the reason for the visit in order to allot sufficient time for the visit – Select a date and time that works for the patient.
3.7 Apply procedures to edit demographic information in Prime Suite.	– All information about a patient must be current and correct. – Verification of demographic and administrative information is done by administrative personnel at the time a patient checks in. – Information is edited, added, or deleted as appropriate.

3.8 Follow the steps performed upon patient check-in.	– Knowing where the patient is in the flow through the office is important to maintain efficiency.
	– Typical flow:
	  • Patient checks in at reception desk.
	  • Patient is called back to the exam room by the healthcare professional.
	  • Patient is seen and examined by the provider.
	  • Patient checks out.
	  • Claim process begins.

3.9 Apply procedures to capture insurance information in Prime Suite.	– Capturing complete, correct insurance information is vital to cash flow and financial success. – Require patients to present their insurance card on every visit. – Information in the practice management system must match what is on the insurance card.

3.10 Locate the Help feature in Prime Suite.	– Help feature is available in any software.
	– User's manual includes
	  • Getting Started and Navigating Prime Suite Help
	  • Prime Suite Topics
	  • Frequently Asked Questions
	  • Work Flow Solutions

chapter review

MATCHING QUESTIONS

Match the terms on the left with the definitions on the right.

_____ 1. **[LO 3.6]** chief complaint

_____ 2. **[LO 3.2]** ICD-10-CM

_____ 3. **[LO 3.1]** CMS-1500

_____ 4. **[LO 3.1]** administrative data

_____ 5. **[LO 3.1]** Clinical Documentation Architecture

_____ 6. **[LO 3.4]** Master Patient Index

_____ 7. **[LO 3.1]** UB-04

_____ 8. **[LO 3.1]** Continuity of Care Documents

_____ 9. **[LO 3.1]** library

_____ 10. **[LO 3.1]** data dictionary

a. information, such as a patient's insurance information, marital status, employer

b. list of correct definitions for a facility's unique terms and jargon

c. form used to submit insurance claims in an outpatient setting such as physician's office

d. in terms of computer software, a comprehensive listing of related entities to choose from, such as ICD-10 codes

e. form used to submit insurance claims in a hospital setting

f. permanent roster of all patients ever seen in a healthcare setting

g. reason for a patient's appointment; may determine the length of an exam visit

h. HL7 standard that outlines the format of clinical documentation, such as reports and discharge summaries

i. document exchange standard that guides how patient information is shared among providers and healthcare settings

j. alphanumeric diagnosis codes

MULTIPLE-CHOICE QUESTIONS

Select the letter that best completes the statement or answers the question:

1. **[LO 3.1]** _____ data include demographic data.
   a. Clinical
   b. HIPAA
   c. Administrative
   d. Financial

2. **[LO 3.4]** Anna Jacobs presented to the ER of County Hospital three times in the past year. She will appear in County's MPI
   a. once.
   b. twice.
   c. three times.
   d. four times.

 Enhance your learning by completing these exercises and more at http://**connect.mheducation.com**!

3. **[LO 3.1]** Which of the following is NOT an example of demographic data?
   a. full name
   b. primary physician
   c. Social Security number
   d. date of birth

4. **[LO 3.2]** Administrative data are used to satisfy _____ requirements.
   a. CCHIP
   b. HITECH
   c. HIPAA
   d. ONC

5. **[LO 3.5]** Before a patient can be treated at a healthcare setting, she must be
   a. prepped.
   b. registered.
   c. logged.
   d. admitted.

6. **[LO 3.4]** How long should a facility's Master Patient Index be kept?
   a. three years
   b. five years
   c. seven years
   d. permanently

7. **[LO 3.1]** Recording a patient's previous or married name might help with
   a. cross-referencing data.
   b. compiling family history.
   c. legal proceedings.
   d. Privacy Rule compliance.

8. **[LO 3.10]** One of the common Help features is
   a. Work Flow Help.
   b. Quick Start Guide.
   c. Frequently Asked Questions.
   d. Topical Outline.

9. **[LO 3.5]** _____ is part of a patient's administrative information found on a registration form.
   a. Occupation
   b. Chief complaint
   c. Provider number
   d. Co-pay amount

10. **[LO 3.1]** Patient demographic information should be verified
    a. at the initial visit.
    b. at each visit.
    c. once a year.
    d. when the patient initiates a change.

11. **[LO 3.9]** An insurance claim may be denied if the receptionist fails to
    a. collect a patient's co-pay.
    b. make a copy of the patient's insurance card.
    c. enter all data correctly.
    d. have the patient sign the front-desk log.

12. **[LO 3.6]** _____ is part of the appointment scheduling feature of Prime Suite.
    a. Occupation
    b. Chief complaint
    c. Provider number
    d. Co-pay amount

13. **[LO 3.3]** Accountable Care Organizations rely on EHR
    a. data.
    b. functionality.
    c. compliance.
    d. format.

14. **[LO 3.2]** A facility's collection of patient data might be used to satisfy _____ requirements.
    a. data dictionary
    b. Meaningful Use
    c. incentive
    d. interoperability

15. **[LO 3.7]** Editing a patient's mailing address is accomplished by using
    a. drop-down menus.
    b. free-text fields.
    c. Help topics.
    d. patient flags.

16. **[LO 3.4]** In a hospital's health information department, patient records are most often filed by
    a. patient's last name.
    b. number of patient encounters.
    c. provider identification number.
    d. medical record number.

17. **[LO 3.8]** Patient check-in is
    a. essential for claims processing.
    b. important for efficient patient tracking.
    c. done in the patient chart.
    d. an optional function in Prime Suite.

18. **[LO 3.2]** Information such as a policyholder name and insurance plan name appear in the _____ section of a claim form.
    a. payer
    b. provider
    c. services
    d. subscriber

Enhance your learning by completing these exercises and more at http://**connect.mheducation.com**!

SHORT-ANSWER QUESTIONS

1. **[LO 3.3]** What is the role of an Accountable Care Organization?

2. **[LO 3.5]** What is the difference between centralized and decentralized registration centers in a hospital setting?

3. **[LO 3.9]** Explain why it is important to enter insurance information into Prime Suite exactly as it appears on a patient's insurance card.

4. **[LO 3.7]** List at least three ways that an office can obtain updated patient information.

5. **[LO 3.1]** Why is it important that every staff member in a facility uses terminology consistently?

6. **[LO 3.10]** List the four most commonly used features of Prime Suite's Help feature.

7. **[LO 3.6]** Explain why the receptionist needs to ask the reason for a patient visit when scheduling an appointment.

8. **[LO 3.2]** The CMS-1500 form is used to submit claims for _____ encounters, whereas the UB-04 form is used to submit _____ claims.

9. **[LO 3.7]** Discuss the importance of reliable, up-to-date patient information.

10. **[LO 3.10]** Discuss why being able to use Prime Suite's Help feature is so important.

11. **[LO 3.1]** List at least five required pieces of demographic information collected for each patient.

12. **[LO 3.8]** Fields, such as Visit Type, that contain a list of options to choose from are known as what type of menus?

13. **[LO 3.4]** What is a medical record number?

14. **[LO 3.2]** List the five major sections on a standard claim form.

15. **[LO 3.9]** List at least three pieces of data typically found on a patient's insurance card.

16. **[LO 3.9]** List at least three pieces of information typically found on a patient's insurance card.

17. **[LO 3.3]** Define and explain the purpose of MACRA.

APPLYING YOUR KNOWLEDGE

1. **[LOs 3.5, 3.6, 3.7, 3.8, 3.9, 3.10]** Which of the Prime Suite exercises completed in this chapter do you think will be used most often in the office setting? Explain your answer.

2. **[LOs 3.1, 3.2, 3.7]** As the receptionist for Greenway Clinic, you recently mailed an informational letter to all patients listed in your MPI. One morning you come into work and see Alfredo Garza's letter marked "Return to Sender, Address Unknown" sitting on your desk. What do you do?

3. **[LOs 3.1, 3.2]** Discuss why administrative data such as race, ethnicity, and preferred language might need to be reported to satisfy Meaningful Use requirements.

4. **[LO 3.4]** The text mentions that if a MPI were inaccessible or unavailable for any reason, it would be nearly impossible to locate a patient's record. Is that true for paper and electronic health records alike? Explain that statement.

5. **[LOs 3.1, 3.2, 3.4]** One of your colleagues has been asked to update the office's data dictionary. She remarks that she does not see why having the data dictionary is so important, because most terms are easily understood by most people in the office. How would you explain to her, with examples, the importance of a solid data dictionary for your practice?

6. **[LOs 3.5, 3.6, 3.7, 3.8]** Discuss the advantages of using a practice management tool such as Prime Suite to complete tasks such as patient registration and appointment scheduling.

7. **[LOs 3.4, 3.5, 3.7]** Why is it important to search for a patient in the MPI before adding the person as a new patient? Explain the consequences of having a patient entered more than once.

8. **[LO 3.3]** Discuss the potential benefits and risks associated with the use of Accountable Care Organizations.

9. **[LO 3.1]** Visit the Commonwell Health Alliance website, at www.commonwellalliance.org. Discuss how they intend to increase the interoperability of EHR systems. Additionally, explain why interoperability is so important when using EHRs.

10. **[LO 3.3]** The Merit-based Incentive Payment System or MIPS is part of the Medicare Access and CHIP Reauthorization Act (MACRA). Explain how MIPS is linked to incentives.

Enhance your learning by completing these exercises and more at http://**connect.mheducation.com**!

chapter references

Centers for Medicare and Medicaid Services (CMS). *MACRA Delivery System Reform, Medicare Payment Reform.* Retrieved from https://www.cms.gov/Medicare/Quality-Initiatives-Patient-Assessment-Instruments/Value-Based-Programs/MACRA-MIPS-and-APMs/MACRA-MIPS-and-APMs.html

Commonwell Health Alliance. Retrieved from http://www.commonwellalliance.org/

Dimick, Chris. "Exposing Double Identity at Patient Registration" *Journal of AHIMA, 80*(11). (2009, November).

Dolin, R.H., Alschuler, L., Beebe, C., et al. (2001, November-December). The HL7 Clinical Document Architecture. *Journal of the American Medical Informatics Association, 8*(6): 552–569.

EHR Incentive Program. *Eligible Professional Meaningful Use Table of Contents Core and Menu Set Measures.* Retrieved from https://www.cms.gov/Regulations-and-Guidance/Legislation/EHRIncentivePrograms/downloads/EP-MU-TOC.pdf

Mertz, Jon. (2010). HL7 Standards. HL7 Quality Reporting Document Architecture (QRDA) Defined. Retrieved from http:// http://healthstandards.com/blog/2010/01/28/hl7-quality-reporting-document-architecture-qrda-defined/

National Committee on Vital and Health Statistics. (1996). *Core Health Data Elements: Report of the National Committee on Vital and Health Statistics.* Retrieved from http://www.cdc.gov/nchs/data/ncvhs/nchvs94.pdf

Newby, Cynthia. (2010). *From Patient to Payment: Insurance Procedures for the Medical Office* (6th ed.). New York: McGraw-Hill Companies.

SearchHealthIT. Continuity of Care Document (CCD). Retrieved from http://searchhealthit.techtarget.com/definition/Continuity-of-Care-Document-CCD

Washington, Lydia. (2013, March 1). ACO Summit Highlights. *Journal of AHIMA.* Retrieved from http://journal.ahima.org/2013/03/01/aco-summit-highlights/

Content of the Health Record—the Past Medical, Surgical, Family, and Social Histories

At the end of this chapter, the student should be able to:

4.1 Outline the use of forms as data collection tools.

4.2 Execute a step-by-step procedure to document past medical, surgical, family, and social histories in Prime Suite.

4.3 Examine the necessity of properly documenting and correcting inconsistent or unclear information.

4.4 Apply procedures to document vital signs in Prime Suite.

Key **Terms**

Cloning
Family history (FH)
Past medical history
Surgical history

Review of systems (ROS)
Social history
Vital signs

What You Need to Know and Why You Need to Know It

Before patients are seen by the care provider, they first meet with the healthcare professional, such as a medical assistant or nurse, to go over the reason for the visit and to capture historical information about their health status. In this chapter we will cover the types of history collected. We will also cover *why* knowing this information is so important in the care of the patient. As with all documentation in a health record, the history must be accurate because often the past history plays a part in the diagnosis and treatment of the current condition. The history generally begins with the chief complaint, which is documented in the patient's (or legal representative's) own words.

4.1 Forms as Data Collection Tools

Take a moment to think of forms that you have completed recently. Most likely they were on paper, and you can probably think immediately of one that was long and cumbersome and took quite a bit of thought to complete. You can also think of one or two that seemed rather logical, well organized, and easy to complete. The same goes for forms that are on screen rather than on paper. When we speak of paper forms, we refer to "boxes" that we are filling out. On screen, these boxes are called *fields*. In most healthcare settings, at this point in time, much of the information gathered from a patient will continue to be accomplished through use of a paper form, and then that information will be transferred to the patient's EHR. Thus, it is important that the design of paper forms be logical to minimize the amount of time it takes to transfer the information and to minimize the likelihood of having missing or incorrect information end up in the EHR. As the transition to an electronic record progresses, patients will increasingly complete the forms electronically, though paper forms will not disappear completely, since there will always be patients who do not want to complete the forms electronically due to lack of a computer, lack of computer literacy, or privacy concerns, and when the computer system "goes down" we will still need to revert to paper and then enter the data manually into the EHR.

When designing a form, keep in mind the following:

- Name the form—give it a title that correlates to the information gathered on the form.
- The name of the office or facility should be added to the form.
- Each page of a multipage form should include the patient's name, date of birth (DOB), and the medical record number or chart number to guard against intermingling the records of patients with the same or similar names and to guard against documentation errors in general.
- The information collected should be relevant to the purpose of the form. Only data that are necessary should be collected—a medical history form in a dermatologist's office will probably not include the patient's menstrual history, for example. If that information were needed for some reason, it could still be added elsewhere in the patient's record.

- Related pieces of data should be adjacent—for instance, the street address, city, and ZIP code of a patient's address should be located adjacent to one another on the form.
- Clearly mark the field names (also called labels) by use of bolding, colored font, or italics.
- If the form is lengthy, separate the form into sections.
- Completion of the form should be easy for the person completing it; in other words, it should be obvious whether the answer to each field should be written on the same line as the field heading or needs to go in the line below.
- Each piece of data should be requested only once on a given form.
- Provide sufficient space for the answer to each field.
- Typically, do not duplicate questions that are answered on other forms; an exception to this is a question about medication allergies—this question is often asked on more than one form due to the importance of the information. It may slip a patient's mind when completing a form at home, but he or she will recall the allergy later in the interview process.

Paper forms are often the source documents used to enter data into the EMR. If that is the case, office policy must reflect what is considered the primary record—paper or EMR—and what will be done with the paper once the data are entered into the EMR: Will it be kept for a period of time and then destroyed, or will the paper be destroyed as soon the data is entered? And, of course, how will the paper be destroyed? Some paper forms may be ordered from an outside company and an inventory of each form kept on hand in the office; in other offices, each form is developed internally and the forms are printed as needed. That decision is often based on available storage space.

Following these guidelines will make it easy for the patient to complete the form. A thoroughly completed form will benefit the care provider as well. Care providers need complete, accurate information quickly, so proper development of data collection tools—whether on paper or on screen—should be an important task in any healthcare setting.

The registration form used in the administrative data chapter is an example of a form that has individual fields in block format. The medical history form in Figure 4.1 is an example of one that has a more free-form format rather than individual fields.

Many "paperless" offices ask their patients to complete history forms online. Think of the last time you applied for a job or when you applied to the college you are attending. Most likely you did so online rather than with a paper application. The rules noted here about ease of completion apply to online forms as well as paper forms.

> **for your information** (fyi)
>
> In some offices, the registration form and the history form are one document rather than individual documents.

4.2 The Past Medical, Surgical, Family, and Social Histories

A patient's **past medical history (PMH)** often contains information that is pertinent to his or her current health status. It is important that the care provider be aware of the patient's past medical history, which includes

- Medical conditions (past and current) for which the patient has been treated or that the patient is experiencing

> **Past medical history (PMH)**
> Previous medical condition(s) for which the patient has been treated.

GREENSBURG MEDICAL CENTER   MEDICAL HISTORY FORM

PATIENT NAME	DOB	MEDICAL RECORD NUMBER

PLEASE ANSWER THE FOLLOWING QUESTIONS THOROUGHLY. IF A QUESTION DOESN'T APPLY, PLEASE ENTER N/A OR PLACE A LINE IN THAT AREA.

PRESENT MEDICAL CONDITION (*why are you being seen today*)

_____

_____

_____

ALLERGIES/REACTIONS TO MEDICINES/FOODS:

NAME OF MEDICATION/AGENT	TYPE OF REACTION

MEDICATIONS: Enter all prescription _and_ non-prescription medicines, herbal remedies, vitamins, or birth control medications here:

MEDICATION	DOSE	HOW OFTEN?	TAKEN FOR?

PERSONAL MEDICAL HISTORY: Please check all conditions you have had (with approximate date or year)

Heart Disease ____ _____   Cancer ____ _____   Type _____

Heart attack ____ _____   Diabetes ____ _____   Type _____

Hypertension ____ _____   Thyroid ____ _____   Type _____

Stroke ____ _____   Bleeding Disorder ___ _____   Type _____

High cholesterol ____ _____   Other ___ _____

Depression/Suicide Attempt ___ _____   Other ___ _____

Alcoholism _____   Other ___ _____

1

Patient Name _____ DOB _____ Med. Record Number _____

SURGICAL HISTORY: Please indicate all procedures or surgeries you have had (with approximate date or year)

Type of surgery	Date (year)	Name of surgeon

FAMILY HISTORY: Please place a check under the family member who has had any of the conditions:

CONDITION	Mom	Dad	Sib.	Child	Other	CONDITION	Mom	Dad	Sibling	Child	Other
Alcoholism						Environmental allergies					
Anemia						Loss of hearing					
Anesthesia problem						Heart problems (heart attack, coronary artery disease, congestive heart failure)					
Arthritis						Hypertension					
Asthma						High cholesterol					
Bleeding problem						Mitral valve disorders					
Cancer, breast						Lupus					
Cancer, colon						HIV/AIDS					
Cancer, melanoma/basal cell						Kidney disease					
Cancer, ovarian						Mental health disorders					
Cancer, prostate						Migraine headaches					
Cancer, other						Osteoarthritis					
Depression						Rheumatoid arthritis					
Type I Diabetes						CVA (stroke)					
Type II Diabetes						Cerebral hemorrhage					
Eczema						Thyroid disorder					
Seizure disorder or epilepsy						Other					
Glaucoma						Other					

IMMUNIZATION HISTORY: Please indicate date (or best guess) of last immunization for:

Hepatitis A ____   Hepatitis B ____   Measles ____   Mumps ____   Rubella ____   Pneumovax (pneumonia) ____

Tetanus (Td) ____   MMR ____   Chicken pox ____   Flu ____ Other _____

SOCIAL HISTORY

Tobacco Use

Cigarettes (current use) ☐ yes ☐ no   If yes, packs per day ____ for ____ years

Cigarettes (past use) ☐ yes ☐ no   If yes, no. of years ____; quit when? _____

2

Patient Name _____ DOB _____ Med. Record Number _____

Other current tobacco use: ☐ snuff/chew ☐ pipe ☐ cigar

Other past tobacco use: ☐ snuff/chew ☐ pipe ☐ cigar

Alcohol Use

Do you drink alcohol? ☐ yes ☐ no   If yes, no. of drinks per week ____

Recreational Drug Use

Do you use any recreational drugs? ☐ yes ☐ no   If yes, what and how often? _____

_____

Physical Activity

How often do you exercise? _____ times/week

Are you relatively active (engage in recreational sports, take stairs daily, job involves standing, walking often, etc.)? ☐ yes ☐ no

SOCIOECONOMIC HISTORY

Occupation _____   Student status ☐ Full time ☐ Part time

Education Completed : ☐ High School graduate   ☐ College graduate   ☐ Graduate School

Marital Status   ☐ Single ☐ Married ☐ Separated ☐ Divorced ☐ Widowed

REVIEW OF SYSTEMS   Answer the following questions for any _current_ problems you are experiencing:

Constitutional: Are you experiencing?

___ Fever/chills/nigh-sweats   ___ Tiredness/weakness

___ Unexpected weight gain/loss   ___ Excessive thirst or urination

___ Tiredness/weakness   ___ Difficulty falling or staying asleep

Eyes, Ears, Nose, Throat and Mouth   *Skin*

___ Change in vision   ___ Rash

___ Difficulty hearing/ringing in ears   ___ Change in moles

___ Teeth/gum problems

___ Hay fever or allergies

Cardiovascular   *Respiratory*

___ Chest pain or discomfort   ___ Cough/wheeze

3

Patient Name _____ DOB _____ Med. Record Number _____

___ Leg pain during exercise   ___ Difficulty breathing/shortness of breath

___ Palpitations (racing heart)

Gastrointestinal   *Genitourinary*

___ Abdominal pain   ___ Frequent urination during night

___ Blood in stool   ___ Leaking urine

___ Nausea/vomiting/diarrhea   ___ Vaginal bleeding (not related to period)

Musculoskeletal   ___ Discharge from penis

___ Muscle/joint pain   *Breasts*

Neurological   ___ Lump or discharge

___ Headaches   *Psychiatric*

___ Dizziness/light-headed   ___ Anxiety/stress

___ Numbness   ___ Depression

___ Memory Loss   *Blood/Lymphatic*

                                      ___ Lumps

                                      ___ Easily bruises/bleeding

Is there anything you want the doctor to address with you today? _____

_____

WOMEN'S HEALTH HISTORY

No. pregnancies ____ No. deliveries ____ No. abortions ____ No. miscarriages ____

Date of last menstrual period _____ Frequency of periods _____ Length _____

_____   _____

Patient's Signature   Date

FOR INTERNAL USE ONLY (ENTER DATE REVIEWED AND INITIALS) ANY CHANGES, ADDITIONS, DELETIONS SHOULD BE DOCUMENTED ABOVE, DATED AND INITIALED.

_____

_____

_____

4

Figure 4.1   Medical History Form

- Date of onset and date resolved for each medical condition
- Known allergies (particularly to medications) as well as the actual reaction
- Immunization status, particularly in children
- Current list of medications, including name, dosage, frequency, and reason it is being taken
- **Review of systems (ROS)**, that is, a body-system inventory of symptoms he or she is having

Many offices include the patient's current condition on the history form, or the particulars of the current condition may be documented in the progress note for the visit. The information about the current condition includes

- Chief complaint (the reason the patient is being seen that day—generally speaking, the reason for the appointment)
- History of present illness: location of the condition (for example, pain in the right shoulder); type of pain (ache, sharp pain, etc.); severity (mild, severe); duration (how long the complaint has been present); and any associated signs and symptoms (for example, difficulty raising arm above head when pain is present)

The **surgical history** includes information about procedures the patient has undergone. If a patient, Carolyn Wright, is experiencing right lower quadrant pain yet her history shows she had an appendectomy 14 years ago, the care provider will concentrate diagnostic testing on other possibilities. Surgical history includes

- Name of the operation or procedure
- Reason for the procedure
- Date the procedure was performed (may be approximate)
- Name of the surgeon who performed the procedure
- Anesthesia reactions or complications, if any

The **family history (FH)** includes information that will alert the care provider to any conditions that may affect the patient's overall health now or in the future. For example, Neil Alexander is a 45-year-old patient who has been experiencing chest pains and shortness of breath. He notes that his father and paternal grandfather both had a myocardial infarction (heart attack) before the age of 50. In this case, that information is important to the care provider in order to make diagnostic and treatment decisions for the patient. Past family history includes

- Name of the condition(s)
- Family member(s) who had the condition(s)
- Sometimes, whether immediate family members (parent, sibling) are still alive and, if not, the date/cause of death

The **social history (SH)** is important because the care provider needs to know the patient's habits in order to assess possible causes of conditions or potential health concerns that could arise as a result of the patient's habits or lifestyle. An example is a patient who is overweight, works in a sedentary

Review of systems (ROS) A body-system-by-body-system inventory of any symptoms the patient is having or has had based on a series of questions asked by the care provider.

Surgical history Previous surgical procedure(s) the patient has undergone, the approximate date(s), name of surgeon, reason for procedure(s), and complications, if any.

Family history (FH) Documentation of conditions and diseases found in immediate family members (e.g., diabetes mellitus, cancer, or heart disease).

Social history (SH) Lifestyle or social habits of the patient. Examples include smoking history or current use, use of alcoholic beverages and frequency, patient's profession, etc.

job, and has noted that she does not exercise or participate in any other strenuous activity. That patient would be at risk for heart disease, stroke, and other serious medical conditions. Elements of a social history include

- Smoking history—past or current use
- Other tobacco use (snuff, pipe, or cigar, for example)
- Alcohol use—current or past
- Recreational drug use
- Socioeconomic data—occupation, education, marital status
- Sexual activity and use of protection
- Exercise and physical activity

cloning (copy and paste) Used in an electronic environment, copying similar or identical information from a previous encounter of the same or a different patient.

Unlike a written record, an EMR lends itself to being copied from one encounter to the next relatively easily, particularly the past medical, surgical, family, and social histories. This is known as **cloning** or more commonly as **copy and paste**. The reason providers and practitioners clone parts of a record is speed and efficiency. Let's say Dr. Ingram is reviewing the social history of a 58-year-old established patient, Mary Cay Gregory. Dr. Ingram goes over the social history that is already in the previous record with Mrs. Gregory, and she says that nothing has changed, and she has nothing to add. Rather than type those notes again, the physician simply copies them from the previous record and pastes them into the current record. A patient's social history may contain sensitive information, and care should be taken to ensure that the copied information is verified. In the scenario I just described, the information is being copied from and to the same patient's health record. Although the practice of copying information between different patients' records is discouraged, some medical offices choose to do so. In these instances, it is imperative to pay attention to detail, and ensure accuracy and completeness of the documentation.

Even copying from encounters belonging to the same patient has its dangers. Let's say that for the same patient, Dr. Ingram copies and pastes the diagnosis of pneumococcal pneumonia from her last visit into the current problem list. Mrs. Gregory's last visit was two years ago, and she no longer has pneumococcal pneumonia. Including pneumococcal pneumonia as an active condition on this visit is not accurate; it is not an acute condition and therefore should not appear as such on this current record. Doing so brings into question the validity of the record in general.

Though it may seem efficient, cloning entries can be dangerous, particularly if incorrect medications, prior or current treatments, or past histories are incorrectly carried over to a patient's record. Before the cloning feature of an EMR is used, it is imperative that the providers, practitioners, and staff understand the serious nature of incorrect information within the record. They must remember the importance of the health record; it serves as a basis for medical decision making, and it is a record upon which legal decisions are based in cases of medical malpractice, liability (such as in the case of a car accident), and Workers' Compensation. Additionally, reimbursement is tied to the documentation found in the health record—as proof of what is wrong with the patient, what was done to or for the patient, and the quality of care provided to the patient (Haugen).

The documentation of the past medical and surgical histories, the family and social history, along with the findings of the physical examination

Enter a Patient's Past Medical History

In this exercise, we will be following the past medical history of a patient, Amy Peterson. She has arrived and checked in for her appointment with Dr. Rodriguez at Greensburg Medical Center. The healthcare professional has called Mrs. Peterson back to the exam room for the initial portion of the visit. Mr. Peterson has accompanied the patient to the appointment and is in the exam room as well. The healthcare professional begins by accessing Amy Peterson's Facesheet screen in Prime Suite, as noted in Figure 4.2.

The healthcare professional will verify Mrs. Peterson's information and change it if necessary before going on to the Past Medical History. The healthcare professional clicks on the Past Medical History screen from the Facesheet.

Though some information may be entered previously, the healthcare professional should ask about any other conditions. Mrs. Peterson's husband confirms she has osteoporosis, and osteoarthritis, but no other medical conditions. The healthcare professional asks about any previous surgeries. Mr. Peterson responds that she had an appendectomy back in 1971 and she had a cataract removed from her right eye in 2007. They are the only surgical procedures Mrs. Peterson has had, but she does have one child, so the healthcare professional asks Mrs. Peterson about her reproductive history. Mrs. Peterson says she was pregnant once and has one child. The pregnancy was a full-term pregnancy.

Follow these steps to complete the exercise on your own once you have watched the demonstration and tried the steps with helpful prompts. Use the information provided in the scenario to complete the information.

1. Click the Past Medical History radio button.
2. Click Musculoskeletal.
3. Check Osteoarthritis.
4. Check Osteoporosis.
5. Click PSHx.
6. Check Appendectomy.
7. Click details.
8. Type "1971".

Prime Suite Tip

When the action is to click on a heading that has a radio button to the left of it, click on the radio button, NOT the words.

Figure 4.2 **Amy Peterson's Facesheet**

(continued)

9. Click OK.
10. Check Cataract Surgery.
11. Click details.
12. Type "2007".
13. Click Notes field.
14. Type "Right Eye".
15. Click OK.
16. Click RHx.
17. Click Pregnancy.
18. Click the Total Preg field.
19. Type "1".
20. Double-click the Full Term field.
21. Type "1".
22. Click Close.

✔️ **You have completed Exercise 4.1**

EXERCISE 4.2 EHR Go to http://connect.mheducation.com to complete this exercise. McGraw Hill Education connect®

Enter a Patient's List of Current Medications

In this exercise, the patient's current medications are entered. Part of the functionality of Prime Suite is the differentiation between those medications prescribed by Greensburg Medical Center and those prescribed by another provider or bought over the counter.

This process begins by accessing Mrs. Peterson's Facesheet in Prime Suite and then selecting Medication List (Figure 4.2). Mrs. Peterson shares with the healthcare professional that she takes ibuprofen for her osteoarthritis. She takes 800 mg tablets, three times a day. She also takes glucosamine chondroitin every day. These are tablets as well, and she takes the 750–600 mg tablets. She is also taking alendronate, which is a drug for post-menopausal osteoporosis prevention. These are taken in tablet form as well, 35 mg one time a week.

Follow these steps to complete the exercise on your own once you have watched the demonstration and tried the steps with helpful prompts. Use the information provided in the scenario to complete the information.

1. Click the Medication List radio button.
2. Click Record Medication.
3. Click Search By Name.
4. Click the Medication Name field.
5. Type "ibuprofen".
6. Click ibuprofen.
7. Click Osteoarthritis.
8. Click Oral.
9. Click 800 mg oral tablet.
10. Click "take 1 tablet (800 mg) by oral route 3 times per day with food."

11. Click OK.
12. Click Record Medication.
13. Click Search By Name.
14. Click the Medication Name field.
15. Type "Glucosamine chondroitin".
16. Click glucosamine-chondroitin.
17. Click 750-600 mg oral tablet.
18. Type "2" in the take field.
19. Click by oral route field.
20. Click QD.
21. Click Done.
22. Click Add Another.
23. Type "alendronate" in the Medication Name field.
24. Click alendronate.
25. Click Post-Menopausal Osteoporosis Prevention.
26. Click 35 mg oral tablet.
27. Click OK.
28. Click Save.

 You have completed Exercise 4.2

 Go to http://connect.mheducation.com to complete this exercise.   **EHR**   **EXERCISE**   **4.3**

Enter a Patient's Known Drug Allergies

Mrs. Peterson has an allergy to Reglan. Knowing the patient's medication allergies is a very important piece of information. Not knowing her allergies, and prescribing a drug that she is allergic to, could cause a very serious reaction. Her allergy to Reglan will be documented in the Allergies List section of the Facesheet (Figure 4.2).

Follow these steps to complete the exercise on your own once you have watched the demonstration and tried the steps with helpful prompts. Use the information provided in the scenario to complete the information.

1. Click the Allergy List radio button.
2. Click Add.
3. Type "Reg" in the Allergen field.
4. Click Reglan.
5. Click OK.
6. Click the check box next to Reglan to select it.
7. Click close.

 You have completed Exercise 4.3

and the patient's signs and symptoms, which we will discuss in more detail in the next section of the worktext, are all pieces of the puzzle that allow the care provider to accurately diagnose and treat the patient.

4.3   Handling Inconsistent or Unclear Information

As we discussed earlier, a patient's history is gathered by use of a form, as well as through an interview with the patient. Sometimes, what a patient has documented on the history form contradicts what comes out during the interview. When entering any information about a patient—for instance, if you are reviewing a past medical history with the patient, and you see on the past medical history form that the patient had an appendectomy in 1997 yet she tells you verbally that she has never had any surgeries—you need to question the patient to determine the correct answer. Though the patient completed the form, she could have checked the wrong box on the form, or she may have forgotten that she had the surgery. Sometimes, patients choose not to tell the healthcare professional or care provider all of the facts. Often, the healthcare professional senses that the patient is being evasive or is only partly answering questions. It is part of the healthcare professional's role to act in such a way that instills trust; communicating *why* these questions are being asked is often all that is needed for a patient to become more comfortable. The fact that there is a discrepancy (or that information is missing) should never be ignored and should be documented. The medical practice or hospital must have written policies on how to handle such situations.

Following is an example of a policy statement regarding inconsistent information: *In the event that an error or inconsistency is found in a health record or in the information given verbally by a patient/legal representative, an attempt should be made to verify the information and document the same. The circumstances surrounding the discrepancy should be documented sufficiently in the health record to explain the situation thoroughly.*

Documentation in a health record must be accurate, precise, reliable, and consistent, not only because it is a legal document, but also to ensure quality medical care. Prime Suite, like other EHR software, has built-in mechanisms to amend, delete, or add documentation without compromising the integrity of the record. Though a change to documentation may occur, the original version of the documentation is always retrievable. Remember, the health record is a *legal document,* so any written information upon which care may have been based or that may have been released to other care providers, insurance companies, or other third parties must remain retrievable. In the previous example regarding the discrepancy about the patient's surgery, the explanation of the discrepancy can be documented in a details box, found in the past surgical history section of the record. Later in this worktext, when covering data integrity, we will further examine correcting and amending entries and will test your knowledge through Prime Suite exercises.

Vital signs Measurements taken (temperature, heart rate, respiratory rate, blood pressure, height and weight, and sometimes body mass index) to determine the status of basic body system functions.

4.4   Documenting Vital Signs

The patient's **vital signs** are taken by the healthcare professional—some offices take them before completing the history, and others take them after. Prime Suite software includes a very helpful feature: the ability to see a connect Go to http://connect.mheducation.com to complete this exercise.

Enter a Patient's Vital Signs

Prime Suite allows documentation of the position the patient is in when the blood pressure is taken: sitting, standing, or lying down.

In our example, the healthcare professional is in the process of taking Amy Peterson's vital signs. She asks Amy to sit on the exam table and takes her blood pressure. The reading is 110/65. Her heart rate is 68 beats per minute (bpm) and regular, with a respiratory rate of 22. Mrs. Peterson's temperature is 97.6 F. Her weight was taken before coming into the exam room, and she weighed 135 pounds. She is 5 feet 2 inches (62 inches) tall. Her oxygen saturation today is 99%.

Follow these steps to complete the exercise on your own once you have watched the demonstration and tried the steps with helpful prompts. Use the information provided in the scenario to complete the information.

1. Click the Vital Signs radio button.
2. Click Add New Vitals.
3. Type "110" in the Systolic field.
4. Click the Diastolic field.
5. Type "65".
6. Click the Heart Rate field.
7. Type "68".
8. Click the Respiratory Rate field.
9. Type "22".
10. Click the Temperature field.
11. Type "97.6".
12. Click the Weight field.
13. Type "135".
14. Click the Height in inches field.
15. Type "62".
16. Click the Oxygen Saturation field.
17. Type "99".
18. Click Add Vitals.
19. Click Close.
20. Click the Facesheet tab to confirm that you have viewed the screen.

☑ **You have completed Exercise 4.4**

for your information fyi

The body mass index (BMI) is now a standard entry in most health records. BMI is a formula showing body weight adjusted for a patient's height. A healthy BMI is between 18.5 and 24.9. EHR software will automatically compute the BMI once the patient's height and weight are entered in the vital signs field.

patient's vital signs over time. The tracking of the vital signs can be seen graphically or chronologically. This helps the provider assess such conditions as hypertension or significant weight gain or loss.

Like the documentation of the patient's history, entering the vital signs is done from the vital signs section of the Facesheet.

The vital signs include the patient's blood pressure, heart rate, respiratory rate, temperature, height, weight, body mass index (BMI), and oxygen saturation. Technically, height and weight and BMI are not vital signs, but all are taken or calculated about the same time as the vital signs and therefore are included in that section of the record.

At this point in the process, the patient has been taken to the exam room, vital signs have been taken, and she is ready to be seen by the care provider.

APPLYING YOUR SKILLS

1. What is meant by using a paper form as a "source document"?
2. Why is a social history important in the care of a patient?
3. Would a patient's vital signs ever be cloned from one record to another? Explain your answer.

chapter 4 **summary**

LEARNING OUTCOME	CONCEPTS FOR REVIEW

4.1 Outline the use of forms as data collection tools.	– Paper form versus computer screen
	– When designing a form, keep the following in mind:
	  • Name the form
	  • Name of the office or facility
	  • Patient's name on every page
	  • Purpose of the form
	– Keep related information close together on the form.
	– Clearly mark field headings.
	– Lengthy forms should be separated into sections.
	– Ease of completion and of reading
	– Don't duplicate information on the form.
	– Sufficient space for answers on paper forms

4.2 Execute a step-by-step procedure to document medical, surgical, family, and social histories in Prime Suite.	– All histories are important in the assessment of patients. – Past medical history includes current and past medical conditions; allergies; medications; immunization status; chief complaint; history of present illness; review of systems. – Surgical history includes all surgeries or procedures the patient has had and the dates (even if approximate). – Family history is collected to assess whether the patient is predisposed to certain conditions. – Social history is collected to determine if the patient may be at a greater risk for certain conditions. – The use of cloning (copy and paste) in an EMR/EHR
4.3 Examine the necessity of properly documenting and correcting inconsistent or unclear information.	– Office or facility must have clear policies to deal with inconsistent information. – When a discrepancy is found and the patient is present, ask which is correct; amend the record according to policy. – If the correct information is not certain, document that as well.

4.4 Apply procedures to document vital signs in Prime Suite.	– Vital signs include
	  • Blood pressure
	  • Temperature
	  • Heart rate
	  • Respiratory rate
	  • Height
	  • Weight
	  • Body mass index
	  • Blood oxygen saturation
	– Prime Suite will show vital signs over time, which may alert the provider to certain risk factors such as high blood pressure or significant weight loss or gain.

chapter **review**

MATCHING QUESTIONS

Match the terms on the left with the definitions on the right.

_____ 1. **[LO 4.2]** review of systems

_____ 2. **[LO 4.2]** surgical history

_____ 3. **[LO 4.2]** medical history

_____ 4. **[LO 4.2]** social history

_____ 5. **[LO 4.2]** family history

_____ 6. **[LO 4.4]** vital signs

a. patient information such as blood pressure and respiratory rate

b. patient information that includes immunizations and allergies

c. patient information that includes information such as frequency of drinking and smoking

d. comprehensive inventory of patient symptoms such as headaches, vision, heart palpitations, and swelling of joints

e. patient information that includes past procedures and who performed the procedures

f. patient information that includes possibly inherited conditions

MULTIPLE-CHOICE QUESTIONS

Select the letter that best completes the statement or answers the question:

1. **[LO 4.1]** An on-screen item of data is known as a
   a. box.
   b. crate.
   c. carton.
   d. field.

2. **[LO 4.3]** Prime Suite allows you to note discrepancies in the _____ field.
   a. details
   b. discrepancies
   c. information
   d. registration

3. **[LO 4.1]** It is important to keep the design of paper forms
   a. cumbersome.
   b. detailed.
   c. logical.
   d. short.

4. **[LO 4.2]** Which of the following is NOT a required patient history?
   a. family
   b. birth
   c. social
   d. surgical

5. **[LO 4.1]** Of the following, who will benefit from thoroughly completed paper forms?
   a. care providers
   b. patients
   c. receptionists
   d. all of these

6. **[LO 4.2]** The patient's _____ history can help predict a future health condition.
   a. family
   b. medical
   c. social
   d. surgical

7. **[LO 4.4]** A patient's vital signs can be easily viewed via Prime Suite's _____ screen.
   a. Facesheet
   b. Help
   c. Patient
   d. Registration

8. **[LO 4.3]** Which of the following is an acceptable way of gathering a patient's history?
   a. medical/surgical history form
   b. physical exam
   c. provider asks the patient questions
   d. a & c

9. **[LO 4.1]** Which piece of information might be included multiple times on a form?
   a. address
   b. drug allergies
   c. marital status
   d. patient history

10. **[LO 4.1]** What information should you see on all forms in a patient chart?
    a. name
    b. DOB
    c. medical record number
    d. all of these

11. **[LO 4.2]** A patient's surgical history includes the
    a. approximate date of the procedure.
    b. name of the attending physician.
    c. patient's recovery time.
    d. type of sutures used.

12. **[LO 4.1]** For ease of completion, related information should be _____ on a form.
    a. adjacent
    b. duplicated
    c. labeled
    d. separate

Enhance your learning by completing these exercises and more at http://**connect.mheducation.com**!

13. **[LO 4.4]** What does BMI stand for?
    a. basic medical information
    b. body mass index
    c. body matter indicator
    d. base measurement index

14. **[LO 4.2]** Which of the following would include the patient's frequency of alcohol consumption?
    a. family history
    b. medical history
    c. social history
    d. surgical history

15. **[LO 4.3]** Any discrepancies in patient information need to be
    a. detailed.
    b. documented.
    c. filed.
    d. transcribed.

SHORT-ANSWER QUESTIONS

1. **[LO 4.1]** Explain why it is important to keep the design of paper forms logical and orderly.

2. **[LO 4.2]** Explain why a patient's social history is important.

3. **[LO 4.1]** Why is it recommended that a patient's name, DOB, and chart number/medical record number appear on each page of a multipage form?

4. **[LO 4.4]** List the vital signs that are typically taken at each patient visit.

5. **[LO 4.1]** Why, in the age of EHRs, is patient information still gathered mainly through the use of paper forms?

6. **[LO 4.2]** Differentiate between the social and family histories.

7. **[LO 4.3]** Why does a medical office need to have clear policies in place for dealing with discrepancies in patient information?

8. **[LO 4.4]** Prime Suite includes a feature to allow the provider to view the patient's vital signs in different ways. Explain the benefit of this feature.

9. **[LO 4.2]** Why might so many patient histories need to be taken?

10. **[LO 4.2]** Dr. Stephens copied and pasted the physical exam from Jeanie Lopez's visit for strep pharyngitis to the physical exam of Shelly Lopez's visit for strep pharyngitis. Could that cause any problems with the care rendered to Shelly Lopez? Explain your answer.

APPLYING YOUR KNOWLEDGE

1. **[LO 4.2]** Stephanie Lewis comes to your office for her annual wellness checkup. As the healthcare professional who will be doing her initial interview, create a list of questions you might ask Stephanie to obtain her social history.

2. **[LO 4.4]** How can the Prime Suite tracking feature assist you in analyzing a patient's vital signs over time? Give a specific example.

3. **[LO 4.1]** As an office manager for a large healthcare practice, you have been asked to design a new patient intake form. Sketch out your form's layout, keeping in mind the best practices discussed in the chapter.

4. **[LO 4.3]** Bob Larks is a new patient in your practice, and he brought his informational form with him on his first visit. During the patient history portion of his exam, he says that he does not drink, but while entering that information in Bob's chart you notice that his initial history stated that he was a "social drinker." What should you do?

5. **[LOs 4.2, 4.3]** As a healthcare professional, you are attempting to obtain the medical history of your patient, Lisa Sanchez. However, you are having difficulty because Lisa is evading your questions and is refusing to respond. What can you do?

 Enhance your learning by completing these exercises and more at http://**connect.mheducation.com**!

chapter references

Booth, K.A., Whicker, L.G., Wyman, Terri D., and Moany Wright, Sandra. (2011). *Administrative Procedures for Medical Assisting* (4th ed.). New York: McGraw-Hill Companies.

Green, M.A., and Bowie, M.J. (2016). *Essentials of Health Information Management: Principles and Practices* (3rd ed.). Clifton Park, NY: Delmar, Cengage Learning.

Haugen, Heather. (2014, June). Overcoming the Risks of Copy and Paste in EHRs. *Journal of AHIMA, 85*(6): 54–55.

Newby, C. (2010). *From Patient to Payment: Insurance Procedures for the Medical Office* (6th ed.). New York: McGraw-Hill Companies.

chapter five

Content of the Health Record— the Care Provider's Responsibility

Learning Outcomes

At the end of this chapter, the student should be able to:

5.1 Explain each element of a SOAP note.

5.2 Identify elements of the history of present illness (HPI).

5.3 Identify elements of the review of systems (ROS).

5.4 Identify elements of the physical exam (PE).

5.5 Describe the process of traditional dictation and transcription.

5.6 Illustrate the advantages of speech recognition technology.

5.7 Outline the benefits of ePrescribing.

5.8 Evaluate the benefits of computerized physician order entry (CPOE).

5.9 Support the necessity to track physicians' orders.

5.10 Examine the benefits of a problem list.

Key Terms

Computerized physician order entry (CPOE)

Discharge summary

ePrescribing

History & Physical (H&P)

History of present illness (HPI)

Interface

Physical exam (PE)

Point of care (POC)

Problem list

Review of systems (ROS)

Scribe

SOAP note

Speech recognition technology

Voice recognition technology

What You Need to Know and Why You Need to Know It

In this chapter, the EHR is assessed from the care provider's perspective. In the Prime Suite demonstrations, we will illustrate how a care provider captures clinical information.

Knowing where in a record certain information resides is important because it is often necessary for the medical assistant, coder, biller, or other healthcare professional to access a care provider's documentation to answer a question for another care provider or for an insurance company, or to complete forms.

SOAP An acronym for the documentation used in a care provider's office to record the patient's symptoms, signs, assessment (diagnosis), and plan of care.

5.1 The SOAP Note

SOAP stands for **S**ubjective, **O**bjective, **A**ssessment, and **P**lan. It is a format for documentation that reflects a patient's visit (typically an office visit) in an orderly fashion—from the time the visit begins to the time it ends. A SOAP note consists of four distinct areas of documentation. They are

Subjective (S): This is the information the care provider learns from the patient. The subjective findings are the patient's description of his or her symptoms. For instance, Philip James is seen in Dr. Connors' office today; he tells the doctor that he has had a "cold and terrible headache" for three days. He also states that he "has been achy and has pressure over both eyes." These are all sensations that only the patient can feel and therefore are subjective. They are not measurable.

Objective (O): Objective findings include information the care provider gathers from performing a physical exam. These are measurable findings. For example, upon conducting a physical exam on Philip James, the physician notes that the patient flinches when he palpates the area above the patient's eyebrows and his cheekbones; because the patient flinches, the physician knows that the patient is experiencing discomfort. The patient also has a green nasal discharge. Mr. James is an established patient of Dr. Connors' and he has had three sinus infections in the past two years, as noted in the patient's past medical history, which is based on the documentation from his prior encounters. Objective findings also include measurable test results such as an x-ray finding or lab results.

Assessment (A): At the assessment stage, the care provider *assesses* the patient's signs and symptoms and the results of his physical exam in order to make a diagnosis or diagnoses. In many cases, it is necessary to await test results to determine a diagnosis; in the meantime, a diagnosis may be considered "probable," "possible," or "suspected." In the case of Philip James, the physician has documented the diagnosis as acute sinusitis.

Plan (P): The plan is also known as the *plan of care.* The care provider will order any tests he feels are medically necessary, prescribe medications or recommend over-the-counter medications, order consultations with other care providers if necessary, educate the patient about his condition, and advise the patient of follow-up instructions. So in Mr. James' case, Dr. Connors wrote an order for a CT scan of the sinuses. His instructions to Mr. James included drinking plenty of fluids and taking the next two days off from work. A prescription for a Z-Pak was ordered and he was given printed educational material about sinusitis (from the EHR software). He was told to schedule a follow-up appointment for 10 days from now.

An example of an instruction screen for a patient is found in Figure 5.1. In a paper record, the physician would handwrite the patient's record, as seen in Figure 5.2.

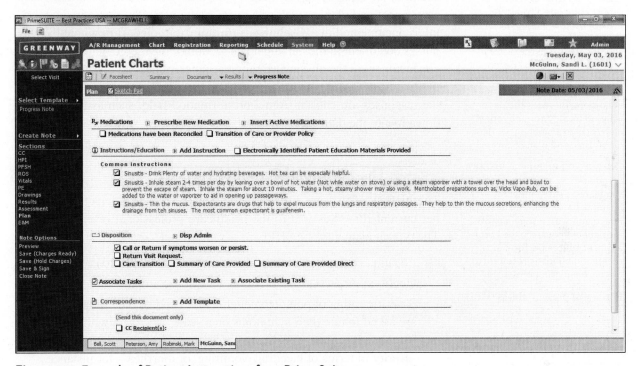

Figure 5.1   Example of Patient Instructions from Prime Suite

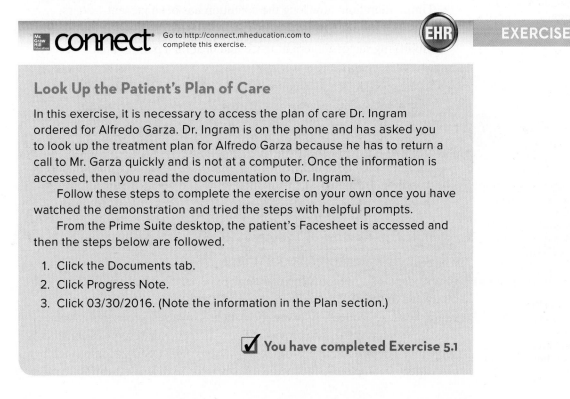

Go to http://connect.mheducation.com to complete this exercise.

EXERCISE   5.1

Look Up the Patient's Plan of Care

In this exercise, it is necessary to access the plan of care Dr. Ingram ordered for Alfredo Garza. Dr. Ingram is on the phone and has asked you to look up the treatment plan for Alfredo Garza because he has to return a call to Mr. Garza quickly and is not at a computer. Once the information is accessed, then you read the documentation to Dr. Ingram.

Follow these steps to complete the exercise on your own once you have watched the demonstration and tried the steps with helpful prompts.

From the Prime Suite desktop, the patient's Facesheet is accessed and then the steps below are followed.

1. Click the Documents tab.
2. Click Progress Note.
3. Click 03/30/2016. (Note the information in the Plan section.)

✓ **You have completed Exercise 5.1**

History &Physical (H&P) A report completed by a care provider that includes the reason(s) the patient is being seen or admitted; the history of present illness; the pertinent past medical, surgical, social, and family histories; other current conditions/diseases the patient is being treated for; the report of a physical examination; working diagnoses; and plan of care.

Discharge summary A report completed by a care provider that summarizes a patient's stay in the hospital. It generally includes the final diagnoses, a summary of the patient's course in the hospital, any procedures performed, a recap of diagnostic results, and discharge instructions.

History of present illness (HPI) The patient's description of current complaints such as when the symptoms started, the location of the condition, quality of the symptoms, severity of the symptoms, anything that makes the symptoms better or worse, and additional symptoms the patient is experiencing.

for your information

Some typical questions asked during a ROS are Have you been having any unusual headaches? Have you been having any blurry or double vision? Have you had any change in bowel habits? Have you had any swelling of your joints?

Review of systems (ROS) A body-system-by-body-system inventory of any symptoms the patient is having or has had based on a series of questions asked by the care provider.

In an electronic health record, these elements are documented, but rather than being handwritten, a combination of free-text writing and use of drop-down menus and standard text makes documentation more thorough, consistent, easily retrievable, and legible. As you complete the exercises later in this chapter, you will see that the SOAP elements just described are present in the EHR.

When a patient is admitted to a hospital, the care provider documents the subjective and objective findings, along with the results of a physical exam, in the **History & Physical** report, otherwise known as an **H&P**. The assessment and plan, as well as a recap of the patient's course in the hospital, is documented in a **discharge summary** (or note). Throughout the stay, nurses document in the nursing notes section of the record, and care providers document in the physicians' progress notes. When handwritten or typed, these are *unstructured data;* when an electronic health record is used and the responses are chosen from a pre-formatted field, such as from a drop-down menu, the data are *structured*.

5.2 The History of Present Illness (HPI)

The **history of present illness,** or **HPI**, is the patient's depiction of his or her current illness as told to the healthcare professional or care provider. The typical elements of an HPI are

- Location of the condition (abdomen, arm, leg, head, etc.)
- Quality: pain is sharp, dull, or an ache, for example
- Severity: rating of pain/itch/cough/nausea and so on. Often, patients are asked to rate their symptoms on a scale of 1 to 10, with 1 being barely noticeable and 10 being intolerable. This may also mean the severity in terms of bleeding, vomiting, or diarrhea—for instance, profuse bleeding from a laceration versus a small amount of bleeding.
- Timing/duration: how long the condition has been present—hours, days, weeks, months, for example
- Modifying factors: alternating ice and heat on a painful area, effect of pain medication, and so on
- Associated signs and symptoms: for instance, the cold symptoms described by Philip James in Figure 5.2

Read Philip James' SOAP note in Figure 5.2 again. Match the information listed in the subjective portion of the note to the typical elements of an HPI. Not all elements are collected on all visits—only those that are necessary based on the patient's chief complaint would be documented.

5.3 The Review of Systems (ROS)

The **review of systems (ROS)** is a body-system-by-body-system assessment of any signs or symptoms the patient is experiencing that may or may not be related to the reason for the visit. The ROS is not the same as a physical exam, because the ROS refers to the patient's own responses, not an objective assessment by the care provider. Thus, the patient's responses constitute subjective content in the health record. Often, the ROS is accomplished by the patient's completing the medical history form, discussed earlier. Or the

Patient: Philip James	DOB: July 31, 1991 **Date of Service:** 05/03/2016
S	Mr. James presented today because he has had a headache for the past three days. He has not received any relief from OTC decongestants or antihistamines. He describes the pain as more of an ache, though when he pushes on his forehead, it is painful. He has had cold symptoms for about a week, but his symptoms are getting worse, and on a scale of 1 to 10, he says that his pain is an 8. He has also noted that he has had two minor nose bleeds in the past two days.
O	Vital signs noted in his chart. All within normal limits. Head and face: physical exam of nasal passages reveals a moderate amount of green discharge from both nares. The patient is tender to the touch above each eyebrow and cheek bone. Chest is clear to percussion and auscultation. Heart: Regular rate and rhythm. Abdomen: Non-tender. This is the third time Mr. James has been diagnosed with a sinus infection in the past 18 months.
A	Acute sinusitis.
P	CT scan of sinuses to be done today or tomorrow at Memorial Hospital (order given to patient). Instructed to drink plenty of fluids and bedrest for two days. To return to office in 10 days for follow-up. Z-Pak single-dose pack was sent to The Corner Pharmacy via ePrescribe. Patient was given sinusitis literature.
	Jared Connors, MD 05/03/2016

Figure 5.2 **Written SOAP Note**

EHR **EXERCISE** **5.2**

connect Go to http://connect.mheducation.com to complete this exercise.

Locate Alfredo Garza's Blood Pressure

In this exercise, Alfredo J. Garza stopped by the office and wants to know what his blood pressure was on his last visit. To look this up, you will access Alfredo Garza's health record.

You will start by going to Alfredo J. Garza's Facesheet. The vital signs are found there, and you do not need to leave the Facesheet to find his blood pressure readings.

Follow these steps to complete the exercise on your own once you have watched the demonstration and tried the steps with helpful prompts.

From the Prime Suite Desktop, access the patient's Facesheet and then follow these steps:

1. Click the Vital Signs radio button.
2. Click the 03/30/2016 blood pressure reading to highlight it.
3. Click Close.

Once you locate the vital signs, you will tell Mr. Garza that on his visit of March 30, 2016, his blood pressure reading was 160/80.

 You have completed Exercise 5.2

care provider may use that as a starting point and ask questions based on the patient's responses on the form. The completion (or review) of the ROS is an integral component in assessing the patient's overall health as well as gaining a better picture of any additional signs or symptoms that may be related to the patient's chief complaint. In addition, the ROS plays a role in how much the patient will be charged for the visit, since it takes into account the

Prime Suite Tip **PS**

Click on the radio button next to the words "Vital Signs," *not* on the words themselves.

care provider's time and medical expertise during an office visit. Regardless of whether (1) the history form is already completed and the care provider reviews it or (2) the care provider completes the form during an office visit, there must be some form of documentation to show that the ROS was done or reviewed in order to receive reimbursement for it. The particulars of procedure coding, charging, and reimbursement will be covered briefly in the financial management chapter.

Usually, a care provider will start at the head and work down through the body to the lower extremities. Following are the organs and/or body systems that are typically reviewed, as well as examples of questions that may be asked for each:

- General, also referred to as constitutional (how the patient is feeling in general, any complaints or concerns, and a recap of vital signs)
- Skin (any rashes or wounds that will not heal, any unusual moles or markings that have appeared, and so on)
- Head, eyes, ears, nose, and mouth (headaches, double vision, blurring of vision, ringing of ears, earache, nosebleeds, dry mouth, dental issues)
- Throat (persistent sore throat, difficulty swallowing)
- Breasts (whether monthly self-exams are done; any changes, lumps, nipple discharge)
- Respiratory (difficulty breathing, shortness of breath)
- Cardiovascular (any chest pain, palpitations, or fluttering)
- Gastrointestinal (problems with stomach pain, constipation, diarrhea; changes in stool, signs of blood in stool)
- Genitourinary (problems voiding, cloudiness of urine, changes in color or odor of urine, difficulty starting to urinate, nighttime urination, signs of blood in urine)
- Musculoskeletal (pain in joints or extremities, difficulty walking)
- Neurologic (dizziness; light-headedness; difficulty with memory, cognition, coordination; severe headaches)
- Endocrine (if female, problems with menses, swelling of the thyroid)
- Psychological (depression, changes in mood)
- Hematologic/lymphatic (unexplained or profuse bleeding, swelling of lymph glands)
- Allergies (problems with environmental allergies, known allergies or reactions to medications)

In Prime Suite and most EHR software, the ROS choices are determined by the patient's chief complaint or the corresponding body system. Not every ailment requires a thorough ROS. For instance, for a patient being seen with cold symptoms, the care provider may review just the head, eyes, ears, nose, and throat (HEENT) and the chest (which essentially makes up the respiratory system). The care provider would typically have no need to review the breasts or the neurologic, psychological, or reproductive system.

Figure 5.3 shows the master ROS file in Prime Suite, and Figure 5.4 shows the full ROS.

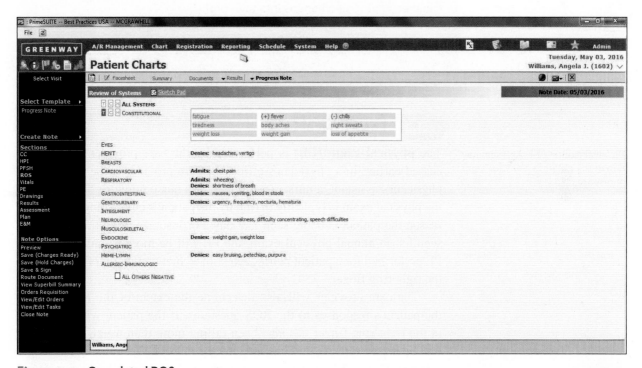

Figure 5.3 Prime Suite Review of Systems Admin Screen—Constitutional Section

Figure 5.4 Completed ROS

Each office must construct a master ROS file; however, each care provider chooses the content of each ROS screen and how it displays. Thus, in Prime Suite the ROS screens are user-based and can be customized to each user's needs or preferences. (Figure 5.4 shows a completed ROS in narrative form.)

Prime Suite Tip PS

When documenting the ROS in Prime Suite, a check mark means the question is active, but the answer is neutral. A negative sign means the patient denies the complaint; a plus sign means that the patient admits to having the complaint.

Add New Options to the ROS

Even though the Prime Suite ROS Admin function is comprehensive, your practice may want to customize specific sections by adding new choices or adjusting existing ones. This is done through the ROS Admin screen.

1. Click the Chart drop-down menu.
2. Click Review of Systems Admin.
3. Click Edit Options.
4. Type "Stomach cramps" in the Add New Option field.
5. Click the plus sign.
6. Click the scroll bar.
7. Double-click malaise.
8. Type "tiredness".
9. Click OK.
10. Click Save.

You have now customized your ROS Admin screen. If you are the office manager in charge of customizing the practice's screens, you can click Export at the bottom of the screen to share it with other users; those users can then import the changes into their profiles.

☑ **You have completed Exercise 5.3**

5.4 **The Physical Exam**

Physical exam (PE) An examination of the patient's body for signs of disease.

The **physical exam (PE)** is performed by the care provider. As we discussed earlier, in a physician's office, the care provider is the physician, a physician's assistant, a nurse practitioner, or a nurse midwife. The extent of the physical exam is typically driven by the patient's chief complaint, or the reason the patient is being seen that day. For instance, if a patient is being seen for an annual physical exam, the PE will be more extensive than the PE performed for a patient being seen with a chief complaint of a splinter in the right ring finger.

The care provider will also determine the extent of the PE based on the patient's responses to the ROS questions. If the patient with a splinter in the right ring finger has also been falling more than usual, then the PE will be more extensive and may include the musculoskeletal and neurologic systems. Figure 5.5 depicts a written physical exam similar to one found in a paper health record. Figure 5.6 shows a physical exam as documented using Prime Suite.

The healthcare professional who needs to know the results of a patient's physical exam to answer questions, complete forms, or handle insurance issues will need to access the patient's physical exam.

Though an EHR results in more detailed, timely documentation, it is still labor intensive for the care provider, and patients might leave with the perception that the physician was more interested in the computer than in them. To counter this, many physicians, hospitals, emergency departments,

PHYSICAL EXAM

Alexis Shaw is a 25-year-old African American female being seen today for her annual physical. Her ROS has been reviewed; and is unremarkable.

HEENT: Scalp clear; eyes and ears within normal limits; Nose: Some congestion noted; Throat: post-nasal drip noted.

Chest: Lungs clear to auscultation, no wheezes or rales.

Cardio: Heart rate and rhythm normal; no murmurs.

Abdomen: Soft, non-tender, no guarding or rebound noted.

Skin: No rashes, broken skin, or open wounds. Nails: bites her nails, but otherwise unremarkable.

Breasts & Genitalia: Deferred - she has an appointment with her GYN in two months. Her LMP was April 15 of this year. Periods are normal.

Extremities: Range of motion intact; no swelling.

Neuro: Within normal limits.

Figure 5.5 Written PE

Figure 5.6 PE as Seen in Prime Suite

and clinics are utilizing **scribes** to enter data into the EHR. A scribe is not a clinician and does not have to have any clinical education. The qualifications differ by setting (hospital, physician's practice, urgent care, long-term care facility, etc.) and individual facility. For all scribes, however, excellent keyboarding skills, including speed and (most importantly) accuracy, are a must. In addition, the scribe works only under the supervision of the care provider and must have knowledge of medical terminology, human disease, and pharmacology. The care provider is ultimately responsible for the information entered into the EHR. The entries made by the scribe are electronically signed or attributed to the scribe, but the care provider must countersign the documentation. Best practice dictates that the care provider not countersign any notes until after reading them and verifying their accuracy.

Scribes not only enter information into the health record as the physician or other healthcare provider is examining the patient but also locate information in the EHR that the physician asks for while seeing the patient.

Scribe An assistant who enters data either in writing or electronically into the health record as the care provider verbally dictates recent findings.

For instance, the physician may need to know when a patient was started on a particular medication or how long the patient has been seen for a particular condition.

Regulations covering the use and responsibilities of scribes vary from state to state and by accrediting agency; thus, it is important to do a thorough search of regulations and standards prior to implementing the use of scribes in your organization (AHIMA).

The use of scribes is not an entirely new practice. Many care providers have long used scribes to document in their paper or electronic records. Dermatologists, for example, are not only examining skin with their eyes but also must hold measuring tools and a magnifier and therefore cannot stop to document each lesion. A scribe is needed to document as the dermatologist verbally describes each lesion. The same applies to an ophthalmologist, who uses instruments to examine a patient's eyes and therefore cannot stop to write or type in findings. However, the general use of scribes is a relatively new practice. Even so, a good deal of research has been done regarding the effectiveness of the use of scribes on productivity, reimbursement, quality of documentation, and patient (and provider) satisfaction. So far, results are showing positive outcomes in all areas (Shultz and Holmstrom).

5.5 Medical Dictation and Transcription

With a manual record system, care providers choose to handwrite their charts. That has often been problematic, because handwriting is often illegible. A record that is not legible can cause safety concerns and negative patient outcomes, and it wastes time for the healthcare professional who cannot read the writing and has to track down the care provider for clarification. You have no doubt read or heard horror stories of wrong medications or wrong dosages being given to patients because of illegible handwriting. Health insurance companies may also deny payment based on illegible handwriting.

One solution many physicians used in the past was to dictate their notes into a recorder (hand-held or a larger system via telephone), and a transcriptionist then transcribed the physician's words into a typed document. Dictation used as a business tool dates back to the early 20th century, when Thomas Edison, Inc., and Columbia Graphaphone Company distributed their first versions of voice recorders, known as the Ediphone and Dictaphone, respectively. Dictation has evolved considerably—from hand-held machines to less cumbersome systems that require the use of only a telephone.

The use of dictation and transcription software resulted in greater accuracy (because of better recording quality), faster turnaround time than the original dictation systems, and more advanced reporting capabilities, which allowed physicians' offices and hospitals to analyze the cost of dictation and transcription as a means of documentation.

The cost of dictation, and the required transcriptionists who translate the spoken word into the written word, is not negligible. As the technology progressed, so did the price of dictation systems. As the requirements of government agencies and insurance companies rose, as well as escalating malpractice and negligence cases, the need for better, faster documentation grew. But recording a physician's words on paper also needed to be done in a timely manner. The need for qualified transcriptionists grew, but they were often in short supply.

Voice and Speech Recognition Technologies

Over the past 25 years or so, voice and speech recognition technologies have replaced traditional dictation to a great degree. **Voice recognition technology** is software that "learns" as it is used. In other words, it learns the voice and tone inflections of the dictator, and accuracy improves with time. **Speech recognition technology**, on the other hand, does not recognize individual voices. Many of you may already be using voice recognition technology and do not even realize it. For instance, your cell phone has a feature that allows you to voice dial, or you call your local cable company and go through a series of questions to which you respond by "saying or pushing 3." Both are forms of voice recognition. In these two examples, a command is carried out based on your speech response. With voice recognition used in the medical environment, as the care provider dictates, the words appear on the computer screen. In true voice recognition systems, the software "learns" the dictator's voice. The words that end up on screen are not perfect; for instance, "there" may be typed rather than "their" or Xanax may be heard as Zantac. But, since medicine requires accurate information, the transcriptionist's role has become more that of an editor than that of a transcriptionist. The transcriptionist may listen to the entire piece of dictation and compare it against what appears on the screen, or, once the system learns that physician's voice and becomes more accurate, the transcriptionist may only read what is on the screen to look for obvious errors.

The quality of transcription is higher with voice recognition (if the software recognizes the words correctly). Once physicians are comfortable with the use of voice recognition software, it may be less time consuming than dictation. Also, long-term costs are lower, since in most instances the transcription costs are lower (especially if a transcription service has been utilized in the past). The greatest advantage, though, is speed of documentation. With traditional transcription, days could pass between the time a chart note was dictated and the time it was transcribed (known as turn-around time). With voice recognition, the documentation is instant—as the words are spoken, they are documented in the chart. Of course, the record should be reviewed and edited before the care provider authenticates (signs) the note, but the fact that there is a draft copy in the record so quickly is a strong benefit.

Most EMR/EHR software solutions have a voice recognition component.

Voice recognition technology Software that recognizes the words being said by the person dictating and converts speech to text; differs from speech recognition because voice recognition "learns" the voice of the dictator and is therefore more accurate.

Speech recognition technology Software that recognizes the words being said by the person dictating and converts the speech to text.

for your information **fyi**

Nuance is a popular service provider of speech recognition technology. This YouTube video gives you a physician's perspective and shows the dictation process using speech recognition: http://www.youtube.com/watch?v=5FOVFVh_Nuw&list=TLw0-tV2ksT50

Electronic Prescribing (ePrescribing)

ePrescribing software is another component of the Meaningful Use requirements of HITECH. With ePrescribing, the care provider sends prescriptions to the patient's pharmacy electronically, at the **point of care (POC)** (occurring at the time the patient is being seen). Electronically sending prescriptions speeds up the process for the patient, as opposed to the traditional method in which the care provider hands the patient a written prescription and the patient takes it to the pharmacy and waits for it to be filled (or returns at a later time). Even if the office calls in the prescription, the process takes longer than using ePrescribing.

Most important, quality of care is greatly improved with electronic prescribing; not only does the prescription itself go directly to the pharmacy, but also the patient demographics, insurance information, allergies,

ePrescribing Electronically transmitting prescriptions from care provider to pharmacy.

Point of care (POC) Documentation, dictation, ordering of tests and procedures that occur at the same time the patient is being seen.

and medication history are sent as well. Care providers and pharmacists are alerted to possible food and drug interactions between medications that are currently prescribed or that the patient is already taking, and drug allergies and sensitivities are flagged. Also, medication dosing errors are avoided—for instance, if the care provider orders 250 mg of a particular drug for a 15-year-old patient, but the recommended dosage for that drug is 25 mg for a 15-year-old, an alert message automatically appears, so that the care provider can make the correction before the prescription is sent through to the pharmacy. Prescription renewal requests are handled more efficiently, too, since they are received electronically, with no need to manually update the patient's chart. And, of course, there are no more legibility issues—pharmacists do not have to make phone calls to the office to ask what the care provider had written, and the office staff does not have to take the time to track down the care provider or chart.

Go to http://connect.mheducation.com to complete this exercise.

Using ePrescribe

Before we look at the steps involved in using ePrescribe, we will cover the parts of a prescription. They are

Drug name: The name of the drug in brand or generic form. For instance, HydroDIURIL is a brand name for hydrochlorothiazide (the generic name).
Dosage: The measurement of the amount of drug that is being administered. HydroDIURIL is prescribed in 25 or 50 mg doses to treat adult hypertension.
Sig: The "label," or instructions that the pharmacist needs to list on the prescription label. A common Sig for HydroDIURIL is "Take one tablet by mouth, once daily."

In our scenario for ePrescribe, Alfredo J. Garza has called in for a refill of his prescription for Caduet (a medication for high blood pressure and angina).

Since this information is found in the clinical part of the chart, Alfredo J. Garza's Facesheet is first accessed, then the Medication List. The care provider typically carries out these steps unless he or she has given the healthcare professional a verbal order to do so.

Follow these steps to complete the exercise on your own once you have watched the demonstration and tried the steps with helpful prompts. Use the information provided in the scenario to complete the information.

1. Click the Medication List radio button.
2. Click View Medication History.
3. Click Caduet 10-10 mg oral tablet.
4. (Note the refill sent via ePrescribe.) Click Close.

✓ **You have completed Exercise 5.4**

5.8 Computerized Physician Order Entry (CPOE)

No treatment, diagnostic test, or medication administration is performed on any patient without a care provider's order. Using paper records, orders were traditionally either written by the care provider or given verbally and written in the patient's record by a nurse. Orders may be in written form or electronically submitted via **computerized physician order entry (CPOE)**. Prime Suite's functionality is called *Orders Requisition*. Through this function, orders can be printed or electronically submitted to an outside laboratory, a medical equipment company, or a hospital with **interface** capabilities with Prime Suite. The interface capability means that one computer system (or component) can accept and receive data from another system. The systems may be at different locations or within the same facility. Your office may have Prime Suite software for PM and EHR, but your laboratory system may be manufactured by a different vendor. If the computer programs for each are configured to exchange data without having to re-enter the data, orders can flow directly to the laboratory system and the results can flow directly back to the EHR in Prime Suite.

A major advantage of CPOE functionality is built-in clinical decision support. Alerts appear when orders are entered for medications or treatment that may cause an adverse reaction to a drug or drugs previously ordered for that patient. The same applies to dosing errors. If a care provider has ordered 250 mg of a drug for a 10-year-old patient, but the maximum dosage is 100 mg for that age group, then an alert appears, and a potentially serious situation is averted because the alert occurs before the drug is administered. Through the use of CPOE, as long as the facility's data dictionary includes a comprehensive listing of medications and abbreviations used, the probability of medication errors is greatly reduced.

Regarding orders for diagnostic tests, once the order is carried out—for instance, a complete blood count (CBC)—the results are electronically sent to the care provider who ordered the lab test. Using CPOE is safer in this case as well, because there is no questionable handwriting or error in transcribing physicians' verbal orders—improving overall patient care.

Computerized physician order entry (CPOE) Entering physician orders electronically rather than on paper. The order is transmitted directly to the appropriate department; for instance, an order for an x-ray would go directly to the radiology department, whereas an order for a CBC would go directly to the laboratory.

Interface The ability of one computer system or component to accept or send data to another system without loss of integrity or meaning.

5.9 Tracking Physicians' Orders

If a test is important enough to order, then learning the results of that test is equally important. Tests that are not carried out and reported in a timely manner can delay necessary care and cause inefficiency in the business processes of an office. Having this functionality in an EHR system prevents communication breakdowns and unnecessary rework.

When an order has been completed and the results are ready for the care provider's review, he or she receives notification on the Desktop. In Figure 5.7, note on the left side of the screen that the Lab Flowsheet tab shows one resulted order and has a red star next to it, meaning it is high priority. The care provider would click on the Orders tab to review the returned results.

Once the care provider clicks the Orders tab, all resulted orders will appear on the screen. In Figure 5.8, you can see that one order has been resulted, and it is for a metabolic panel on Dr. Ingram's patient Tom Gunn.

If, based on the results of the lab test, Dr. Ingram wants to order additional tests, prescribe a particular medication, or follow up with the patient soon, he will give additional orders to the healthcare professional to handle the situation accordingly.

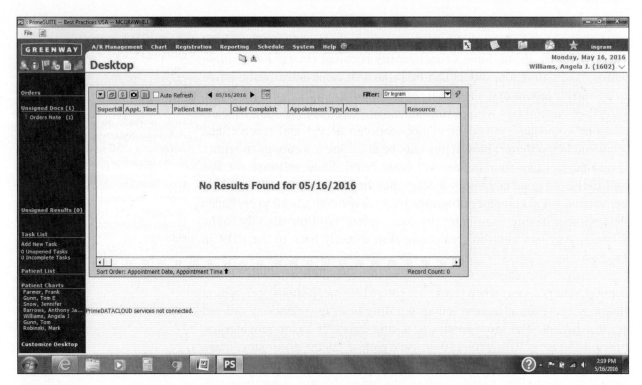

Figure 5.7   Results Ready for Review

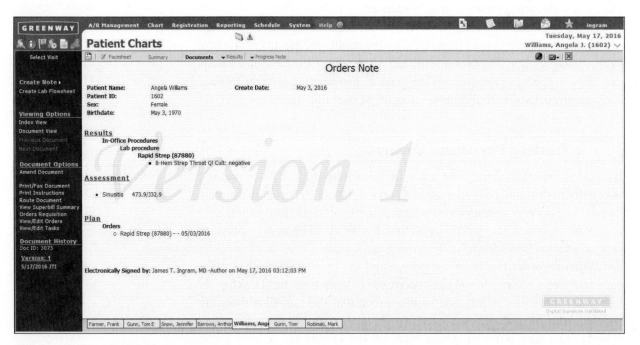

Figure 5.8   Resulted Order

Figure 5.9 represents the final screen the care provider sees. From it, he or she can note whether the results were normal or abnormal or were a specific assessment. The care provider can also send a follow-up task to one of the healthcare professionals in the office or to another care provider in the practice for review. These tasks can be done directly from the Order screen without having to exit that function and find another.

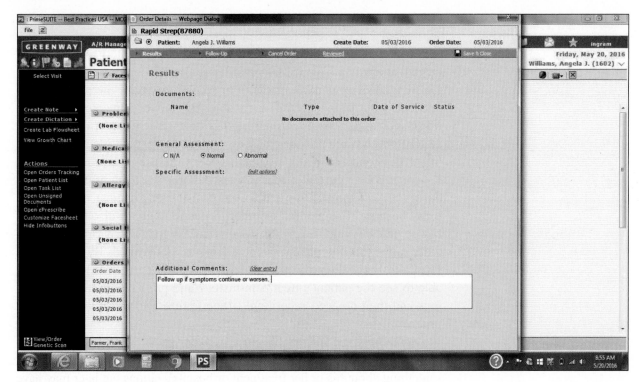

Figure 5.9   Order Details Screen

EHR   EXERCISE   5.5

Locate the Status of an Order

In this exercise, Dr. Ingram is asking you about the results of Alfredo Garza's lab and radiology work. You will again go to the Facesheet of Alfredo J. Garza, but find the section titled Order Tracking History, since our goal is to find out if Alfredo had the tests done and if the results are in his chart.

Once the Facesheet is accessed, follow these steps to complete the exercise on your own once you have watched the demonstration and tried the steps with helpful prompts.

1. Click the Orders Tracking History radio button.
2. Click Category.
3. Click Imaging procedure.
4. Click Lab procedure.
5. Click OK.
6. Click View/Edit.
7. Click Imported - Document - Radiologic examination, chest X-Ray PA and Lateral.
8. Click the Scroll down button.
9. Click Close Note.
10. Click Save & Close.

✓ You have completed Exercise 5.5

Problem list A listing kept in the patient's health record of all of his/her current (active) and resolved medical conditions.

Another requirement of Meaningful Use is an up-to-date **problem list** of current and active diagnoses. Providing quality care means following current diagnoses or conditions on an ongoing basis until the problems are resolved, or at least until they are stable. Of course, some medical conditions, such as asthma or coronary artery disease, may never resolve completely, but the care provider must ensure that the patient is stable and that his or her condition is not worsening. With the use of a problem list, as long as it is kept current, necessary testing or assessment of the condition does not "fall through the cracks." For instance, a patient may be seen today because of an upper respiratory infection but has also been treated by the care provider for hypertension, and on today's visit the care provider notes that the patient's blood pressure is elevated. By clicking on Hypertension in the problem list of diagnoses, the care provider is quickly able to see the patient's treatment history and prior blood pressure readings and then proceed accordingly. (See Figure 5.10 for an example of a problem list.)

Sometimes the information in a problem list is helpful to the patient as well as the care provider. The patient may have told the care provider something about his or her treatment or hospitalizations but later may have forgotten the details. By having this complete history, the medical office has the information readily available when needed.

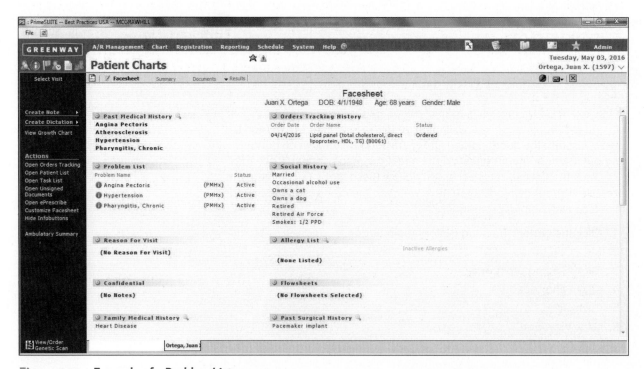

Figure 5.10   **Example of a Problem List**

Go to http://connect.mheducation.com to complete this exercise.

Utilizing the Problem List

In the scenario we are about to view, Alfredo J. Garza has been treated for angina over the past few years. He was first diagnosed in 2012 and has been hospitalized at Memorial Hospital twice for it—once on June 15, 2014, and once on August 10, 2015. Mr. Garza has asked the office staff to complete a form he must give his employer, who needs to know if Mr. Garza has ever been hospitalized for angina and, if so, when. He does not recall the dates but does remember giving that information to Dr. Ingram on his last visit, so he hopes the information can be found in his record.

From the Facesheet of Alfredo J. Garza, the healthcare professional will click on angina from the Problem List area in order to get Mr. Garza the information he needs.

Once the Facesheet of the patient's chart is accessed, follow these steps to complete the exercise on your own once you've watched the demonstration and tried the steps with helpful prompts.

1. Click Angina (Under the Problem List section).
2. Click OK. (Note the hospitalization dates.)

☑ **You have completed Exercise 5.6**

APPLYING YOUR SKILLS

In this chapter, we covered the usual contents of a SOAP note. Following are random sentences likely to be found in a provider's office note. After each sentence, note whether the sentence should be in the **S**ubjective, **O**bjective, **A**ssessment, or **P**lan portion of the office note. Again, these are random sentences and will not come together to form a note for one particular patient.

1. A chest x-ray performed in the office showed an infiltrate in the right lower lobe of the lung.
2. Grace has been complaining of a pain in her right side, which is stabbing in nature.
3. The patient was given an order for an ultrasound of the kidneys and bladder, which she should have done in the next week or so.
4. Nephrolithiasis
5. The patient's blood pressure is 145/95.
6. "I am here because I've had a headache for three days that just won't go away."
7. The patient should continue physical therapy for two more weeks.
8. Right lower lobe pneumonia
9. Both pupils are equal and reactive.
10. The patient states she has tried Aleve, but her right knee pain has not improved.

chapter 5 **summary**

LEARNING OUTCOME	CONCEPTS FOR REVIEW
5.1 Explain each element of a SOAP note.	– Subjective—the patient's description of the problem – Objective—the care provider's results of physical examination – Assessment—the diagnosis or diagnoses – Plan—the diagnostic tests or treatment plan for the patient
5.2 Identify elements of the history of present illness (HPI).	– Location of the condition (abdomen, arm, leg, head, etc.) – Quality of the symptoms – Severity of the symptoms – Duration/timing of the symptoms – Context under which symptoms occur – Modifying factors – Associated signs and symptoms
5.3 Identify elements of the review of systems (ROS).	– Body-system-by-body-system assessment of any signs or symptoms the patient is experiencing that may or may not be related to the reason for his or her visit – Not the same as the physical exam
5.4 Identify elements of the physical exam (PE).	– The extent of the exam is dependent on the patient's presenting symptoms (the chief complaint). – The physical exam relates to the findings of the care provider, not the patient, as in the ROS; for example, the patient complains of pain in the right lower abdomen, yet when the care provider presses on the right lower abdomen, the patient does not express feelings of pain. – The advantages of using a scribe, particularly during the physical exam
5.5 Describe the process of traditional dictation and transcription.	– The physician dictates medical notes into a recording device. – A transcriptionist types the words using word processing software. – Often takes days for the transcribed report to be filed in the patient's record
5.6 Illustrate the advantages of speech recognition technology.	– The provider's documentation immediately appears in the patient's record, with no lag time between dictation and transcription. – In the long term, it may be less expensive than traditional dictation and transcription. – Quality is higher than with traditional transcription (in most cases).
5.7 Outline the benefits of ePrescribing.	– Less chance for medication errors – Potential food/drug interactions identified – Fewer man-hours to complete the process – More convenient and less wait time for patients – Overall, better-quality care

LEARNING OUTCOME	CONCEPTS FOR REVIEW
5.8 Evaluate the benefits of computerized physician order entry (CPOE).	– Fewer errors in carrying out orders because they are no longer handwritten – Orders sent directly from the office to the laboratory or hospital – Safer for the patient—the order is sent by the care provider rather than verbally given to another healthcare professional to send on to the laboratory or hospital – If an interface exists, the results automatically come back to the ordering physician.
5.9 Support the necessity to track physicians' orders.	– Patient care—knowing the results of the test in a timely manner, proper treatment can be started quickly
5.10 Examine the benefits of a problem list.	– Timely follow-up of conditions – Serves as a reminder to the care provider to address problems on the patient's problem list – Information about each problem is located in one place.

chapter **review**

MATCHING QUESTIONS

Match the terms on the left with the definitions on the right.

_____ 1. **[LO 5.1]** SOAP note

_____ 2. **[LO 5.8]** interface

_____ 3. **[LO 5.4]** scribe

_____ 4. **[LO 5.6]** voice recognition technology

_____ 5. **[LO 5.8]** computerized physician order entry

_____ 6. **[LO 5.2]** history of present illness

_____ 7. **[LO 5.7]** point of care

_____ 8. **[LO 5.10]** problem list

_____ 9. **[LO 5.7]** ePrescribing

_____ 10. **[LO 5.6]** speech recognition technology

a. patient's description of current symptoms

b. EMR feature that is part of HITECH's Meaningful Use requirements

c. software that recognizes spoken words and converts them into text

d. immediate, real-time documentation of patient procedures

e. comprehensive record of a patient's complaints and conditions

f. documentation format that allows healthcare professionals to capture all aspects of a patient encounter

g. ability to access another provider's practice management software for patient care purposes

h. assistant who enters the dictation of a care provider into a patient record

i. software that automatically turns spoken words into text and learns voice inflections the more it is used

j. electronic entry of care provider orders for direct transmission to appropriate departments

MULTIPLE-CHOICE QUESTIONS

Select the letter that best completes the statement or answers the question:

1. **[LO 5.2]** Which of the following statements would *not* be included in the history of present illness?
    a. Blood pressure is 130/84, right arm, sitting
    b. Pain radiate down the left leg
    c. Productive cough for one week
    d. Symptoms improved after taking ibuprofen

2. **[LO 5.3]** Which of the following would most likely require a complete review of systems?
    a. annual exam
    b. headache
    c. mole on back
    d. sore throat

3. **[LO 5.1]** Notes about a prescription ordered for a patient would appear in the _____ section of a SOAP note.
   a. subjective
   b. objective
   c. assessment
   d. plan

4. **[LO 5.3]** An ROS covers information likely documented in the
   a. history of present illness.
   b. medical history form.
   c. physical exam.
   d. SOAP note.

5. **[LO 5.9]** Prime Suite has the capability to _____ the status of an order.
   a. assign
   b. generate
   c. query
   d. track

6. **[LO 5.6]** The biggest advantage of voice recognition software over manual transcription is
   a. clarity.
   b. cost.
   c. ease.
   d. speed of turn-around time.

7. **[LO 5.1]** Information gathered during a provider's physical exam would appear in the _____ section of a SOAP note.
   a. subjective
   b. objective
   c. assessment
   d. plan

8. **[LO 5.6]** The more voice recognition software is used, the
   a. faster it corrects mistakes.
   b. quicker it gets.
   c. more it learns voice inflections.
   d. slower it gets.

9. **[LO 5.8]** There must be a _____ to perform any tests or treatments.
   a. diagnosis
   b. referral
   c. care provider order
   d. SOAP note

Enhance your learning by completing these exercises and more at http://**connect.mheducation.com**!

10. **[LO 5.5]** A person hired to manually record a physician's spoken words is known as a
   a. dictator.
   b. recorder.
   c. stenographer.
   d. transcriptionist.

11. **[LO 5.2]** Which of the following elements of an HPI are collected at a visit?
   a. all of them
   b. duration, quality, and severity
   c. location and severity
   d. only those that apply to the patient's chief complaint

11. **[LO 5.4]** The extent of a physical exam largely depends upon which of the following?
   a. age of the patient
   b. amount of time available
   c. patient's chief complaint
   d. patient's medical history

12. **[LO 5.10]** Meaningful Use regulations require the keeping of an up-to-date
   a. exam registry.
   b. order queue.
   c. problem list.
   d. provider note.

13. **[LO 5.7]** The use of ePrescribing is part of the requirements for
   a. HIPAA.
   b. HITECH.
   c. HIM.
   d. HPI.

SHORT-ANSWER QUESTIONS

1. **[LO 5.2]** List the typical elements of a history of present illness.

2. **[LO 5.5]** List at least three drawbacks of handwritten patient charts.

3. **[LO 5.3]** In order for a practice to receive reimbursement for an ROS, what must happen?

4. **[LO 5.4]** Explain the factors that might influence the extent of a physical exam.

5. **[LO 5.1]** List the four sections of a SOAP note and give an example of each.

6. **[LOs 5.5, 5.6]** Why is there still a need for medical transcriptionists in an age of voice recognition software?

7. **[LO 5.3]** List the typical organs and body systems that would be covered in a complete review of systems.

8. **[LO 5.10]** List one reason a provider might use a patient's problem list.

9. **[LOs 5.3, 5.4]** Contrast an ROS with a PE.

10. **[LO 5.4]** List four types of medical providers who might perform a physical exam.

11. **[LO 5.8]** Explain what it means to have interface capabilities with Prime Suite. What benefits does interfacing have?

12. **[LO 5.9]** List three benefits of Prime Suite's order tracking capabilities.

13. **[LO 5.4]** Based on Alexis Shaw's physical exam as documented in the text, what is her chief complaint?

14. **[LO 5.6]** Contrast voice recognition with speech recognition.

APPLYING YOUR KNOWLEDGE

1. **[LOs 5.1, 5.2, 5.3, 5.4]** Patient James Frank presents for his appointment. He is complaining of fatigue and headaches. When Dr. Ingram examines him, he finds that James has an enlarged lymph node on the right side of his throat; his lungs are clear; his blood pressure is a little low at 100/68. Dr. Ingram suspects anemia or an underactive thyroid as the causes of James' fatigue, so he orders that a comprehensive blood panel be done. Create a SOAP note that properly documents each piece of James Frank's visit with Dr. Ingram.

2. **[LO 5.6]** Your office is preparing to implement new voice recognition technology, and you have been tasked with creating some talking points and benefits to share with your peers. How could you go about explaining the benefits of voice recognition software?

3. **[LOs 5.7, 5.10]** Why would ePrescribing and an up-to-date problem list be addressed under Meaningful Use requirements?

4. **[LOs 5.7, 5.8, 5.9, 5.10]** Of the following Prime Suite capabilities—ePrescribing, CPOE, order tracking, and the problem list—which do you think is the most beneficial? Explain your answer.

5. **[LO 5.7]** Create two flowcharts: one that shows the progression of a manually written prescription and one that shows the progression of a prescription entered using ePrescribing.

6. **[LO 5.4]** What are the benefits of using a scribe to document a patient's visit?

Enhance your learning by completing these exercises and more at http://connect.mheducation.com!

chapter references

American Health Information Management Association (AHIMA). (2012, November). Using Medical Scribes in a Physician Practice. *Journal of AHIMA, 83*(11): 64–69 [expanded online version].

Recording History: The History of Recording Technology. Retrieved from http://www.recording-history .org/HTML/dicta_tech5.php

Recording History: The History of Recording Technology. The 1970s and the Decline of Dictation. Retrieved from http://www.recording-history.org/HTML/dicta_biz7.php

Recording History: *The History of Recording Technology*. Retrieved from http://www.recording-history. org/HTML/dicta_tech2.php

Shultz, C. G., and Holmstrom, H. L. (2015, May–June). The Use of Medical Scribes in Health Care Settings: A Systematic Review and Future Directions. *Journal of the American Board of Family Medicine, 28:* 371–381.

Wiedemann, Lou Ann. (2010, October). CPOE Lessons Learned. *Journal of AHIMA, 81*(10): 54–55.

Financial Management: Insurance and Billing Functions

At the end of this chapter, the student should be able to

6.1 Illustrate the need for a claims management process.

6.2 List the information contained in an encounter form (Superbill).

6.3 Apply procedures to update a patient's account in Prime Suite.

6.4 Demonstrate coding using ICD-10-CM/PCS and CPT codes in Prime Suite.

6.5 Examine the correlation between documentation and code assignment.

6.6 Describe Accountable Care Organizations.

6.7 Describe the information contained in a remittance advice, or explanation of benefits.

6.8 Apply procedures to manage accounts receivable in Prime Suite.

6.9 Demonstrate the need for a compliance plan.

Abuse

Accountable Care Organization (ACO)

Accounts payable

Accounts receivable

Adjudication

Affordable Care Act (ACA)

Code linkage

Coinsurance

Compliance plan

Co-payment (co-pay)

Deductible

Evaluation and Management (E&M)

Explanation of benefits (EOB)

Fee schedule

Fraud

Healthcare Common Procedure Coding System (HCPCS)

Insurance plan

Insurance verification

Managed care plan

Medical necessity

Remittance advice (RA)

Subscriber

Transactions

What You Need to Know and Why You Need to Know It

Physicians, hospitals, and any other healthcare facilities are in business to take care of patients, first and foremost. However, they are also businesses. They have bills to pay, just like any other business—payroll, rent or mortgage, utilities, supplies, insurance, and, yes, the providers themselves need to be paid. The efficiency we have discussed in terms of providing patient care also applies to collecting monies owed to the office. The billing and collections process will be discussed in this chapter. Remember, though, that this is not a course on billing procedures. From this chapter, you will gain an awareness of how billing and EHR applications are intermeshed using Prime Suite. The specifics of *how* to complete and file insurance claims, manage accounts, collect unpaid bills, and handle financial management in general will be covered in another course. The coding of diagnoses and procedures will also be covered in other classes, but when you finish this chapter, you will understand how documentation, coding, and reimbursement are related.

6.1	Claims Management—Why and How

Every patient seen in a healthcare facility is charged for the care he or she receives. Yes, some accounts are "written off"; in other words, the patient does not pay, but there still needs to be an accounting of the visit and the charges that were incurred for the visit. If this is not done, the business profile of the office will show an inaccurate picture of the number of patients seen, the procedures carried out, the charges incurred, and the amount of money collected. In other words, the statistics collected for that medical practice will not be valid, because not all of the patients are included in the practice's database.

The financial well-being of a medical office is of great importance if the practice is to stay in business. Therefore, a process—or, to be specific, a written claims management process—is necessary. Each step of the process must be carried out efficiently and effectively. This process includes written policies—how much is charged per service (**fee schedule**), the timing of filing claims, follow-up on unpaid claims, and collections procedures when claims are not paid must all be in writing. The importance of written policies will be addressed in the compliance section of this chapter.

The use of practice management (PM) software greatly improves the efficiency of a claims process, because it allows for more accurate capturing of charges, submits automatic reminders, offers a variety of reporting options, and provides automatic follow-up of each account. There is far less chance of missed charges, missed payments, and payments posted to the wrong account with a computerized system than with a manual one. Just the ability to run reports on daily charges, daily payments, and accounts in collections increases the efficiency of the business processes.

Remember that each patient is entered only once in the practice's database of patients, but each patient may have more than one encounter (visit) attached to that master entry (Figure 6.1). Each visit has an account attached to it, and therefore the claims process must be fulfilled for each of those accounts. Without PM software, just tracking insurance payments on one patient who is seen a couple of times a month would be a daunting task!

Fee schedule The amount charged for services rendered in a physician's office by Current Procedural Terminology (CPT) code.

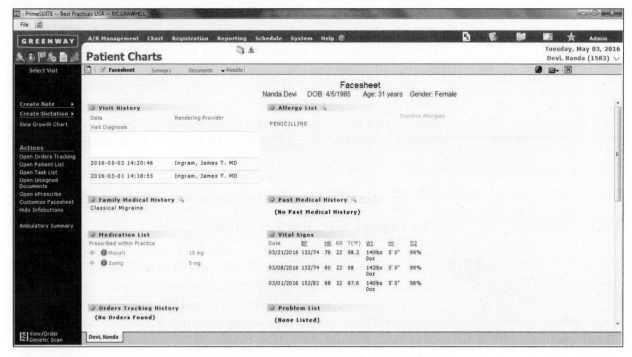

Figure 6.1 Multiple Visits for One Patient

The patient's account for each visit begins when the patient makes the appointment. It is important to ask the patient for at least two personal identifiers, such as name and date of birth, upon scheduling the appointment. This will ensure that the correct patient account is being pulled up for the appointment and that new accounts will not be made for established patients. The healthcare professional also asks for the expected source of payment at that time. If the patient is going to be paying out of pocket (no insurance), the office's payment policies are discussed with the patient.

Many patients have some type of insurance coverage, whether it be Medicare, Medicaid, TRICARE, private insurance, or group insurance, including managed care plans. **Managed care plans** promote quality, cost-effective healthcare through monitoring of patients, preventive care, and performance measures of providers. Physicians contract with managed care plans to provide care at a predetermined rate that is paid out per member per month or in one predetermined payment. If the patient is covered by insurance, **insurance verification** is completed by the office staff, usually before the patient arrives for the appointment, so that the office is reasonably sure that the patient is covered and that payment will come from some source. Verifying insurance is the process of contacting the insurance carrier and receiving validation of coverage for that patient, whether he or she owes a co-pay amount (due from the patient at the time of the visit) or co-insurance (percentage that the carrier pays and the patient pays), whether the visit and services ordered are covered by the insurance, and whether the patient has met the **deductible**.

Once the patient, George Jones, for example, arrives for his appointment, he checks in at the front desk. He is then seen by a healthcare professional, such as a medical assistant or nurse, who takes the patient's vital signs and begins the documentation for the visit, including chief complaint, history of present illness, medication review, and perhaps history. Mr. Jones

Managed care plan Insurance plan that promotes quality, cost-effective healthcare through monitoring of patients, preventive care, and performance.

Insurance verification The process of contacting the insurance carrier and receiving validation of coverage for that patient, deductible status, and co-pay amount.

Deductible The out-of-pocket payment amount that a policyholder must meet before insurance covers the service(s).

is seen next by the care provider, and charges are applied to his bill. When the visit is complete, he checks out (in a hospital, this is called *discharge*). George Jones now has an account for that visit, to which charges have been applied.

In a hospital setting, all of the preceding tasks are performed; however, specific rules apply to insurance verification, especially if the patient presents through the emergency department and/or is in labor. Hospital billing is beyond the scope of this worktext, but a claim is filed with insurance.

6.2 | Use of an Encounter Form

The Paper Encounter Form (Superbill)

A document that is often used in medical offices to capture the diagnoses and services or procedures performed, either as a hard-copy piece of paper or computer generated by the PM system, is known as an encounter form, a routing slip, or a Superbill (this concept was introduced earlier in the worktext in the Prime Suite overview chapter). The information on the Superbill will be transferred to a form known as the CMS-1500 claim form and used to bill an outpatient encounter.

Typically, a hard-copy Superbill (Figure 6.2) includes the following information, though it may contain more elements than these:

- Name and address of the medical practice
- Provider's National Provider Identification (NPI) number
- Patient's name
- Patient's chart number
- Date and time of visit
- CPT codes for common procedures performed in that office
- Diagnosis narrative (as written by the care provider)
- ICD-10-CM codes corresponding to each written diagnosis (not on all Superbills)

On this form, the provider documents the services that were rendered during the encounter. Even if a PM system is computerized, the paper form may still be printed. The patient's identifying information is already completed for the provider, who checks off the CPT codes for the procedures that were performed and writes in the diagnosis or diagnoses the patient was treated for during that visit.

The Electronic Encounter Form

Medical necessity The fact that there is a medical reason to perform a procedure or service. Documentation exists in the patient's record to show there are sufficient signs, symptoms, or history to warrant the services provided.

Code linkage On an insurance claim, this is the relationship between each procedure (CPT code) and a diagnosis (ICD-10 code) to demonstrate medical necessity.

Figure 6.3 shows a Superbill Summary in Prime Suite for a patient, Mark Robinski, who is being seen for cholelithiasis (gallstones).

Notice that the charges are listed just under the *charge* section of the Superbill. There are five CPT codes listed; these were introduced earlier and will be discussed in more detail later in this chapter. Each CPT code must "map" to a diagnosis code, because the diagnosis code shows **medical necessity** (the fact that there is a medical reason to perform that procedure). This is called **code linkage**, and it is necessary that the relationship between the procedure and the diagnosis be shown, so that the insurance company will not deny the claim due to lack of medical necessity. To the left of the

ENCOUNTER FORM

11/11/2016	11:15 am
DATE	TIME
Edwin Hsu	HSUEDWI0
PATIENT NAME	CHART #

OFFICE VISITS - SYMPTOMATIC NEW		
99201	OF--New Patient Minimal	
99202	OF--New Patient Low	
99203	OF--New Patient Detailed	
99204	OF--New Patient Moderate	
99205	OF--New Patient High	
ESTABLISHED		
99211	OF--Established Patient Minimal	
99212	OF--Established Patient Low	X
99213	OF--Established Patient Detailed	
99214	OF--Established Patient Moderate	
99215	OF--Established Patient High	
PREVENTIVE VISITS NEW		
99381	Under 1 Year	
99382	1 - 4 Years	
99383	5 - 11 Years	
99384	12 - 17 Years	
99385	18 - 39 Years	
99386	40 - 64 Years	
99387	65 Years & Up	
ESTABLISHED		
99391	Under 1 Year	
99392	1 - 4 Years	
99393	5 - 11 Years	
99394	12 - 17 Years	
99395	18 - 39 Years	
99396	40 - 64 Years	
99397	65 Years & Up	
PROCEDURES		
12011	Simple suture--face--local anes.	
29125	App. of short arm splint; static	
29540	Strapping, ankle	
50390	Aspiration of renal cyst by needle	
71010	Chest x-ray, single view, frontal	

PROCEDURES		
71020	Chest x-ray, two views, frontal & lateral	
71030	Chest x-ray, complete, four views	
73070	Elbow x-ray, AP & lateral views	
73090	Forearm x-ray, AP & lateral views	
73100	Wrist x-ray, AP & lateral views	
73510	Hip x-ray, complete, two views	
73600	Ankle x-ray, AP & lateral views	
LABORATORY		
80048	Basic metabolic panel	
80050	General health panel	
80061	Lipid panel	
82270	Blood screening, occult; feces	
82947	Glucose screening--quantitative	
82951	Glucose tolerance test, three specimens	
83718	HDL cholesterol	
84478	Triglycerides test	
85007	Manual differential WBC	
85018	Hemoglobin	
85651	Erythrocyte sedimentation rate--non-auto	
86580	TB Mantoux test	
87040	Culture, bacterial; blood	
87076	Culture, anaerobic isolate	
87077	Bacterial culture, aerobic isolate	
87086	Urine culture and colony count	
87430	Strep test	
87880	Direct streptococcus screen	
INJECTIONS		
90471	Immunization administration	
90703	Tetanus injection	
96372	Injection	
92516	Facial nerve function studies	
93000	Electrocardiogram--ECG with interpretation	
93015	Treadmill stress test, with physician...	
96900	Ultraviolet light treatment	
99070	Supplies and materials provided	

FAMILY CARE CENTER
285 Stephenson Blvd.
Stephenson, OH 60089
614-555-0000

☐ DANA BANU, M.D.
☐ ROBERT BEACH, M.D.
☒ PATRICIA MCGRATH, M.D.

☐ JESSICA RUDNER, M.D.
☐ JOHN RUDNER, M.D.
☐ KATHERINE YAN, M.D.

NOTES

REFERRING PHYSICIAN	NPI	AUTHORIZATION #

DIAGNOSIS
J06.9, Acute URI

PAYMENT AMOUNT
$20 copay, check #1066

Figure 6.2   Paper Encounter Form (Superbill)

Source: Sanderson, Susan M. (2013). *Computers in the Medical Office* (8th ed.). New York: McGraw-Hill Companies.

CPT code column (highlighted in Figure 6.3), notice that there are symbols. There are many coding rules set down by Medicare and Medicaid, and most insurance companies have additional rules as well. The symbols you see are an advantage of using PM software; cash flow is not adversely affected

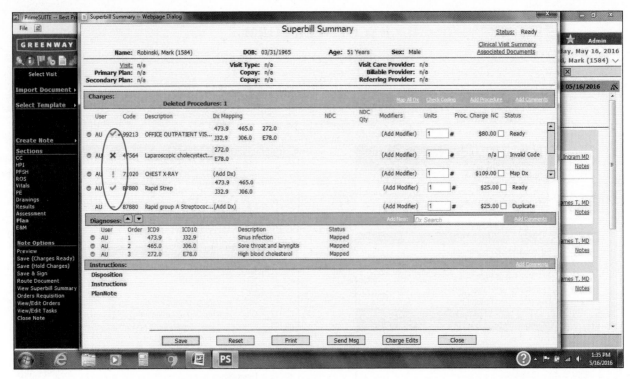

Figure 6.3 Prime Suite Superbill Summary

✗	Indicates An Invalid Code! This Procedure Code Is Not Found In The Prime Practice Procedure Master File. The Red Light Must Be Resolved Before The Charge Can Be Posted On The Charges Page. Click The Red X To Open The Procedure Maintenance Page To Add Your Code To The Master File.
!	Indicates That No Diagnoses Are Currently Mapped To This Procedure Code. The Yellow Indicator Must Be Resolved Before The Charge Can Be Auto Posted On The Charges Page. The Charge Can Be Marked As Manual Post If Necessary. Click The Yellow Exclamation Point To Display The Diagnosis Mapping Window.
✓	Indicates That Everything Associated With This Charge Line Is Ready Or Marked As Manual Post And May Be Posted.
✓*	The Asterisk Indicates That The Charge Is Ready But There Are Alternate Billing Codes Associated And Available For Selection With This Procedure Code. Click The Green Check With Asterisk To Display The Alternate Code Selection Window.
—	Indicates That This Charge Line Will Not Be Posted. The Status Of This Procedure Code Is Either "Hold", "Duplicate", "Posted", "Not Billable" Or "Delete".

Figure 6.4 Symbols Used on Prime Suite Superbill Summary

when potential coding problems leading to denied claims are taken care of before the claim is filed. In Figure 6.4, you will find the legend for these symbols. For instance, a green check mark denotes that there are no problems with that code and charges can be posted. A yellow exclamation point, on the other hand, means that no diagnosis code is mapped to that procedure code to justify payment of the claim; until that is resolved, cash flow will be affected, because the insurance company might deny or return the claim for more information. A red "X" indicates that an invalid code appears on the Superbill and that payment would be denied or returned for more information.

6.3 The Claims Process Using Prime Suite

As noted, the process begins when the patient makes an appointment. But the charges do not start accruing until the patient presents for the appointment and services are rendered.

The first step, if the patient has insurance, is to collect the **co-payment**, otherwise known as the **co-pay**. In managed care plans particularly, this is the portion of the bill that is the responsibility of the patient. Because co-payments are fixed amounts, they do not change from visit to visit, so they are often due at the time of the office visit. Many offices collect the co-pay at the time of arrival; others collect it when the patient checks out at the conclusion of the visit. For inpatient hospital visits, co-pays do not exist. Some

Co-payment (co-pay) The amount due from the patient at the time of the office visit; typically a requirement of managed care plans.

types of insurance plans may require **coinsurance**, in which the insurance carrier and the patient are both responsible for a percentage of the charges. In cases such as these, the amount due is relative to the amount charged, because it is based on a percentage, so patients are often billed for the remaining balance after the insurance carrier has paid its portion. Medicare, for example, often has an 80-20 coinsurance. This means that the insurance carrier (Medicare) will pay 80% of the charges (based on the Medicare fee schedule) and the patient will be responsible for the remaining 20% of the charges.

You will recall that one of the benefits of using PM software is the alerts that are generated. An alert is a reminder to do something. These alerts are generated based on the patient's **insurance plan**. For instance, a patient who has Medicare Part B might not need to pay a co-pay, so no alert appears, but a patient with a managed care plan will most likely have one, so the reminder appears. Many offices refuse to see patients who do not pay their co-pay at the time of the visit. Look at Figure 6.5 for an example of the co-pay reminder in Prime Suite.

Coinsurance A form of cost-sharing in which the insurance carrier pays a percentage of the claim and the patient pays the remaining percentage. Medicare, for example, has an 80-20 coinsurance, in which Medicare pays 80% and the patient pays 20% of the charges.

Insurance plan The medical insurance contract under which a patient is covered; the extent to which services are covered. Also referred to as "the plan."

Figure 6.5 Co-pay Alert in Prime Suite

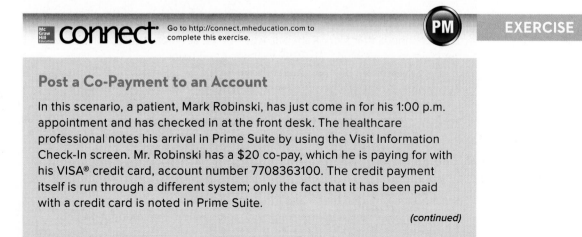

Go to http://connect.mheducation.com to complete this exercise.

EXERCISE 6.1

Post a Co-Payment to an Account

In this scenario, a patient, Mark Robinski, has just come in for his 1:00 p.m. appointment and has checked in at the front desk. The healthcare professional notes his arrival in Prime Suite by using the Visit Information Check-In screen. Mr. Robinski has a $20 co-pay, which he is paying for with his VISA® credit card, account number 7708363100. The credit payment itself is run through a different system; only the fact that it has been paid with a credit card is noted in Prime Suite.

(continued)

Follow these steps to complete the exercise on your own once you have watched the demonstration and tried the steps with helpful prompts in practice mode. Use the information provided in the scenario to complete the information.

1. Click Registration.
2. Click Visit Information: Check-In.
3. Click Robinski, Mark to select him.
4. Click Close.
5. Click Check-In.
6. Click Post Co-Pay.
7. Click the Method drop-down menu.
8. Click Credit Card.
9. Click the Supplier drop-down menu.
10. Click Visa.
11. Click the Additional Info field.
12. Type "7708363100".
13. Click the Amount field.
14. Type "20.00".
15. Click Save.
16. Click Yes.
17. Click OK.
18. Click Save.

☑ **You have completed Exercise 6.1**

In the next exercise, we will check on the status of a claim for Mark Robinski for an earlier appointment he had at Greensburg Medical Center. This might be done for any number of reasons—the patient may be inquiring, the billing staff may be investigating because his name and visit date appeared on an unpaid accounts report, or an office manager may be doing a quality check of the work performed by a member of the staff.

EXERCISE 6.2 PM   Go to http://connect.mheducation.com to complete this exercise.

Given a Scenario, Look Up the Status of an Insurance Claim

The scenario is that Mark Robinski, while being seen on April 4, 2016, asks if the claim from his March 11, 2016, visit has been paid.

The healthcare professional will investigate by accessing the Accounts Receivable (A/R) Management menu, and then the claims management function. Accounts receivable includes money that is received by the medical practice, including insurance payments and payments made by the patient. The patient's identification number (chart number) is needed for this step, and it is found in the upper right corner of every screen. Mr. Robinski's chart (ID) number is 1584.

Follow these steps to complete the exercise on your own once you have watched the demonstration and tried the steps with helpful prompts. Use the information provided in the scenario to complete the information.

1. Click the Search for Patient Icon.
2. Type "Robinski" in the *Last Name field.
3. Click Search.
4. Click Select.
5. Click Claims Maintenance.
6. Click the Patient ID field.
7. Type "1584".
8. Click Search.
9. Click the Scroll Bar.
10. Click U - Paid In Full: Closed to note the claim status.

In this exercise, we have seen how to perform the co-pay posting function as well as how to find the status of a patient's claim using Prime Suite.

 You have completed Exercise 6.2

6.4 Diagnosis and Procedure Coding Using Prime Suite

In the medical field, care providers diagnose patients using medical terms—for instance, a myocardial infarction (heart attack), an upper respiratory infection (a common cold), or cholelithiasis (gallstones). They also perform tests to make a diagnosis, such as an EKG (heart test), a strep screen (for strep throat), or a lower GI series (x-rays to detect abdominal conditions). Therapeutic procedures (those that are done to alleviate symptoms or correct a condition) are done as well—for example, suturing a laceration, packing the nose to stop a severe nosebleed, or removing a cyst. Supplies are necessary to complete procedures or for treatment purposes. For instance, a suture kit is used to suture a laceration, serum is used to administer an injection, and a sling may be ordered for a patient with a sprain.

Though the care provider documents the diagnoses, procedures, or services in words, those words have to be converted to a numeric form in order to file claims to insurance companies and to keep statistics of the conditions treated and procedures performed at the office or facility. These codes are also nationally recognized to ensure that providers and insurance carriers across the nation are "speaking the same language," which prevents miscommunication. Additionally, *code linkage*, or showing the relationship between a procedure that was performed and the diagnosis to support medical necessity, is an important aspect of the billing process. For example, if an appendectomy is performed, the medical necessity for that procedure must be linked to a diagnosis—typically, acute appendicitis. Alternatively, improper code linkage will result in a denial of a claim. For example, if a patient is seen by a physician for ankle pain, there is no justification to charge for an ear irrigation procedure. To ensure payment and claim approval, all procedure codes must be linked to an appropriate diagnosis code during the billing process.

The legacy classification system, the International Classification of Diseases, 9th revision, Clinical Modification, ICD-9-CM, was in use for 36 years but eventually was no longer serving the needs of the medical community or public health. To the extent possible, it was updated yearly to reflect new diagnoses, remove obsolete ones, and capture the advances in technology, but it was far overdue for a complete revision, because it was simply not up to date with current medical diagnoses or available treatment options. The World Health Organization (WHO), in 1990, endorsed the newest version, ICD-10, and since 1994 it has been used in the majority of industrialized nations, with the United States being one of the exceptions. That changed on October 1, 2015, when ICD-10-CM and ICD-10-PCS were adopted as the classification systems to capture diagnostic and procedural data in the U.S. health system.

At the time of this writing, you may encounter three different ICD classification systems. The legacy system, ICD-9-CM, was in use from October 1, 1979, to September 30, 2015, to code diagnoses and procedures in hospitals and diagnoses in other healthcare settings. Those codes will continue to be seen on healthcare claims as they are paid, audited, or disputed over the next several months and to gather healthcare statistics for several years. The current classification system includes ICD-10-CM, which is used to code diagnoses in healthcare settings as of October 1, 2015, and ICD-10-PCS, which is used to code procedures in hospital inpatient settings as of October 1, 2015. In the example of an appendectomy necessitated by acute appendicitis, under ICD-10-CM the diagnosis code for acute appendicitis is K35.80 and the procedure code for the appendectomy is 0DTJ4ZZ. Using ICD-9-CM, the diagnosis code would have been 54.1 and the appendectomy code 47.01.

The International Classification of Diseases (ICD) is used to classify diseases and conditions diagnosed in any healthcare setting. It is also used to record cause of death on death certificates. The United States began using ICD-10-CM and ICD-10-PCS—International Classification of Diseases, 10th revision, Clinical Modification and International Classification of Diseases, 10th revision, Procedure Coding System— on October 1, 2015. Only hospitals are required to use ICD-10-PCS, but the two are often referred to as ICD-10-CM/PCS.

The United States had lagged behind in the adoption of ICD-10 in healthcare settings, due in large part to the high cost of converting current computer systems to accept ICD-10 rather than ICD-9 codes, the time and cost involved in training staff in the use of ICD-10, and general questions of whether or not ICD-10 would meet the needs of the U.S. healthcare system. In the United States, coding enables the storage and retrieval of diagnostic information for clinical, epidemiological, and quality purposes as well as the compilation of morbidity and mortality statistics. This is its use in other nations as well, but in this country ICD-9 had also been used for reimbursement purposes, and now that ICD-10-CM and PCS have been adopted, they also will be used for reimbursement purposes. The amount a hospital is reimbursed per inpatient hospital stay is tied in part to each patient's diagnosis and procedure codes, or combination thereof. In hospital outpatient and freestanding outpatient settings, the ICD code correlates to the medical necessity of the procedures and services being done to or for patients. ICD-9 did not address the severity of a patient's condition, whereas ICD-10, though not perfect, does a better job of capturing a truer picture of the resources needed to care for a patient during a particular stay or encounter.

Another glitch that held up implementation in this country was the coding of procedures in hospital settings, which was done using ICD-9-CM. The CM means "clinical modification" and includes procedure codes. In other countries, the CM portion is not used. With ICD-10-PCS, the PCS stands for "procedure coding system" and contains the procedure codes that, as of October 1, 2015, hospitals use for inpatient procedure coding. Outpatient facilities—for instance, outpatient diagnostic laboratories, outpatient surgery in hospitals, physicians' offices, and other freestanding outpatient surgery centers—will continue to code procedures with Current Procedural Terminology (CPT).

The following table shows a comparison of how common diagnoses were coded in ICD-9-CM and how they are now coded in ICD-10-CM.

Narrative Diagnosis	ICD-9-CM Code	ICD-10-CM Code
Epistaxis (nosebleed)	784.7	R04.0
Allergic urticaria (hives)	708.0	L50.0
Chest pain	786.50	R07.9
Diabetes mellitus, Type II	250.00	E11.9
Routine general medical exam	V70.0	Z00.00
Streptococcal pharyngitis	034.0	J02.0
Subarachnoid hemorrhage (stroke)	430	I60.9
Acute anterior wall myocardial infarction (heart attack)	410.11	I21.09
Cholelithiasis (gallstones)	574.20	K80.20

In Prime Suite, on the Assessment screen, both the ICD-9 and the ICD-10 diagnosis codes will be displayed. ICD-10-CM codes can capture a level of specificity that ICD-9-CM could not. In the figures that follow, pay attention to the Barton's fracture codes in ICD-9-CM as well as ICD-10-CM. Figure 6.6 reflects more vague diagnostic codes.

Figure 6.7, however, demonstrates how the care provider can select a more specific code by checking appropriate diagnostic descriptors or modifiers.

Figure 6.8 shows the codes after all diagnostic modifiers (initial fracture, open, type 1, and right-side fracture location) have been documented by the care provider. Notice that the Barton's fracture code has stayed the same in ICD-9-CM but is now S52.561B in ICD-10-CM.

Patients will have at least one diagnosis code, or many, for each encounter. Any conditions that were diagnosed, were treated, or required more nursing or care provider attention should be documented in the patient record and coded. Remember, if there is no supporting documentation, then a provider cannot bill for a service or procedure. The first listed diagnosis

Figure 6.6   ICD-9 and ICD-10 Diagnosis Codes Displayed for a Patient's Active Problems

Figure 6.7   Increasing the Specificity of the Diagnosis of Barton's Fracture

is most closely related to the reason the patient was seen for that encounter (the chief complaint).

The second code set we will discuss is Current Procedural Terminology, or CPT. It is Level 1 of the **Healthcare Common Procedure Coding System**, known as **HCPCS**.

In the physician's office setting, CPT codes are used to code procedures or services given to a patient. In a hospital setting, they are used for outpatient coding (emergency room, outpatient diagnostic testing, or ambulatory surgery, for example).

Healthcare Common Procedure Coding System (HCPCS) Coding system required by Medicare and Medicaid to document services and procedures (Level 1, Current Procedural Terminology, CPT) and equipment, supplies, and transport (HCPCS Level 2).

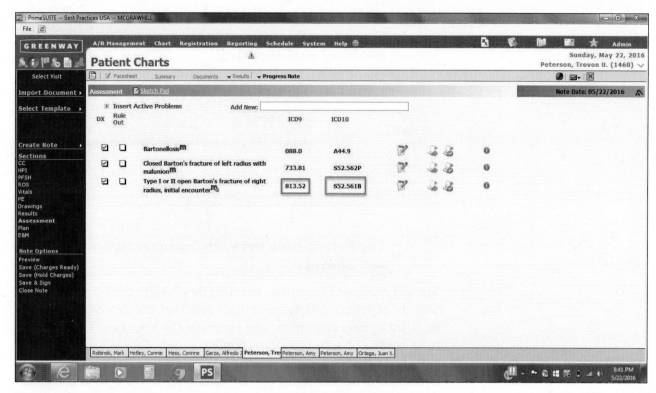

Figure 6.8 The Final ICD-9-CM and ICD-10-CM Codes for Barton's Fracture

Examples of CPT codes in a physician's office include

Code	Description
87430	Strep test
90703	Tetanus injection
71010	Chest x-ray
11100	Skin biopsy
99213	Detailed office visit of an established patient
99202	Low complexity office visit of a new patient

For procedure coding using ICD-10-PCS, these are used only in the hospital setting. The following are comparisons of ICD-10-PCS procedure codes to ICD-9-CM procedure codes. As you can see, ICD-10-PCS procedure codes are very different in ICD-10 than they were in ICD-9. Much more specificity can be coded in ICD-10 than could be captured in ICD-9 procedure codes. Again, in an outpatient setting, such as a physician's office, CPT is used to code procedures.

Narrative Procedure	ICD-9-CM Code	ICD-10-PCS Code
Splenectomy (removal of spleen)	41.5	07TP4ZZ
Salpingectomy (removal of fallopian tubes), bilateral	66.51	0UT74ZZ
Cholecystectomy (removal of gallbladder)	51.22	0FT40ZZ

HCPCS Level 2 codes are used to show tangible items provided, such as suture kits, ambulance services, and orthotic devices (cane, splint, etc.). They are used in any healthcare setting.

Examples of HCPCS level 2 codes include

Code	Description
A0998	Ambulance response and treatment without transport
E0105	Cane, triple or quad
A6453	Self-adherent elastic bandage

6.5 The Relationship between Documentation and Coding

Services rendered to a patient—whether they involve the face-to-face time with the physician, treatment, or diagnostic tests and procedures—cannot be billed to insurance unless they are medically necessary. That is to say, there need to be sufficient signs, symptoms, or history to warrant the services given. Again, this is the purpose of code linkage in the billing process. In addition to demonstrating the relationship between diagnosis and procedure codes, the documentation in the record must support the need for any and all services and procedures. The EHR has been instrumental in making it possible for care providers to spend beneficial face-to-face time with their patients rather than spend time completing their records. Of course, documenting the patient's record while the patient is in the room also takes some finesse. The provider does not want to appear to be paying more attention to the computer screen than to the patient, but the longer the provider uses the computer to document, the more easily she is able to document, listen attentively, and converse with her patients at the same time.

Performing services that are not necessary and coding services that were not actually performed both constitute insurance (including Medicare and Medicaid) **fraud**. Fraud is intentional deception, which in healthcare takes advantage of a patient, an insurance company, or Medicare or Medicaid.

Fraud Intentional deception, which in healthcare takes advantage of a patient, an insurance company, Medicare, or Medicaid.

Whether you are studying to become a health information professional, a medical assistant, or a medical coder and biller, you will take courses that are specific to coding, and you will spend a significant amount of time discussing accurate, appropriate coding as well as the guidelines that apply to the coding and billing functions.

In the next exercise, you will see how ICD-10 and CPT coding are assigned using the Prime Suite software.

EXERCISE 6.3 (PM) (EHR) (HIM) Go to http://connect.mheducation.com to complete this exercise.

Enter Diagnoses and Procedures to Locate ICD-10 and CPT Codes

Once a patient has been seen and examined by the care provider, a diagnosis is made. The written diagnosis is then transformed into a numeric code. In our example, it is done using a function of Prime Suite, but it can also be done manually, using code books. As we mentioned earlier, the diagnosis coding is done using ICD-10-CM, and the procedures or services are coded using CPT and/or HCPCS Level 2.

In the example that follows, Dr. Ingram has just seen a patient, Mark Robinski. Remember, only the care provider can make a diagnosis. So, from the Patient Notes Progress Note screen, Dr. Ingram will be using the Assessments tab (found on the left side of the screen) to add a diagnosis for Mark Robinski.

Mark Robinski's diagnosis is diabetes mellitus, type 2, and Dr. Ingram orders a fasting blood sugar. A diagnosis code (ICD-10-CM) and a procedure code (CPT) will be assigned in the following exercise. The software will automatically assign the codes, but it is important to read the description of the codes and compare it to the narrative diagnosis the care provider has made. You should never code more than what the care provider has documented, and if information is missing in the documentation, it is important to query the provider to determine if the documentation is accurate or if a procedure should not be billed for.

Follow these steps to complete the exercise on your own once you have watched the demonstration and tried the steps with helpful prompts in practice mode. Use the information provided in the scenario to complete the information.

for your information

An assessment is synonymous with a diagnosis or diagnoses (plural).

1. Click Assessment.
2. Click Add Diagnosis (Magic wand icon).
3. Click Search.
4. Type "diabetes".
5. Click Search.
6. Click "Diabetes Mellitus, Type II (Endocrine/Metabolic/Immune)".
7. Click OK.
8. Click MAP ICD10.
9. Click Controlled type 2 diabetes mellitus without long-term current use of insulin.
10. Click Plan.
11. Click Add Order.
12. Click Name Search.
13. Type "Fasting Blood" in the Orders field.
14. Click Search.
15. Click Fasting blood glucose measurement (82947).
16. Click the Category drop-down menu.
17. Click Lab procedure.
18. Click OK.

 You have completed Exercise 6.3

6.6 Accountable Care Organizations

The model of healthcare reimbursement for patients enrolled in the original Medicare program has been fee-for-service for years, although there are some managed care models of Medicare. In other words, services are rendered and hospitals and physicians are paid as long as the services were considered medically necessary. In the latest healthcare reform legislation, through a portion of the **Affordable Care Act (ACA)**, however, providers and hospitals are required to show that they are providing high-quality, coordinated care and are seeking patient input regarding their experience. In addition, positive patient outcomes and less redundancy of services are expected. In other words, reimbursement is tied to quality and efficient use of healthcare services as well as overall patient satisfaction.

When hospitals, doctors, and other healthcare providers formally work together to provide this high-quality care, the result is an **Accountable Care Organization (ACO)**.

Accountable Care Organizations are groups of doctors, hospitals, and other healthcare providers (home health agencies or durable medical equipment companies, for example) who form a voluntary partnership that results in coordinated, high-quality care to their Medicare patients.

As of this writing, Medicare has provided the following six ACO models:

1. The *Medicare Shared Savings* program, which transitions current Medicare fee-for-service providers to the ACO model

2. The *ACO Investment Model,* which is for Medicare Shared Savings program ACOs to test pre-paid savings in rural areas and areas that are underserved in healthcare

3. The *Advance Payment ACO Model,* which is a supplementary incentive model that is open only to providers in the Shared Savings program

4. The *Comprehensive ESRD Care Initiative,* which was designed for beneficiaries who are in end-stage renal disease receiving dialysis

5. The *Next Generation ACO Model,* which is for ACOs that are experienced in managing care for various populations of patients

6. The *Pioneer ACO Model,* which is for healthcare organizations that are currently experienced in the coordination of care for patients

Participation is voluntary, and Medicare patients will not see any changes to their coverage because of a physician's or hospital's choice to become part of an ACO.

In order for care to be "coordinated," the hospital(s), provider(s), and ancillary service providers within the ACO must be able to share patient information. The EHR and interoperable systems make the sharing of these data possible. Approximately 30 quality measures will be monitored and are related to the patient's experience, care coordination, and patient safety. The higher the quality of care delivered, the higher the shared savings earned by the ACO.

Structured data (through ICD-10, CPT, and HCPCS codes) are necessary to measure quality, and the exchange of health information between and among members of the ACO is necessary to achieve coordination of care. Both are made possible through the electronic health record.

6.7 Accounts Receivable—Getting Paid

You may have heard the terms **accounts payable** and **accounts receivable** at some point in time. Accounts payable is money going out—paying the bills. Accounts receivable, on the other hand, is money coming in—in this context, it is the insurance companies' payment of claims that have been filed by Greensburg Medical Center and any monies owed by patients. Of course, it is imperative that what is billed is paid, and that there is an accurate accounting of all **transactions**. Transactions are the posting of charges and the payment of claims.

Insurance companies submit payments to care providers and hospitals electronically (electronic claims transactions or submissions), by check, or by automatic deposit into the bank account of the office. But the amount of the payment may be for more than one patient's care. The insurance company submits the payment with a detailed accounting of the claims for which payment is being made. The document that accompanies the payment is called a **remittance advice (RA)** (Figure 6.9). A similar document, sent to the patient to provide details about the insurance claim, is called an **explanation of benefits (EOB)**. Many insurance companies use the term *remittance advice* to describe the document that accompanies payment to the provider, and the explanation of benefits is generally the form the **subscriber** (the primary person covered by the insurance) receives to notify him or her of what was billed, what was paid, and what the subscriber owes.

Regardless of what it is called, the following information is typically included on an RA or EOB. Again, this is not a billing class; there will be more than one patient included, typically, and many insurance companies include more information than is listed here:

- Provider's name and National Provider Identification (NPI) number
- Patient's name
- Claim number
- Medical record number
- Date(s) of service
- Claim status (open, denied, more information needed, paid, etc.)
- Electronic Transaction Number (if RA and payment have been sent via electronic means)
- Service detail
  - Each CPT code billed (as submitted on the claim form)
  - Amount charged for each code
  - Allowed amount (amount the insurance carrier has agreed to pay) for each code
  - Co-pay paid by patient
  - Adjusted amount (difference between what was charged and the allowed amount)
- Recap of charges and payments
  - Total reported charges amount
  - Charges not covered amount
  - Charges denied amount
  - Covered charge amount
  - Glossary of explanation codes

It is important to have a good understanding of the entire process involved in submitting an insurance claim and receiving payments. The process begins after the patient has completed services or procedures. A healthcare professional will complete the insurance claim, based on the

Transactions Posting of charges and the payment of claims in the practice management system to update patients' accounts.

Remittance advice (RA) A detailed accounting of the claims for which payment is being made by an insurance company. The remittance advice accompanies the payment from the insurance company.

Explanation of benefits (EOB) An explanation of the charges for services, the amount paid by the insurance company, and the amount due by the subscriber, which is sent to the subscriber (and to the provider, in some instances).

Subscriber The primary person covered by an insurance plan.

Figure 6.9 Remittance Advice

PHYSICIAN PERFORMING SERVICES

JOHN GOLDMAN, MD
SUITE 206
85 HARRISON STREET
NEWARK, NJ 07697-1234

PROVIDER NUMBER: 0004120000

PATIENT	INSURANCE CLAIM CONTROL NO.	1 PROCEDURE CODE	2 NO. SVCS / FROM DATE / THRU DATE / POS / SERVICE CODES TYP	3 AMOUNT BILLED	4 AMOUNT APPROVED	5 AMOUNT APPLIED TO DEDUCTIBLE	6 CO-INSURANCE	7 MEDICARE PAYS 80% OF THIS AMOUNT	8 SERVICES PAID IN FULL	9 WITHHELD FOR OFFSET	10 MEDICARE PAID PATIENT	11 MEDICARE PAID PROVIDER	12 MEDICARE DOES NOT PAY FOR THESE SERVICES
MARY DOE 123-45-6789A	1131101414-00	99214	001 0909 0909 11 1	55.57	55.57								
		81000	001 0909 0909 11 5	4.37	4.37								
		78730	001 0909 0909 11 4	76.80	76.80								
				136.74	136.74								
		CLAIMS TOTALS				0.00	26.47	132.37	4.37	0.00	0.00	110.27	
JANE JONES 555-44-3211A	1131101415-00	99244	001 0905 0905 11 3	131.03	131.03								
		81000	001 0905 0905 11 5	4.37	4.37								
		52000	001 0905 0905 11 2	150.68	150.68								
		78730	001 0905 0905 11 4	76.80	76.80								
				362.88	362.88								
		CLAIMS TOTALS				0.00	71.71	358.51	4.37	0.00	0.00	289.17	
JACK SMITH 987-65-4321A	1131101436-00	99214	001 0912 0912 11 1	55.57	55.57								
		81000	001 0912 0912 11 5	4.37	4.37								
		78730	001 0912 0912 11 4	76.80	76.80								
				136.74	136.74								
		CLAIMS TOTALS				0.00	26.47	132.37	4.37	0.00	0.00	110.27	

PAYMENT FOR THE LABORATORY TEST IS BASED ON A FEE SCHEDULE. A COPY OF THIS CLAIM DETERMINATION WILL BE FORWARDED TO THE BENEFICIARY'S SUPPLEMENTAL INSURER WITHIN THE NEXT 30 DAYS. QUESTIONS REGARDING PAYMENT OF SUPPLEMENTAL BENEFITS SHOULD BE DIRECTED TO THAT INSURER.
PAYMENT FOR THIS SERVICE IS BASED ON THE MEDICARE FEE SCHEDULE.

TOTAL	NUMBER OF CLAIMS	AMOUNT BILLED	AMOUNT APPROVED	AMOUNT APPLIED TO DEDUCTIBLE	MEDICARE PAYS 80% OF THIS AMOUNT	COINSURANCE	MEDICARE PAYS 80% OF THIS AMOUNT	AMOUNT OF 80% PAYMENT	SERVICES PAID IN FULL	WITHHELD FOR OFFSET	MEDICARE PAID PATIENT	MEDICARE PAID PROVIDER
PAGE-	3	636.36	636.36	0.00		124.65	623.25	498.60	13.11	0.00	0.00	511.71
CHECK-												

SUMMARY ▶ WEEK ENDING: 10/11/12   CHECK NUMBER: 0475607806   DATE PAID: 10/15/12

NUMBER OF CLAIMS INCLUDED IN STATEMENT

NUMBER OF CHECK ENCLOSED

TOTAL AMOUNT OF CHECK PAID TO PROVIDER

Callout labels:
NAME OF PATIENT (SUBSCRIBER) AND ID NO. — CLAIM NO. — AMOUNT BILLED BY PROVIDER — DATES AND TYPES OF SERVICES (CODED) — AMOUNT ALLOWED ACCORDING TO POLICY — THE 20% MEDICARE COPAYMENT — MEDICARE PAYS 80% OF THIS AMOUNT — MEDICARE PAYS 100% OF THIS AMOUNT — AMOUNT PAID BY MEDICARE TO DOCTOR — NOTATION FOR SERVICES NOT COVERED

Figure 6.9 Remittance Advice

Source: Booth, K.A., Whicker, L.G., Wyman, Terri D., and Moany Wright, Sandra. (2011). *Medical Assisting* (4th ed.). New York: McGraw-Hill Companies. Reprinted by permission.

information listed on the Superbill (also known as a routing slip or encounter form), as well as the provider's documentation. Special attention is paid to ensuring that procedure codes are appropriately linked to diagnostic codes (code linkage) to demonstrate medical necessity. Once the claim is completed and double-checked for accuracy, it is submitted to the insurance carrier. After receipt by the insurance carrier, the claim undergoes a process called **adjudication**.

Adjudication The process of reviewing claims to determine payment.

Adjudication is the process in which claims are reviewed to determine if they should be paid, denied, or partially paid based on the completeness, accuracy, and code linkage of the claim. Once a determination of payment has been made, the insurance carrier will send a payment to the provider along with a remittance advice (RA) that identifies the payment decisions and any items that may need to be resubmitted or corrected. The patient also receives a similar document, an explanation of benefits (EOB), to provide the same information. When the RA has been received with the payment, the practice must post the payments to specific charges (CPT codes) in the patient's account. Any unpaid charges or remaining balances, such as coinsurance charges, will then be sent to the patient in a statement. In some cases, the patient may have a secondary insurance that will be billed for excess charges before the patient statement is generated.

Ensuring that claims are correct before sending them to insurance carriers will provide the best payment results and save the practice the time and expense required to correct and resubmit them. Understanding the claims process is essential to maintaining a healthy revenue and positive cash flow for the practice.

   Go to http://connect.mheducation.com to complete this exercise. **PM** **HIM** **EXERCISE 6.4**

Investigate an Unpaid Insurance Claim

A patient, Mark E. Shaw, calls the billing office because he has received an EOB from his insurance company that his office visit of April 11, 2016, was not covered and therefore the charges are his responsibility to pay. He contacted his insurance company and was told that the diagnosis submitted was for history of kidney stones (Z87.442) and is not covered. He recalls that his office visit on April 11 was for a follow-up of his diabetes mellitus. He asks the biller to check the account. The biller finds that indeed, the documentation on his record shows that his chief complaint was for follow-up of diabetes, which should be a first listed diagnosis on the claim for April 11. This exercise will take you through looking up the diagnosis codes that were filed on the insurance claim for the April 11 visit and correcting the first listed diagnosis to read E11.9, diabetes mellitus, type 2.

1. Click Search for Patient.
2. Type "Shaw" in the *Last Name field.
3. Click Search.
4. Click Select.
5. Click Patient Charts.
6. Click Documents.
7. Click Progress Note (1).
8. Click 04/11/2016.

(continued)

9. Click View Superbill Summary.

10. Click the radio button next to the E11.9 diagnosis code.

11. Click the up arrow.

12. Click OK.

13. Click the up arrow again.

14. Click OK.

15. Click Save.

A corrected claim may now be sent to the insurance company.

☑ **You have completed Exercise 6.4**

6.8 | Managing Accounts Receivable in Prime Suite

The management of patient accounts, from charging patients for services to tracking accounts receivable and collections, begins by setting up the parameters of each insurance carrier and each plan within the insurance. The plan is the extent of coverage offered. For instance, 400 patients in your office may have Blue Cross/Blue Shield insurance, but for those 400 patients, there may be more than 20 plans. Plans differ regarding

- Co-pay and coinsurance requirements: Some plans require a co-pay or coinsurance, others do not, and the dollar amounts vary by plan. Let's look at an example: Neil Holt is an engineer for Johnsontown Analytics, and his insurance is McGraw-Hill Prime. He is responsible for a $20 co-pay, and he is responsible for 20% of all outpatient service charges. Lisa Haver also works for Johnsontown Analytics; she, too, has McGraw-Hill insurance, but she works at a different location in a different state, and her plan requires a $25 co-pay, plus 20% of all outpatient services.

- Extent of coverage and whether or not services are covered at all: For example, Neil Holt's plan covers outpatient mental health services, whereas Lisa Haver's does not.

- Rules regarding filing of claims: These rules may differ from plan to plan, and they certainly differ from insurance company to insurance company.

Because of these differences, it is imperative that the medical office or hospital use a system that efficiently applies the various policies to the correct patients.

When a medical office purchases any type of software, in this case PM software, an administrative staff member (the office manager, office administrator, or business manager) works with an installation specialist from the software company to build libraries and databases that are used to perform functions within the different applications (accounts receivable, patient chart, etc.).

Common libraries include

- Insurance company library—includes all of the insurance companies and the individual plans that are represented by the patients in the practice. These can be created, edited, or deleted within Prime Suite.

- ICD-10-CM, CPT, and HCPCS Level 2 code tables—must be maintained every year to account for additions, deletions, and amendments to codes. In order to get paid in a timely manner, a practice must submit only active, valid codes; otherwise, the claim will be rejected.

- Fee schedule—listed by CPT code and done for Medicare, for group insurance, and by individual contracts for managed care plans. The charge for each service is documented in a fee schedule.

- Reports—in particular, aging reports (length of time a claim has remained unpaid) are set up to allow for timely tracking and follow-up of claims.

- Alerts—reminders to the office staff related to the billing functions. Some examples are co-pay alerts, write-offs, and overdue balances, just to name a few. Alerts assist the staff in collections processes in particular.

Using PM software to accomplish the filing, follow-up, and collection of claims also allows electronic remittance of claims as well as electronic receipt of payment from insurance carriers. The healthcare professional can see at a glance exactly what is happening with a claim or claims at any time in the process. Collections procedures are also streamlined using PM software. Many offices use an outside collections agency to collect overdue balances. With the use of PM software, a report of accounts ready for collections is sent electronically, the office is able to see the status of the account, and paid claims are sent to the office, often electronically.

Greater billing accuracy is an advantage of using PM software, and there is less chance of lost charges and therefore lost revenue. Each time a patient is seen, and the care provider documents the progress note in Prime Suite and orders tests that are done on-site, she is prompted to select the ICD-10 code and the CPT codes that correspond to the diagnosis and procedures (code linkage).

The face-to-face time between a patient and the care provider is charged with a CPT code known as an **Evaluation and Management (E&M)** code. It is generated based on documentation made by the care provider. The E&M code is dependent on whether the patient is new to the practice (not seen by any provider in the practice within the past three years) or an established patient (seen by any provider in the practice within the last three years); the level of history (including chief complaint and review of systems); the level of physical exam performed; the depth of medical decision making necessary; and other contributory factors.

Evaluation and Management (E&M) The CPT codes used to capture the face-to-face time between a patient and the care provider; takes into consideration the extent of the history, the extent of the physical exam, and the level of medical decision making required.

Two examples of E&M codes are

99213 An office visit for an established patient, 20 years old, who was seen for exercise-induced asthma

99203 Initial office visit for a 30-year-old patient who has recently been complaining of rectal bleeding

In your CPT coding class, you will learn the intricacies of assigning E&M codes, but at this point it is important to know that E&M codes are CPT codes that reflect the professional services rendered to a patient.

Enter Documentation to Alter E&M Coding Level

The level of E&M code, and therefore the amount charged for the face-to-face time of a visit, is tied to the extent of history, review of systems, and physical exam documented as structured data in Prime Suite. In this exercise, you will change the level of E&M code by editing documentation in the medical record of Ashley Murray.

1. Click E&M.
2. Click Calculate.
3. Click PE.
4. Click Modify PE Document Structure (Magic wand icon by Note Date:).
5. Click Chest to add it to the physical exam.
6. Click OK.
7. Click Chest.
8. Click Modify PE Document Structure (Magic wand icon by Note Date:).
9. Click Skin.
10. Click OK.
11. Click Skin.
12. Click Plan.
13. Click Add Order.
14. Click Name Search.
15. Click the Orders field.
16. Type "Rapid Strep".
17. Click Rapid Strep (87880) at the top of the list.
18. Click OK.
19. Click E&M.
20. Click Calculate.

✓ You have completed Exercise 6.5

Once the claim has been filed and payment has been sent to the office (either by mail, by direct deposit into the practice's account, or electronically), the payment for each procedure is posted to the patient's record for that date of service.

We will now follow the steps to post a payment using Prime Suite.

connect Go to http://connect.mheducation.com to complete this exercise.

Post an Insurance Payment to an Account

In our scenario, Dr. Ingram's office has received an RA, which includes payment to cover the claim for Mark Shaw for date of service April 11, 2016. There are two charges for this account. They are CPT code 99213, which is an Evaluation and Management code for the face-to-face time he spent with the doctor, and code 82947, which is for a glucose tolerance test. The total amount of the remittance for Mark Robinski is $64. Forty-eight dollars of the $64 is for the services under the 99214 code. Sixteen dollars of it is for the services billed under code 82947. We will be working in the A/R Management module under the insurance transactions function. The objective is to mark the services as paid, based on the amount of money received.

Follow these steps to complete the exercise on your own once you have watched the demonstration and tried the steps with helpful prompts in practice mode. Use the information provided in the scenario to complete the information.

1. Click Search for Patient.
2. Type "Shaw" in the *Last Name field.
3. Click Search.
4. Click Select.
5. Click Insurance Transactions.
6. Click the Amount field for the 99213 line.
7. Type "48.00".
8. Click the Amount field for the 82947 line.
9. Type "16.00".
10. Click Save.

✔ You have completed Exercise 6.6

The Revenue Cycle with Medical Documentation is shown in Figure 6.10. Some steps may be repeated two or three times, but the goal is payment of the claim.

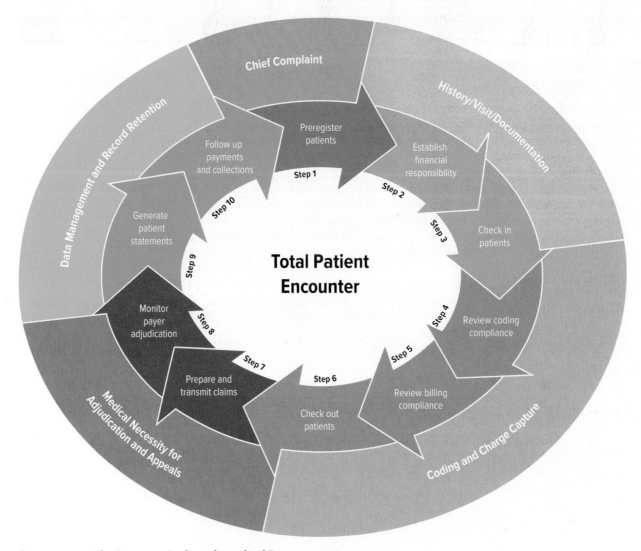

Figure 6.10 **The Revenue Cycle with Medical Documentation**

Source: Sanderson, Susan M. (2011). *Computers in the Medical Office* (7th ed.). New York: McGraw-Hill Companies. Reprinted with permission.

6.9 Compliance

Medicare, Medicaid, TRICARE, Workers' Compensation, group health insurance, and managed care plans are all examples of types of insurance coverage. Each has rules and regulations related to the coding, billing, and collection of healthcare claims. Intentionally not following those rules and regulations can result in allegations of fraud or, at the very least, **abuse**. Abusive coding and billing practices are inconsistent with typical coding and billing practice. Being found guilty of either can result in monetary fines or, in the worst-case scenario, a sanction from any one or more of the insurance plans. If a care provider is sanctioned by Medicare, that means the provider is forbidden to accept Medicare patients into his or her practice. If it is an internal medicine practice, Medicare enrollees most likely make up a good percentage of the patient population in the practice. Needless to say, being sanctioned by Medicare will impact a practice to the point that it may put the provider out of business.

Managed care plans that find a care provider or practice engaging in fraudulent activity may drop that office from their preferred provider list, resulting in a negative impact on the practice's income.

Abuse Coding and billing that is inconsistent with typical coding and billing practices.

For federal programs, the Office of Inspector General (OIG) investigates suspected cases of fraud. In order to defend the practice in the event of a visit from the OIG, a **compliance plan** should be in place in every medical office and hospital. Not only should it be in place, but it should also be followed. If the OIG does audit your practice, showing that you have a compliance plan and demonstrating that it is followed will be an advantage; having one and *not* following it may not be. The requirements of a compliance plan are

Compliance plan A formal, written document that describes how the hospital or physician's practice ensures rules, regulations, and standards are being adhered to.

- Conducting audits and monitoring work performed by the office staff
- Developing and implementing standards of practice to be followed by office staff (including care providers) that are uniformly and consistently applied
- Appointing a compliance officer
- Training new staff immediately after hire on office policies and procedures and offering periodic in-services to all staff (including care providers)
- Fixing any problems that are found, investigating the reason for problems, and retraining staff as necessary
- Encouraging staff to bring any compliance issues to the office administration
- Enforcing the office's policies and procedures and not making exceptions

Having, following, and referencing a practice's written policies, procedures, and compliance plan will assure sound fiscal practices within a practice or facility, and may be a sound defense, should the practice ever be involved in fraud or abuse allegations.

APPLYING YOUR SKILLS

Accountable Care Organizations are part of the largest healthcare reimbursement reform in years. You have been given basic information about ACOs. Now, research on your own to find the following answers:

1. The Centers for Medicare & Medicaid Services (CMS) is responsible for ACOs. List and describe four participation requirements.
2. Why will it be so important to accurately code diagnoses and procedures as this relates to ACOs?
3. Do an Internet search of Accountable Care Organizations and describe an ACO that you find.

chapter 6 **Summary**

LEARNING OUTCOME	CONCEPTS FOR REVIEW
6.1 Illustrate the need for a claims management process.	– Though the primary purpose of a medical office is to provide patient care, it is still considered a business. – Written policies are necessary to run the office effectively and efficiently. – Use of PM software improves efficiency. – A patient account for a visit begins when the appointment is made. – Insurance verification should be completed—either before the day of the visit or when the patient arrives (beforehand is preferred). – Patient check-out occurs once the visit is complete.

6.2 List the information contained in an encounter form (Superbill).	– A Superbill is otherwise known as an encounter form or a routing slip and includes at least
	  • Name and address of medical practice
	  • NPI number
	  • Patient's name
	  • Patient's charge number
	  • Date and time of visit
	  • CPT codes
	  • Diagnosis narrative by care provider
	  • ICD-10-CM diagnosis codes.
	– It can be hard-copy or electronic.
	– The information on the Superbill transfers to the CMS-1500 claim form.
	– It includes some identifying information about the encounter as well as the diagnosis and procedure codes using ICD-10 and CPT code sets.
	– Code linkage is the relationship between the diagnosis and procedure codes to demonstrate medical necessity.

6.3 Apply procedures to update a patient's account in Prime Suite.	– Patients share costs with insurance carriers by paying co-payments and coinsurance. – Co-payments are fixed amounts that are paid for each encounter. – Coinsurance payments are based on a percentage of the patient's healthcare costs. – Co-payment may be collected at the time of check-in or check-out, depending on office policy. – Financial alerts appear when the patient is checked into Prime Suite at the time of arrival. The insurance plan entered in the system determines which, if any, alerts appear. – Once paid, the co-pay is immediately posted in Prime Suite. – Charges start to accrue once the patient is taken to the examining room and is seen by a healthcare professional. – Insurance status may be looked up at any time.

(continued)

LEARNING OUTCOME	CONCEPTS FOR REVIEW
6.4 Demonstrate coding using ICD-10-CM/PCS and CPT codes in Prime Suite.	– The provider's assessment is otherwise known as the diagnosis (or diagnoses, plural). – Services rendered may be diagnostic (x-rays, lab tests) or therapeutic (sutures, cleansing of a wound, injections). – Diagnoses are coded using the ICD-10-CM code set and are used in both hospital and outpatient (physicians' offices) settings. – The first listed diagnosis is the one most closely related to the reason the patient was seen. – Any conditions that were diagnosed, treated, or required more nursing or provider attention should be documented. – Procedures are coded using CPT in the physician's office. – Procedures are coded using ICD-10-PCS in the hospital setting. – Code linkage shows the relationship between the procedure code and the diagnostic code to demonstrate medical necessity. – HCPCS Level 2 codes are used to code equipment or supplies. – Coding is done for statistical and reimbursement purposes.
6.5 Examine the correlation between documentation and code assignment.	– All services and procedures performed must be medically necessary. – The diagnoses support the medical necessity for the procedure(s) and service(s) through code linkage. – Performing services that aren't medically necessary and billing for them are considered fraud.
6.6 Describe Accountable Care Organizations.	– New reimbursement model for Medicare patients – Came about through the Affordable Care Act (ACA) – Goal is high-quality care, patient satisfaction, decreased redundancy of services, and coordination of care. – Voluntary partnership among physicians, hospitals, and other healthcare providers – Six current models: Medicare Shared Savings Program; ACO Investment Model; Advance Payment ACO Model; Comprehensive ESRD Care Initiative; Next Generation ACO Model; and Pioneer ACO Model – Dependent on measurable outcomes through reporting based on ICD-10, CPT, and HCPCS codes as well as the ability to share patient information between and among members of the ACO
6.7 Describe the information contained in a remittance advice, or explanation of benefits.	– Accounts receivable—money paid to the office by insurance carriers – Transactions—documentation of all money paid and applying it to the correct patient's balances – Remittance advice (RA), also referred to as an explanation of benefits (EOB), accompanies the payment and explains the claims to which the payments apply. – The subscriber is the person who is covered under the group insurance plan.

(continued)

LEARNING OUTCOME	CONCEPTS FOR REVIEW
6.8 Apply procedures to manage accounts receivable in Prime Suite.	– Efficiency and effectiveness of managing the financial aspects start with accurately setting up the parameters of each insurance carrier and the plans within each in the PM software.
	– The type of plan a patient has determines the extent of coverage and the co-pay requirements.
	– Each insurance carrier (and the plans within) has rules and regulations regarding filing of claims.
	– Libraries are built within the PM software for each insurance carrier.
	– The revenue cycle with medical documentation demonstrates the process for sending claims and receiving payments.
6.9 Demonstrate the need for a compliance plan.	– All offices should have written policies and procedures for all processes in the office but, in particular, for the financial aspects.
	– All policies should be complied with uniformly and consistently.
	– Each insurance carrier also has rules and regulations that must be followed.
	– Not following the rules and regulations may constitute fraud or abuse.
	– The Office of Inspector General enforces the rules and regulations set forth by any federal insurance plans.
	– The office should have a compliance plan to assure all rules and regulations are being followed. The plan should include
	• Conducting internal audits of work performed
	• Developing standards of practice
	• Appointing a compliance officer
	• Training new personnel, updates for experienced personnel
	• Correcting any known problems, retraining staff as necessary
	• Encouraging open communication from staff regarding compliance issues
	• Enforcing all policies and procedures.

chapter review

MATCHING QUESTIONS

Match the terms on the left with the definitions on the right.

_____ 1. **[LO 6.5]** fraud

_____ 2. **[LO 6.7]** transaction

_____ 3. **[LO 6.1]** managed care plan

_____ 4. **[LO 6.7]** accounts receivable

_____ 5. **[LO 6.8]** Evaluation and Management codes

_____ 6. **[LO 6.1]** fee schedule

_____ 7. **[LO 6.7]** subscriber

_____ 8. **[LO 6.9]** compliance plan

_____ 9. **[LO 6.3]** co-payment

_____ 10. **[LO 6.7]** explanation of benefits

_____ 11. **[LO 6.3]** coinsurance

_____ 12. **[LO 6.2]** code linkage

a. list of how much is charged per service by CPT code

b. document sent from an insurance company to a subscriber outlining payment decisions

c. portion of a bill that is usually the responsibility of the patient, typically collected upon check-in

d. the primary individual covered under an insurance plan

e. formal, written guidelines that describe how a healthcare office intends to follow established rules and regulations

f. actions, such as posting payments or processing claims, done in a practice management system to update patient accounts

g. codes representing the face-to-face time spent with a provider

h. monies coming into a medical practice

i. act of deception that takes advantage of another person or entity

j. form of insurance that monitors patients, care, and performance to ensure quality

k. using the diagnostic and procedure codes together to show medical necessity

l. form of cost sharing with an insurance carrier in which the patient pays a percentage of medical expenses

MULTIPLE-CHOICE QUESTIONS

Select the letter that best completes the statement or answers the question:

1. **[LO 6.2]** The information contained in the encounter form is eventually transferred to the _____ for submission.
   a. claim form
   b. encounter form (Superbill)
   c. insurance form
   d. registration form

Enhance your learning by completing these exercises and more at http://connect.mheducation.com!

2. **[LO 6.5]** Only services deemed medically _____ can be billed to insurance.
   a. necessary
   b. progressive
   c. restorative
   d. useful

3. **[LO 6.4]** What does the "CM" stand for in ICD coding?
   a. care management
   b. clinical modification
   c. code management
   d. coding methodology

4. **[LO 6.8]** The amount of a patient's co-pay may vary by
   a. care provider.
   b. insurance plan.
   c. office location.
   d. visit type.

5. **[LO 6.3]** Charges begin to accrue once the
   a. appointment is made.
   b. patient checks in at the reception area.
   c. medical assistant or care provider interacts with the patient.
   d. claim has been filed.

6. **[LO 6.7]** A remittance advice is typically given to a/an _____, whereas an explanation of benefits is typically given to a/an _____.
   a. patient; provider
   b. provider; patient
   c. insurance company; patient
   d. provider; insurance company

7. **[LO 6.2]** When submitting claims to insurance carriers, providers show medical necessity by
   a. including a glossary of terms in the claim.
   b. using code linkage.
   c. writing a claim summary.
   d. sending copies of patient charts with the claim.

8. **[LO 6.9]** To avoid negative consequences, a compliance plan should be _____ in every hospital and medical office.
   a. ignored
   b. followed
   c. used as a suggestion
   d. discarded

9. **[LO 6.8]** The _____ is usually the person to set up information libraries within practice management software programs.
   a. care provider
   b. healthcare professional
   c. medical assistant
   d. office manager

10. **[LO 6.5]** Who is the only person authorized to make a diagnosis?
    a. care provider
    b. healthcare professional
    c. medical assistant
    d. office manager

11. **[LO 6.3]** To check if a claim has been paid, which menu will the healthcare professional look at?
    a. Accounts Payable
    b. Accounts Receivable
    c. Claims Processing
    d. Claim Updates

12. **[LO 6.6]** Which of the following is true of the advance payment ACO model?
    a. It is based on fee for service.
    b. It is an incentive model.
    c. It is the largest Accountable Care Organization.
    d. It requires participation by hospitals and medical vendors.

13. **[LO 6.1]** Depending on the terms of a patient's insurance coverage, the balance remaining after insurance has paid may be
    a. written off as paid in full.
    b. removed from the Master Patient Index.
    c. sent to collections.
    d. written off as paid in full or sent to collections.

14. **[LO 6.1]** Expected methods of payment are discussed when a patient
    a. checks in.
    b. is seen by the provider.
    c. is discharged.
    d. makes an appointment.

SHORT-ANSWER QUESTIONS

1. **[LO 6.1]** List four ways practice management software improves claim management.

2. **[LO 6.7]** Contrast accounts receivable with accounts payable.

3. **[LO 6.8]** What is the difference between an insurance provider (carrier) and an insurance plan?

4. **[LO 6.2]** List at least five items that are typically included on a hard-copy Superbill.

5. **[LO 6.3]** What is an alert?

6. **[LO 6.5]** How have EHRs improved the face-to-face time between patients and care providers?

7. **[LO 6.2]** Explain how the icons available in practice management software make claim management easier and more accurate.

 Enhance your learning by completing these exercises and more at http://connect.mheducation.com!

8. **[LO 6.6]** Summarize the goal of Accountable Care Organizations in one or two sentences.

9. **[LO 6.5]** Explain fraud in terms of the healthcare profession.

10. **[LO 6.3]** List three reasons that you might need to check the status of an insurance claim.

11. **[LO 6.8]** What is an aging report?

12. **[LO 6.7]** What four items are included in the recap of charges and payments found on an EOB?

13. **[LO 6.4]** List the three types of codes used in a clinical setting and give an example of how each is used.

14. **[LO 6.4]** Discuss at least three benefits of moving to ICD-10.

15. **[LO 6.9]** What is the difference between fraud and abuse?

APPLYING YOUR KNOWLEDGE

1. **[LO 6.3]** Discuss why many healthcare practices refuse to see patients who do not pay their co-pays at the time of their visit.

2. **[LOs 6.5, 6.9]** Research two recent cases of medical/insurance fraud (an Internet search of medical insurance fraud will take you in the right direction) and discuss the outcome of each case. Provide specifics about your sources (Internet, medical journals, textbooks, etc.).

3. **[LOs 6.1, 6.8]** Why might an office need to use a collections agency to pursue overdue accounts?

4. **[LO 6.7]** Why is there so much information contained on an RA or EOB form?

5. **[LOs 6.4, 6.5, 6.9]** Anna Devlan is a healthcare professional. Recently, she posted some patient claims; when performing the coding process, Anna could not find a code that exactly matched the diagnosis made by the care provider, so she found the closest match and coded that. Did Anna commit fraud and/or abuse? Explain your answer.

6. **[LO 6.6]** Paul Donovan, a Medicare patient, suffers from Crohn's disease and rheumatoid arthritis. Recently, he presented to County Hospital complaining of hip pain. How will the interoperability offered under Accountable Care Organization models impact Mr. Donovan's care?

chapter references

Booth, K.A., Whicker, L.G., Wyman, Terri D., and Moany Wright, Sandra. (2011). *Administrative Procedures for Medical Assisting* (4th ed.). New York: McGraw-Hill Companies.

Centers for Medicare and Medicaid Services (CMS). *Accountable Care Organizations.* Retrieved from http://www.cms.gov/Medicare/Medicare-Fee-for-Service-Payment/ACO/index.html?redirect=/aco/

Current Procedural Terminology. (2016). Chicago: American Medical Association.

Examples of CPT codes based on CPT 2016.

Examples of HCPCS codes based on HCPCS 2016.

Examples of ICD-9-CM codes based on ICD-9-CM 2013.

Content related to Greenway Health™, Greenway Prime Suite™, or other related products retrieved from http://www.greenwayhealth.com (or earlier iterations of the website) from 2011–2016.

ICD-10-CM/PCS codes based on ICD-10: Version 2016.

ICD-10-CM Codebook. (2016). Salt Lake City, UT: Contexo Media.

ICD-9-CM, Volumes I, II, & III. (2013). Ingenix. Salt Lake City, UT

Newby, C. (2010). *From Patient to Payment: Insurance Procedures for the Medical Office* (6th ed.). New York: McGraw-Hill Companies.

White, S., et al. (2011, June). An ACO Primer. *Journal of AHIMA, 82*(6): 48–50.

World Health Organization. (2013). International Classification of Diseases. Retrieved from http://www.who.int/classifications/icd/en/

Privacy, Security, Confidentiality, and Legal Issues

	Key **Terms**

What You Need to Know and Why You Need to Know It

No matter what type of healthcare professional you become—a nurse, medical assistant, health information manager, coder, biller, registration clerk, receptionist, or care provider—you will come in contact with patients' health information. In healthcare, and particularly with electronic healthcare, privacy and security are on everyone's mind—the patients', the providers', the media's, and the government's. There is concern that computer hackers and personnel who work in healthcare facilities will gain access to records that they have no legitimate need to access. The concern is justified, but even in a paper system, frequent privacy breaches have occurred. It is just as easy for a healthcare professional to look in a patient's chart at the nurses' station as it is to sit down at a computer that is left open to a patient's record and read it. The difference is that it is far easier to change information within the record or records without the change(s) being detected until it may be too late, and it is far easier to share that patient's or thousands of patients' health information without authorization and for unethical and unlawful reasons when an electronic health record system is hacked. In this chapter we will discuss laws that protect privacy and security as well as methods to lessen the chances of privacy breaches occurring. It is the responsibility of all healthcare professionals and care providers to maintain patient privacy and confidentiality and to access the health information only on a need-to-know basis.

7.1 The HIPAA Privacy and Security Standards

HIPAA was passed in 1996 and contains several rules, though for our purposes in this chapter, we will be concentrating on the privacy and security rules. In addition, in 2009, the Health Information Technology for Economic and Clinical Health Act (HITECH) went a step further, making the original privacy and security rules under HIPAA more stringent. HITECH also gives more power to federal and state government authorities to enforce the privacy and security rules.

On March 26, 2013, the Omnibus Final Rule to the HITECH Act went into effect, with compliance required in September 2013. Changes included more enhancements to protecting patient privacy, additions to individual patient rights, and strengthening of the government's ability to enforce the law. HIPAA was expanded to give more control over any covered entity's business associates—for example, external coding consultants and software service providers. The Notice of Privacy Practices has been expanded, and the maximum penalty for violation of the law was increased to $1.5 million per violation. Related to HITECH, the breach notification standards have been enhanced. Examples of the enhancement in patient rights include the requirement that providers who utilize electronic health records must provide patients with their records in electronic form, when requested. In addition, patients who are paying for their services in cash may instruct the provider not to bill their insurance and not to divulge any information about the services to the patient's health insurance carrier.

The intent of both is to ensure that protected health information (PHI) is kept private and secure. They give patients the right to determine who sees their health information, but still give **covered entities** (healthcare providers, clearinghouses, or health insurance plans) the leeway to access

for your information **fyi**

More information about HIPAA can be found at http://www.hhs.gov/ and then searching for "HIPAA for Professionals," and HITECH information can be found at https://www.healthit.gov/ and searching for "HITECH."

Covered entity Any healthcare entity that captures or utilizes health information. These include healthcare plans (insurance companies), clearinghouses that process healthcare claims, individual physicians and physician practices, any type of therapist (mental health, physical, speech, occupational), dentists, hospital staffs, ambulatory facilities, nursing homes, home health agencies, pharmacies, and employers.

the PHI needed to care for patients, collect payment for services rendered, and operate a business. Protected health information is any piece of information that identifies a patient—it includes a patient's name, DOB, address, email address, and telephone number; the patient's employer; any relatives' names; the patient's Social Security number and medical record number; account numbers tied to the patient's account; the patient's fingerprints; any photographs of the patient; and any characteristics about the patient that would automatically disclose his or her identity (for instance, "the governor of the largest state in the United States").

In addition, PHI includes the medical information that is tied to the person, including diagnosis, test results, treatments, and prognosis; documentation by the care provider and other healthcare professionals; and billing information.

HIPAA states (and HITECH enhances) that only persons who have a need to know may have access to a patient's PHI. And, to take it a step further, they are entitled only to access to the **minimum necessary information** required to do their jobs. An example would be a covered entity such as a health insurance company that is working on a claim for a patient who underwent coronary artery bypass three months ago. Unless the insurance company can prove otherwise, the minimum necessary information it needs is the supporting documentation related to the bypass surgery. The fact that the patient delivered a child in 1980 has nothing to do with the bypass surgery, and therefore the company does not need access to those records.

There are many ways that facilities protect the **privacy** and **confidentiality** of their patients. Privacy is the right to be left alone. In other words, no one should infringe upon a patient's time or personal space while being treated; that is why admissions departments and registration areas have partitions or cubicles, so that the patient has some privacy. Confidentiality is keeping a secret; in healthcare, it means keeping information about a patient to oneself. Patients have the right to expect that their medical information is going to be kept confidential. Written policies and ongoing education of staff are two very important aspects of complying with the HIPAA and HITECH rules.

Privacy and confidentiality policies should address, at a minimum,

- Release (disclosure) of information to outside sources. PHI is released to outside entities only upon written authorization of the patient/legal representative (or as required by law) and release to inside sources (access) is only on a need-to-know basis. The policy should also address exceptions. Let's first look at internal access as an example. Cathy Hess was a patient on unit 3E of Memorial Hospital from May 3 to May 5. Suzanne Hess is a nurse who works at Memorial Hospital and is Cathy Hess' sister-in-law. She does not work on 3E and did not take care of Suzanne. She did not have, does not have, and will not have a need to access Cathy's health record. But, let's say two months after Suzanne's hospitalization, Cathy is on a committee that is auditing records for a study and Suzanne's record happens to be one of the records in the sample. Cathy could ask one of the other reviewers to audit that particular record, but if Cathy does review Suzanne's record, she is accessing the record within the scope of her job, and she does have a need know in that case. Internal access does not require an authorization from the patient, if there is a need to know.

Minimum necessary information As required by the Health Insurance Portability and Accountability Act (HIPAA), releasing the minimum information to satisfy the reason the information is needed or the minimum necessary to perform a job function.

Privacy The right to be left alone; the right to expect that one's personal space is respected while undergoing healthcare.

Confidentiality The patient's right to expect that his/her health information will not be released to any person or entity without the patient/guardian's written authorization or as required by law or regulation.

- Outside access without the need for authorization of the patient/personal representative. This includes access by an insurance company (for payment of the bill), by public health officials in cases of mandatory reporting (infectious diseases, for example), and by licensing and accrediting agencies.

- Release of **directory information**. Directory information includes the fact that the patient is in the hospital (or is being treated at an ambulatory facility) and his or her room number. However, if a patient does not want certain individuals (or anyone) to know that he or she is in the hospital or the location within the hospital, then the patient/legal representative would sign an authorization stipulating who can and cannot have access to that information.

- Written guidelines and examples of what is considered minimum necessary information by reason for the request

- Faxing of documentation—information that can and cannot be faxed and the protocol to be followed, should information be faxed to the wrong location

- Computer access and lockdown. Policy requires staff to lock their computers down (sign out) if they are going to be away from their desks for any length of time.

- Password sharing—makes it a disciplinary offense to share one's password with another

- Computer screens—should be kept out of view of the public or anyone else who might have access to areas with computers

- Shredding any hard-copy documents (where applicable) rather than just discarding them in a waste paper basket

- Signing by patients of a **Notice of Privacy Practices** so that patients are aware of how their personal health information will be used. The Notice of Privacy Practices must be in writing and be signed by the patient/legal representative. It informs the patient how his or her health information will be used and the reasons it may be released, notifies the patient that he or she may view or have copies of the health record and may request amendments to it, and states the procedure for filing a complaint with the Department of Health and Human Services.

- Requirement that all staff (including care providers) sign a document committing themselves to keeping private and confidential the information that is written, spoken, or overheard about any and all patients

Once a paper record is converted to an electronic one, the paper copy is no longer needed. It is best practice to destroy the paper copy, if the electronic version is considered the legal document, and the one upon which healthcare decisions are made. The paper record should be destroyed either by incineration or by shredding. An example of a shredding policy statement in an office that no longer keeps hard-copy records (a "paperless environment") is

> The electronic health record is the legal health record at Greensburg Medical Center. Printed copies should only be made when there is a need to refer to the printed document rather than the computerized image. Once the printed document is no longer needed, it is to be placed in one of the marked shred bins immediately. Shred bins are located in the business office and in the secure area of the front

Directory information The fact that a patient is an inpatient (or being treated as an outpatient) as well as his/her location within the facility.

Notice of Privacy Practices A requirement of the Health Insurance Portability and Accountability Act (HIPAA) that patients are made aware (in writing) of their rights under HIPAA including the fact that the patient has the right to view/receive a copy of his/her own record, the fact that amendment to the documentation may be requested, the ways in which their health information will be used and released to outside entities, and the procedure to file a complaint with the Department of Health and Human Services.

office. The only exception to this policy is the printed copies made for patients' requests, or that are to be mailed by the Release of Information Specialist.

In addition to the policies noted above, security-specific policies should address

Password A unique code, known only to the user, that is used to gain access to computer applications.

- Password protection. Every computer user must have a unique code, or **password**, that is known (and used) only by the user. Passwords should not be easily discerned; for instance, the user's birthdate, spouse's name, child's name, phone number, and the like would not be secure passwords. Instead, the password should be a combination of numbers, letters, and special characters (symbols), no less than six and no longer than eight characters in length, and the system should be set up to prompt users to change their password at least every 90 days. Individual offices and facilities will set policies regarding their password configuration requirements. The software system in use will dictate some of the password constraints as well.

- Appointment of a security and/or privacy officer. Someone in the facility must be named as privacy and security officer, though these may be two different individuals. The privacy/security officer is ultimately responsible for setting, monitoring, updating, investigating, and enforcing all privacy and security policies.

- Log-in attempts. The system set-up should include automatic lock-out when a user attempts to log in a certain number of times (usually three) with the wrong password. The policy and procedure should also address how to regain access. No doubt you have already experienced this with online banking, a credit card company, or the learning management system at your college.

Computer virus A deviant program, stored on a flash drive, hard drive, or CD, that can cause unexpected and often undesirable effects, such as destroying or corrupting data.

Malware Malware is short for malicious software and includes deviant software such as worms, viruses, and Trojan horses, all of which attack computer programs.

- Protection from **computer viruses** and **malware**. This should include the facility's policy on downloading music or other attachments that may carry viruses and malware. A virus is a "deviant program, stored on a computer floppy disk, hard drive, or CD, that can cause unexpected and often undesirable effects, such as destroying or corrupting data. Malware comes in the form of worms, viruses, and Trojan horses, all of which attack computer programs" (Williams and Sawyer). In early 2016 several hospitals were plagued by computer malware. Though patient records were not accessed, MedStar Health near Washington, DC, was affected and the system's users were not able to log in. This attack affected 250 outpatient locations and 10 hospitals. As a precaution, the health system sent patients to other facilities until the problem was resolved and the FBI was involved in the investigation (Cox, Turner, and Zapotsky).

- Security audits. A policy should be in place and carried out that requires random security audits to monitor access to patients' records. Often, this may be done on a rotating basis so that all staff members (including providers) are audited periodically, or it may be done based on a random selection of patients in the database. Of course, the investigation of any rumored or known breaches should include a security audit. It is important that internal security audits be carried out, since the Officer of Inspector General (OIG) also carries out random audits of EHR system security vulnerabilities.

- Off-site access. With the use of current technology, many PMs and EHRs can be accessed via the Internet. Policies must dictate who can access remotely as well as what information can be viewed and/or edited remotely.

- Printing policies. The more information that is printed from the EHR or PM software, the greater chance there is of unauthorized disclosure.

- Destruction policies. If paper copies of the electronic record are going to be made, then the destruction of those copies also needs to be addressed. The usual method of destruction is shredding, either externally by a destruction company or internally through use of portable shredders. Regardless of which is used, a policy must be addressed that states when paper copies are destroyed, how, by whom, and when.

- Detailed policies and procedures that address privacy or security incidents. Disciplinary action should be addressed in this policy as well.

- Staff education—requirement that all staff (including care providers) participate in continuing education opportunities to reinforce the laws governing privacy and security.

- Email. It is a part of everyday life, not just in our personal lives but in our work lives as well. Anything written in an email is protected information. However, it is not a secure means of communication, and the facility should adopt policies related to the sending and receiving of email messages, including what, if any, patient-related information can be sent via email. Like faxes, emails can go to the wrong individual, constituting a privacy breach. There must be a policy regarding patient-related emails or emails to or from patients—are they a part of the patient's health record, and if so, how will the email become part of the record? Emails should be **encrypted**, which means the words are scrambled and can be read only if the receiver has a special code to decipher it, but encrypting still does not ensure total security. Encryption applies to any information that is electronically transmitted.

Firewalls should also be used to deter access to the system by unauthorized individuals. Williams and Sawyer define a firewall as "a system of hardware and/or software that protects a computer or a network from intruders."

Hardware also has to be protected, and policies must be written to govern the security of hardware devices. Hardware includes desktop computers, laptop computers, hand-held devices, and the like. These devices are always at risk for loss or theft. But to protect the information on a device, follow these simple rules:

- Always lock down (sign out of) the device when it is unattended, and require a password to log on.

- Never store the passwords to any of your hardware devices or sites on the computer.

- Back up files onto a CD, external hard drive, or flash drive.

- Encrypt PHI if policy allows health records to be stored on the device.

- Use the portable devices in a secure area—using one in the cafeteria and walking away to freshen your coffee is not secure.

- Wipe the hard drives of any computers that are taken out of use before recycling them or placing them in the trash. This is typically a responsibility of the IT department.

for your information fyi

Use caution when authoring or responding to any email concerning a patient in the clinical applications of Prime Suite, since the email will become a permanent part of the patient's EHR.

Encryption A security method in which words are scrambled and can only be read if the receiver has a special code to decipher the scrambled message.

Firewall A system of hardware and/or software that protects a computer or a network from intruders by filtering activity over the network.

Hardware The tangible items that are used in automation (e.g., the processing unit, screen, keyboard, mouse, laptops, hand-held devices).

Privacy and security need to be kept in mind at all times in any healthcare facility or practice. Not doing so, even unintentionally, may result in hefty fines. The new fines, as a result of the Omnibus Final Rule, are as follows:

Category of Violation	Fine per Violation	Total Violation when Breach Involved the Same Provision within the Same Calendar Year
Unknowing (unintentional)	$100–50,000	$1,500,000
Reasonable cause	$1,000–50,000	$1,500,000
Willful neglect (corrected)	$10,000–50,000	$1,500,000
Willful neglected (not corrected)	Minimum of $50,000	$1,500,000

Healthcare organizations using an EHR must meet the HIPAA standards of privacy and confidentiality. In addition, states may have even more stringent rules. The American Recovery and Reinvestment Act of 2009 (ARRA), through HITECH, made the rules regarding privacy and security of electronic systems more stringent yet. **Accounting of disclosures** is a responsibility of healthcare facilities as a result of HITECH. Facilities must be able to provide a patient with a listing of disclosures, if requested; this is known as accounting of disclosures. Also, facilities with an EHR must be able to provide a patient with a listing of people who had access to his or her protected health information internally. This is known as an **access report**. The access report must contain the name of the individuals who accessed that person's record, and also the names of persons who do not work at the facility who had access to the record. For instance, a hospital may grant a local nursing home admissions department the right to view the health record of a patient who is being considered for nursing home placement. This is required to assess whether or not the nursing home has the facilities needed to care for that patient, and it is part of the continuum of care; thus, it is a necessary release. The hospital would note, in the access report, that the patient's PHI was released to a certain nursing home but would not be able to supply the names of the individual(s) who accessed it at the nursing home.

Accounting of disclosures Providing the patient, upon request, with a listing of all disclosures of his/her health information, both internally and externally.

Access report A report of all persons (within the facility) who have had access to a patient's protected health information.

7.2 **Evaluating an EHR System for HIPAA Compliance**

According to the Office of the National Coordinator for Health Information Technology (ONC) website, "Health information technology (health IT) makes it possible for health care providers to better manage patient care through secure use and sharing of health information." Health IT includes the use of electronic health records (EHRs) instead of paper medical records to maintain people's health information.

To better manage patient care using electronic means, however, it is necessary to comply with certain regulations. The HIPAA rules that address electronic health information are listed in Table 7.1.

Regarding passwords, though longer passwords are more secure than shorter ones, the most secure passwords include a combination of letters

TABLE 7.1	Functionality of an EHR as Required by HIPAA Regulations
Functionality	**Meaning**
Password Protection	Passwords must be assigned to all users of an electronic health record system and the passwords must meet certain criteria: length, properties, expiration intervals, and number of log-in attempts before lockout.
User Identification	Each user must have a unique identifier to log in. Often consists of the person's first initial and last name. Allows for tracking and reporting of activity within the system by the user.
Access Rights	Policies are written and adhered to regarding access to functionality within the EHR that is dependent on the person's (or position's) need to know.
Accounting of Disclosures	Upon authorized request, an accounting of all disclosures from a patient's health record, going back a minimum of six years from the date of request, must be provided. The patient's health record must also be made available to the patient, or to an outside entity at the patient's request.
Security/ Backup/ Storage	A backup of the EHR database must be kept in a secure location, and restoration of the backup database must be possible at any given time. Other security requirements include controlled access to the database, use of passwords to access the database, use of firewalls, and antivirus programs.
Auditing	This task provides the ability to run reports by users or by patients that specify the menu, module, or function accessed; the date and time of the access; whether the information was viewed, edited, or deleted; and the user ID of the individual staff member.
Code Sets	The EHR must use ICD-10 codes, CPT codes, and HCPCS codes to store and transmit information.

Source: Sanderson, Susan M. (2013). *Computers in the Medical Office* (8th ed.). New York: McGraw-Hill Companies.

(upper- and lowercase), symbols, and numbers. The password "summerday" is more secure than "summer," for example, yet "summer18$#" is even more secure. Healthcare organizations set their own policies regarding the length and configuration of passwords.

In a medical practice, it may be the office administrator who starts the search for EHR software and keeps in mind the requirements of a compliant system. Other individuals who should also be involved in researching, selecting, and implementing the EHR include a representative of care providers, a member of the front office (reception) staff, a clinical staff representative, health information staff, coding/billing staff, and an information technology (IT) professional who is an expert in the technological aspects of the software and hardware, networking, and interoperability of systems. This group should always keep in mind

- The required components of a compliant EHR
- The needs of the office or facility
- The intended budget for acquiring a system as well as yearly budget requirements
- Staff and training needs
- The intent of the EHR—is it to interface with the existing PM system, or will an entirely new system that accomplishes both be purchased?
- The timeline—what is the target date for implementation?

7.3 The Role of Certification in EHR Implementation

There are many agencies that certify EHR software. Both the information technology (IT) and the health information technology (HIT) aspects of an EHR system must be taken into consideration, and during the process of assessing various systems and vendors, looking at certified EHR systems is a good place to start.

CMS and the Office of the National Coordinator for Health Information Technology (ONC) have established standards and other criteria for structured data that EHRs must use in order to qualify for an incentive program to upgrade an existing EHR or purchase a new one. The ONC, through consultation with the Director of the National Institute of Standards and Technology, recognizes programs for this voluntary certification if they are in compliance with certification criteria (HHS: Proposed Establishment).

The **Healthcare Information and Management Systems Society (HIMSS)** is an independent, nonprofit organization with the mission "To lead healthcare transformation through the effective use of health information technology" (HIMSS: About HIMSS). HIMSS and the **American Health Information Management Association (AHIMA)** are professional associations that are highly respected in the fields of Information Technology (IT) and Health Information Management (HIM). Each has myriad sources, references, guides, best practices, and practice briefs for use in the selection and implementation of an EHR, and both organizations highly value certification.

Other current certifying agencies include InfoGard; Drummond Group, Inc.; and ICSA Labs. The Certified Health IT Product List (CHPL) can be found by performing an Internet search using those exact words.

Selecting a product that is certified is good business practice and will save the office administration much of the legwork necessary to ensure selection of a product that not only meets the needs of the organization but has already been tested and proven to meet regulatory requirements.

It is worth a student's time to view this listing, select one or more products, and view the ONC criteria that have been met by each.

7.4 Applying Security Measures

Assigning passwords, allowing access to only the functions that are necessary to perform a job, and following the other policies outlined in Section 7.1 all play a role in assuring the privacy, confidentiality, and security of the health information stored in your facility's PM and EHR systems.

The next two exercises apply basic security measures in Prime Suite. These functions will usually be set up by the office administrator or manager.

Healthcare Information and Management Systems Society (HIMSS) An association of health informatics and information professionals formed to promote a better understanding of healthcare informatics and management systems.

American Health Information Management Association (AHIMA) A professional association for the field of health information management.

Adding Users to Prime Suite

Add a New Clinical User and Assign a Password

In this scenario, the office manager has just hired a new medical assistant (MA), Patric Olson, and he is going to set Patric up as a user in Prime Suite. Certain information is needed from Patric before the office manager begins the setup process. You will notice that the password "greenway" is used in the initial setup of Patric Olson. In the examples used throughout the worktext, the default password is "greenway." In an actual work setting, this default password would be changed to a password of the user's choice that meets the practice's password requirements.

Field	Value
Full name	Olson, Patric
Username	polson
Email	polson@greenwaymedical.com
Sex	Male
Telephone number	770-555-1234
DOB	07/08/1960
Soc. Security No.	123-45-1234

Follow these steps to complete the exercise on your own once you have watched the demonstration and tried the steps with helpful prompts in practice mode. Use the information provided in the scenario to complete the information.

1. Click User Administration.
2. Click Add New.
3. Type "polson" in the Username:* field.
4. Click the Email: field.
5. Type "polson@greenwaymedical.com".
6. Click the SSN: field.
7. Type "123-45-1234".
8. Click the First Name:* field.
9. Type "Patric".
10. Click the Last Name:* field.
11. Type "Olson".
12. Click the Contact Number: field.
13. Type "770-555-1234".
14. Click the Date of Birth: field.
15. Type "07/08/1960".
16. Click the Sex:* drop-down menu.
17. Click Male.
18. Click the Must Change Password At Next Login check box.
19. Click Save.
20. Type "******" in the *New Password field.

(continued)

21. Click the *Confirm Password field.
22. Type "*****".
23. Click OK.
24. Click OK.

☑ You have completed Exercise 7.1

Setting Up Care Providers

EXERCISE 7.2   Go to http://connect.mheducation.com to complete this exercise.

Set Up a Care Provider

In our next scenario, there is also a new care provider starting this week, Lynette Dean, M.D. The office manager will set her up in the system, assigning a user ID and user rights.

The information necessary before beginning the setup process is

Field	Value
Full name	Dean, Lynette
Sex	Female
Credentials	MD
NPI number	1234567891
State Medical License number	345678
DEA Number	GA456789
On staff at Greensburg Medical Center	Yes
Provides billable services from Greensburg Medical Center	Yes
Assigned User ID	Idean

Follow these steps to complete the exercise on your own once you have watched the demonstration and tried the steps with helpful prompts in practice mode. Use the information provided in the scenario to complete the information.

1. Click Care Providers.
2. Type "Dean" in the *Last Name field.
3. Click the *First Name field.
4. Type "Lynette".
5. Click the Sex drop-down menu.
6. Click Female.
7. Click the *Credentials drop-down menu.
8. Click MD to select it.
9. Click the National Provider Identifier field.
10. Type "1234567891".
11. Click the State License Number field.
12. Type "345678".
13. Click the DEA Number field.

160

14. Type "GA4567890".
15. Click On Staff?
16. Click Billable?
17. Click the Set User ID icon next to the User ID field.
18. Click the *Username field.
19. Type "Idean".
20. Click the *First Name field.
21. Type "Lynette".
22. Click the *Last Name field.
23. Type "Dean".
24. Click Sex drop-down menu.
25. Click Female.
26. Click Add New.
27. Click Yes.
28. Click Save.

✓ **You have completed Exercise 7.2**

Setting User Rights for Staff

We will take security functions a step further by adding **user rights**. Log-on rights simply mean that one is assigned a log-in and password to allow access to the computer software, in our case, Prime Suite. The user is then assigned user rights, which are privileges that limit access to only the functionality of the software needed by that individual. The position held and job description of each staff member (including care providers) dictate what privileges each person has.

User rights The limitations of one's access to the functionality of the software as defined by one's job description or position within the organization.

 Go to http://connect.mheducation.com to complete this exercise.   EXERCISE 7.3

Assign User Rights to a Medical Assistant (MA)

In the scenario that follows, John Greenway is an office manager. He will be setting up the user rights for Patric Olson, an MA who is new to the office. We will start by setting up Chart rights from the action bar on the left side of the screen. Chart rights have to do with viewing, adding, editing, or changing documentation within patients' charts. For instance, Patric will be able to access the Patient Chart page of every patient. He will have access to a very extensive allergy module, which will include setting up a patient's allergy shot schedule, dosage calculations, and similar applications. Of course, *he will do this based only on the physician's orders*. Patric will be able to delete vital signs from a Facesheet; reasons for this may be that the vitals were incorrectly typed into the Facesheet or were put on the wrong patient's chart, or that the healthcare professional who entered the blood

(continued)

pressure, for example, did not get an accurate reading. *These privileges are very sensitive and are only given to appropriate staff members with the expertise and position within the practice to warrant such rights.* But even deleted, the original documentation is not lost forever—hidden is actually a better description for it—there is an **audit trail** that shows the original documentation and then the corrected version. The topic of data integrity and versions of documentation will be covered in more detail later in this chapter.

Custom views of the Facesheet can be set up in many EHR software packages, Prime Suite included. The information displayed is consistent, but the way it looks on the screen is different. Some MAs or nurses are granted the right to sign off on lab results; *that right is determined by office policy (and may vary by care provider) as well as the level of knowledge of the individual.* An example is a standard blood test, such as a CBC, that is completely within normal limits on an established patient; the care provider may feel that an experienced MA or nurse is qualified to sign off on those results without sending them through for review by the care provider. The same applies to some prescriptions. The care provider may give a verbal order to an MA or a nurse for a prescription renewal to be called in to the patient's pharmacy or refilled by ePrescription. For example, Robyn Berkeley is a long-time patient of Dr. Rodriguez. She has a long-standing prescription for metronidazole for treatment of her rosacea, and she has run out; the MA gives Dr. Rodriguez the request, and he then authorizes her to send through a refill via ePrescribe. The MA is able to access and print (or electronically transmit) the prescription renewal with Dr. Rodriguez's digital signature.

User rights for all registration functions are also set up; if the healthcare professional works in the reception and registration areas, she would have user rights to any routine daily functions, including registering a patient for the first time, editing demographic information, scheduling an appointment, checking a patient in or out, viewing alert flags, and so on.

System rights affect just that—the overall system. The rights you will see in this exercise include importing documents that do not originate within Prime Suite and accessing patient tracking.

Follow these steps to complete the exercise on your own once you've watched the demonstration and tried the steps with helpful prompts in practice mode. Use the information provided in the scenario to complete the information.

1. Click User Rights.
2. Click Current User.
3. Click Patric Olson.
4. Click Chart.
5. Click Chart.
6. Click Access the Patient Charts Page.
7. Click Allergy Module-Can modify serum sheet status.
8. Click Allergy Module-Override EP rules.
9. Click Facesheet-Delete vitals.
10. Click Facesheet-Manage problem list custom views.
11. Click Lab Flowsheet-Initial a lab or revoke initials.
12. Click Orders-Add to order favorite list.
13. Click Orders-Edit/delete from orders favorite list.
14. Click Prescriptions-Access ePrescribe.
15. Click OK.
16. Click Prescriptions-Can edit medication alert override.
17. Click OK.

18. Click Prescriptions-If a digital signature other than this user's is saved with a prescription, allow printing of the signature.
19. Click OK.
20. Click Save.
21. Click Registration.
22. Click View Patient or Person Registration Information.
23. Click Modify Patient or Person Registration Information.
24. Click View Patient List.
25. Click Check-In patients.
26. Click Undo Check-Out.
27. Click View and Modify Chart Patient Flags.
28. Click View Clinical Alerts Flags.
29. Click Save.
30. Click System.
31. Click Document Import.
32. Click Access Document Import.
33. Click Save.
34. Click Patient Tracking.
35. Click Access Patient Tracking.
36. Click Save.
37. Click Close (in the top right corner of the Patient Tracking Rights box).
38. Click Close (in the top right corner of the System Categories box).

☑ **You have completed Exercise 7.3**

Setting User Rights for a Manager

  Go to http://connect.mheducation.com to complete this exercise.   **EXERCISE** **7.4**

Assign User Rights to an Office Manager

Office managers or administrators have increased functionality such as setting up files in accounts receivable management, chart configuration and administration, registration screens, research (clinical trial) functionality, reporting, scheduling, and overall system configuration. As you go through the exercise that follows, in which you will assign rights to Diane Baxter, take a look at the entire list of rights that are assigned. The research category pertains to participation in clinical trials that are run by the Food and Drug Administration.

Follow these steps to complete the exercise on your own once you have watched the demonstration and tried the steps with helpful prompts in practice mode.

1. Click User Rights.
2. Click Current User.
3. Click Diane Baxter.

(continued)

4. Click A/R Management.

5. Click Select All.

6. Click Save.

7. Click Chart.

8. Click Chart Admin.

9. Click Select All.

10. Click Save.

11. Click Research.

12. Click Select All.

13. Click Save.

14. Click Registration.

15. Click Select All.

16. Click Save.

17. Click Reporting.

18. Click Select All.

19. Click Save.

20. Click Scheduling.

21. Click Select All.

22. Click Save.

23. Click System.

24. Click Select All.

25. Click Save.

26. Click Close.

☑ **You have completed Exercise 7.4**

Setting Up a Group

    EXERCISE 7.5 PM EHR HIM Go to http://connect.mheducation.com to complete this exercise. McGraw Hill Education connect®

Create a Group

In the previous exercises, we have been working with just one staff member. In this exercise we will set up an entire group within Prime Suite. Setting up groups, such as all medical assistants, all receptionists, or all care providers, allows the office administrator to give rights by group rather than having to set up each person individually. Of course, if some of the users within the group have higher-level rights, then their profiles can be modified by adding rights individually.

In Exercise 7.5 we will be working within the Group Administration module of the Systems Menu. Essentially, a group is formed and the individual staff members are moved into it, and finally the group is named. Or a group may already exist and staff members are moved into it. The other advantage of groups is that if an email needs to be sent to an entire group—for instance, the health records staff—then just one email needs to be sent rather than a separate email to each staff member. An example would be that the health records staff is required to attend an in-service meeting on HITECH regulations at 2:00 p.m. on May 5. Just one message can be sent to the entire group, notifying them of this in-service meeting.

Follow these steps to complete the exercise on your own once you've watched the demonstration and tried the steps with helpful prompts in practice mode.

1. Click Group Administration.
2. Click Allison Tubiak (atubiak).
3. Click the Move highlighted item to selected list arrow.
4. Click Jennifer Brady (jbrady).
5. Click the Move highlighted item to selected list arrow.
6. Click Jared Howerton (jhowerton).
7. Click the Move highlighted item to selected list arrow.
8. Click Patric Olson (polson).
9. Click the Move highlighted item to selected list arrow.
10. Click Save Group.
11. Type "MedAssts" in the Save Security Group field.
12. Click Save.
13. Click Enable Messaging.
14. Click Save Group.

✓ **You have completed Exercise 7.5**

 Go to http://connect.mheducation.com to complete this exercise.   **EXERCISE** **7.6**

Set General Security

General security settings involve password maintenance. To complete the exercise, you will need the following information regarding Greensburg Medical Center's security policies:

Configuration Setting	Value
Password length	7 characters
Password change occurs	Every 90 days
Maximum inactivity before system automatically logs off	15 minutes
No. of days before password can be re-used	364 days
Log-in banner	Good Morning Greensburg!

Follow these steps to complete the exercise on your own once you have watched the demonstration and tried the steps with helpful prompts in practice mode. Use the information provided in the scenario to complete the information. There are already some values that appear in the exercise, so we will not be covering every setting.

1. Click System Configuration.
2. Click the Min Password Chars field.
3. Type "7".

(continued)

4. Click the Days Password Valid field.
5. Type "90".
6. Click the Inactivity Limit field.
7. Type "15".
8. Click the Days Prevent Password Reuse field.
9. Type "364".
10. Click the Practice Defined Login Banner field.
11. Type "Good Morning Greensburg!".
12. Click Save.
13. Click OK.

☑ **You have completed Exercise 7.6**

Audit Trails

EXERCISE **7.7**   Go to http://connect.mheducation.com to complete this exercise.

Run an Audit Trail Report

In this exercise, an audit trail report will be run. This functionality helps to fulfill the HITECH requirement to provide an accounting of disclosures (or, in this case, accesses to a record), or it may be used to monitor activity of a certain staff member or activity in general in a particular area of the EHR software.

Our objective in this exercise is to view the Vitals History accesses over the past month by one of the staff members with the user ID of "admin."

Follow these steps to complete the exercise on your own once you have watched the demonstration and tried the steps with helpful prompts in practice mode.

1. Click Report Selection . . . F7.
2. Click System.
3. Click Audit Log Report.
4. Click the Report Type drop-down.
5. Click Vitals History.
6. Click the User drop-down.
7. Click Admin.
8. Click the Date drop-down.
9. Click Month To Date.
10. Click Immediate View.
11. Click Print.
12. Click Print.
13. Click Close.

☑ **You have completed Exercise 7.7**

A health record contains not only pertinent clinical data but also information about a patient that may be considered embarrassing or make a patient uncomfortable, or is just very private. Examples are personal history data such as history of abortion or having given up a child for adoption, or history of drug or alcohol abuse. In these instances, a record may be marked as sensitive within Prime Suite or other EHR software so that extra care is taken when handling or releasing information.

Though all health information is confidential and is not released unless a proper authorization is on file, as required by law, or for continuity of care, some health information is such that a higher level of confidentiality is vital, even from staff within an office or a hospital. Take, for instance, a patient who is well known to the office and in the community who has a diagnosis of a sexually transmitted disease. In this case, only the care provider and staff who absolutely have a need to know in order to care for the patient, or process the record for the insurance claim, would have access to that record. Perhaps the sister-in-law of that patient is a receptionist in the office—it would not be prudent for her to handle that particular record. Or consider another patient who is on an antidepressant but does not want the record open to the entire staff because one of the medical assistants in the office is a friend of hers. In both of these examples, the record might be marked as "sensitive" within Prime Suite, and access to those records may be limited to only a select few providers and staff within the practice; this is known as "restricted access" within Prime Suite. Many practices mark records of all their staff (and often any family members) as restricted access, and only the office manager controls access to providers and other staff members who have a need to know.

Records of celebrities and other well-known individuals would also be considered sensitive and/or allow restricted access. A well-publicized case of a privacy breach involving George Clooney and his girlfriend occurred in 2007. The two were in a motorcycle accident and were taken to a New Jersey hospital. More than 20 staff members of that hospital were suspended for a month without pay due to accessing the pair's health records without a need to know and without authorization.

 Go to http://connect.mheducation.com to complete this exercise.   **EXERCISE** **7.8**

Mark a Record as Sensitive

Corinne Hess is a 17-year-old patient of Dr. Rodriguez who has been suffering from depression. The record contains information that is of a very personal nature and is going to be flagged as "sensitive."

Follow these instructions to register Corinne and input her insurance information, as well as to mark the record as sensitive. You will need the information on the registration form shown in Figure 7.1.

1. Click Search for Patient.
2. Type "Hess" in the *Last Name field.
3. Click the *First Name field.

(continued)

4. Type "Corinne" in the *First Name field.
5. Click Search.
6. Click the Date of Birth field.
7. Type "05/06/1999".
8. Click the Sex drop-down menu.
9. Click Female.
10. Click the Phone field.
11. Type "770-555-1234".
12. Click Add New.
13. Click OK.
14. Click Registration.
15. Click Information.
16. Click the *Race 1: drop-down menu.
17. Click Caucasian/White.
18. Click the Religion: drop-down menu.
19. Click Protestant.
20. Click the *Ethnicity: drop-down menu.
21. Click Not Hispanic or Latino.
22. Click the Address *Line 1: field.
23. Type "904 Wrigley Road".
24. Click the *Zip: field.
25. Type "30117".
26. Press "Tab".
27. Click the Cell: field.
28. Type "770-555-7881".
29. Click the Email: field.
30. Type "corinne@anywhere.com".
31. Click the *Preferred Communications: drop-down menu.
32. Click Email.
33. Click the Occupation field.
34. Type "Student".
35. Click "Click here to search for plan" icon.
36. Click the Insurance Co: drop-down menu.
37. Click McGraw-Hill HealthMark.
38. Click Search.
39. Click Select.
40. Click the Policy Number field.
41. Type "GAR512374".
42. Click the Policy Holder field.
43. Type "Jared Hess".
44. Click the Group Number field.
45. Type "1600".
46. Click the Effective Date field.
47. Type "05/01/1999".
48. Click the Expiration Date field.
49. Type "12/31/2016".
50. Click Save.
51. Click View/Edit Patient Flags icon.
52. Click Sensitive Chart.
53. Click Save icon (located in the upper right corner).
54. Click the Close button.

 You have completed Exercise 7.8

Greensburg Medical Center
REGISTRATION FORM
(Please Print)

Today's date: *May 4 2016*	Care Provider: **Dr. Rodriguez**

PATIENT INFORMATION

Patient's last name: *Hess*	First: *Corinne*	Middle:	☐ Mr. ☐ Mrs.	☐ Miss ☒ Ms.	**Marital status (circle one)** (Single) / Mar / Div / Sep / Wid

Is this your legal name? ☒ Yes ☐ No	If not, what is your legal name?	(Former name):	Birth date: *05/06/1999*	Age: *19*	Sex: ☐ M ☒ F

Street address: *904 Wrigley Road*	Social Security no.: *887-66-2489*	Home phone no.: *770-555-3450*

P.O.Box:	City: *Carrollton*	State: *GA*	ZIP Code: *30117*

Occupation: *Student*	Employer:	Employer phone no.:

Email address: *corrinne@anywhere.com*	Cell phone: *770-555-8989*	

Race: *White*	Ethnicity: *American*	Primary language: *English*	Religion: *Protestant*

Next of kin: Jared Hess, father Home phone: *770-555-1234*   Work phone: *770-555-5544*   Cell phone: *770-555-7881*

INSURANCE INFORMATION
(Presentation of Insurance Card is required at time of each visit)

Person responsible for bill: *Jared Hess*	Birth date: *07/23/1968*	Address (if different): *Same*	Home phone no.: *Same*

Is this person a patient here? ☒ Yes ☐ No

Occupation: *Teacher*	Employer: *Carrollton Elementary*	Employer address: *900 W. Norfolk Avenue*	Employer phone no.: *770-555-5000*

Is this patient covered by insurance? ☒ Yes ☐ No

Please indicate primary insurance	☒ McGraw-Hill Healthmark Insurance	☐ BlueCross/Shield	☐ [Insurance]	☐ [Insurance]	☐ [Insurance]
☐ [Insurance]	☐ Workers' Compensation	☐ Medicare	☐ Medicaid *(Please provide card)*	☐ Other	

Subscriber's name: *Jared Hess*	Subscriber's S.S. no.: *555-88-1456*	Birth date: *07/23/1968*	Group no.: *1600*	Policy no.: *GAR512374*	Co-payment: *$20.00*

Patient's relationship to subscriber: ☐ Self ☐ Spouse ☒ Child ☐ Other	Effective Date: *05/01/1999*

Name of secondary insurance (if applicable):	Subscriber's name:	Group no.:	Policy no.:

Patient's relationship to subscriber: ☐ Self ☐ Spouse ☒ Child ☐ Other

IN CASE OF EMERGENCY

Name of local friend or relative (not living at same address): *Amanda Jaxon*	Relationship to patient: *Aunt*	Home phone no.: *770-555-8954*	Work phone no.: *770-555-1518*

The above information is true to the best of my knowledge. I authorize my insurance benefits be paid directly to the physician. I understand that I am financially responsible for any balance. I also authorize [Name of Practice] or insurance company to release any information required to process my claims.

Jared H.Hess

Patient/Guardian signature

05/04/2016

Date

Figure 7.1   Corinne Hess Registration Form

Mark a Record as Restricted Access

David Olivetti is the brother-in-law of Kaitlyn, a medical assistant at Greensburg Medical Center, and is good friends with Dr. Rodriguez. Dr. Ingram is his regular physician at Greensburg Medical Center. Because of the relationship with Kaitlyn and Dr. Rodriguez, David does not want either to have access to his EHR. In this exercise, David's record will be marked for restricted access.

1. Click Search for Patient icon.
2. Type "Olivetti" in the *Last Name field.
3. Click Search.
4. Click Select.
5. Click Patient Charts.
6. Click View/Edit Patient Flags icon.
7. Click Restricted Chart.
8. Click Save icon. (A padlock icon will appear on David Olivetti's Facesheet.)

☑ **You have completed Exercise 7.9**

7.6 | Data Integrity

Data integrity Maintaining the accuracy and consistency of data.

Data integrity refers to the accuracy and timeliness of data collection, and the consistency of the definitions used to collect the data. In addition, there is an expectation that there has been no manipulation of the data once the data have been collected and reported. To maintain data integrity, the healthcare facility must have strict policies regarding who may access data, the definition of a complete record, the accuracy of data, consistent applications of data dictionary definitions, and the timeliness of data entry. Think of it this way: If a patient is seen on Wednesday, but the documentation in the health record is not entered until Friday, how accurate do you think it will be? Or if one of the staff members instructs a patient to document his past surgical history but to include only surgeries done under general anesthesia in the past five years, yet the office policy shows a data dictionary definition of surgery as *any* procedure the patient has had while under local, regional, or general anesthetic at any time in the past, then how consistent are the data? What about a healthcare professional who finds a blood pressure reading of 152/80 in a patient yet enters it as 140/80 and knowingly leaves it as is, figuring it is "close enough"? If you were a care provider using the information found in your EHR database, and you knew poor documentation practices were occurring, you would not have much faith in using those data, would you? Or if you were conducting a research study and knew that the data were flawed, how valid would the study be? In other words, any data found within the health record must be accurate, complete, and documented at the time of or as close to the time of occurrence as possible.

Amending a Chart Entry

Integrity also applies to the addition, amendment, or omission of documentation that has already been recorded. Any alteration in the original documentation must be recoverable. With the use of paper records, if an entry in a health record was amended or corrected, it was obvious. See Figure 7.2 for an example of a proper chart correction. You can readily see that the entry was corrected; originally, it read that the patient had sustained a laceration to her right hand, when, in fact, it was the left hand. A single line was drawn through the incorrect word, the correct word was inserted, and the correction was initialed and dated by the person who made the correction.

In an electronic record, original documentation that is found to be incorrect or incomplete may be hidden from view, and the amended information becomes part of the health record. Only the corrected information is viewable to the healthcare professionals or care providers; however, that original hidden documentation can be recovered at any time. Our next exercise illustrates amendment of an entry in Prime Suite.

The patient sustained a 4 cm laceration to her left (mbs 6-10-11) ~~right~~ *hand three days ago.*

Figure 7.2   Example of Correction to Paper Documentation

for your information

The individual who made the original entry/error should be the person to make the correction in the health record whenever possible.

 Go to http://connect.mheducation.com to complete this exercise.   **EXERCISE   7.10**

Amend a Chart Entry

Juan Ortega's record contains an error in the progress note. The care provider documented the HPI of Juan Ortega's, but after she completed documenting and saved the note, she noticed a word was misspelled. She accesses the progress note of the chart and makes the correction. Notice, while going through the exercise, that in order to make the correction, the care provider must enter her password in order to change an entry. This additional step allows the care provider to think twice about amending the entry to be certain it is necessary and that the information she is about to add is correct. The original progress note with the error is known as version 1 and the corrected progress note as version 2.

Follow these steps to complete the exercise on your own once you have watched the demonstration and tried the steps with helpful prompts in practice mode.

1. Click Documents.
2. Click the Progress Note.
3. Click Amend Document.
4. Click HPI.
5. Click the Form radio button.
6. Click the "also presents" error.
7. Click presents.
8. Click Close in dialog box.
9. Click Save & Sign.

✓ **You have completed Exercise 7.10**

Hiding a Chart Entry

Hide a Chart Entry

There are times when documentation is added to the wrong chart, or when misinformation is given or documented. In these cases, we would need to hide an entry. As noted in Exercise 7.10, though the entry is hidden, it is still retrievable at a later time. Our next exercise steps us through hiding an entry on Mark Robinski's chart. In this case, it is a progress note that was intended for another patient's chart. Typically, only certain staff members such as those who are in lead or administrative positions have this user right. This is not a procedure that is done often, nor is it done without a valid reason, such as that the note was put on the wrong patient's chart or the note pertains to that patient but not to that particular visit. Some software vendors use the term *deleting* rather than *hiding,* but regardless, the deleted/hidden entry will *always* be retrievable, should the record be needed in a lawsuit, to verify some sort of inconsistency, or for insurance purposes.

Follow these steps to complete the exercise on your own once you have watched the demonstration and tried the steps with helpful prompts in practice mode.

1. Click Documents.
2. Click Manage Chart Documents.
3. Click 04/04/2016.
4. Click Delete.
5. Click the Yes radio button.
6. Click the Other radio button.
7. Type "wrong patient" in the Other field.
8. Click OK.

✓ **You have completed Exercise 7.11**

Recovery of a Hidden Entry

Recovery of a Hidden Entry

Hiding a document does not mean that it is truly deleted forever. The original documentation can be retrieved by accessing the Documents Menu and then accessing Manage Chart Documents from the action bar.

Follow these steps to complete the exercise on your own once you have watched the demonstration and tried the steps with helpful prompts in practice mode.

1. Click Documents.
2. Click Manage Chart Documents.
3. Click View Deleted Docs.
4. Click 04/04/2016.
5. Click Undo Delete.
6. Click the Yes radio button.
7. Click the Accidental Delete radio button.
8. Click OK.

✓ **You have completed Exercise 7.12**

<table>
<tr><td>7.7</td><td>**Apply Policies and Procedures to Release Health Information Using Prime Suite**</td></tr>
</table>

Another requirement of Meaningful Use initiatives is to share health information with other healthcare professionals when necessary. For instance, Virginia Hill is a patient of Dr. Ingram's, and he is referring her to a specialist. It is important for the specialist to know her medical history and the reasoning behind the referral; therefore, information is released electronically. This reason is known as continuity of care.

Many releases require a written authorization from the patient or legal representative. If the specialist also has an EHR, he or she is able to access the primary care physician's health record of Virginia Hill, but let's say Dr. Ingram's office printed Mrs. Hill's record and mailed it to the specialist. Now, we will be accounting for the disclosure. Release of information in the case of this referral would not require an authorization, nor would release of information to an insurance company for purposes of payment of the claim, nor release of information to public health agencies, as required by law. Written authorization is required for all releases of information to physicians' offices or hospitals that are not a result of a direct referral. Authorization is also required to release health information to attorneys, employers (if not a Workers' Compensation claim), spouse, children, and law enforcement agencies. Also, certain records such as those related to drug and alcohol abuse, mental health, and HIV/AIDS have more stringent release of information regulations; those will be discussed in great detail in another course.

Releasing information without a required authorization is known as a **breach of confidentiality**. Offices and healthcare facilities are required to report breaches, as was discussed earlier in this chapter, as part of the HITECH regulations. Not only is the office or facility held liable for any breaches, but individual staff members may be as well.

Breach of confidentiality Releasing information without a required, properly executed authorization or as restricted by law.

Compose a Correspondence Letter to Accompany the Release of a Patient's Immunization Record

Follow these steps to complete the exercise on your own once you've watched the demonstration and tried the steps with helpful prompts in practice mode. Use the information provided in the scenario to complete the information.

1. Click Search for Patient.
2. Type "ortega" in the *Last Name field.
3. Click the *First Name field.
4. Type "juan".
5. Click Search.
6. Click Select.
7. Click Create Note.
8. Click Correspondence.
9. Click Select Template.
10. Click Lab results - Lipids (Examples V4.7).
11. Click VISIT CARE PROVIDER NAME.
12. Type Hart.
13. Click Albert Hart MD.
14. Click OK.
15. Click Save & Sign.
16. Type "*******" (7 asterisks) in the Password: field.
17. Click the green check mark.
18. Click 04/19/2016.
19. Click Print/Fax Document.
20. Click Print.

✓ **You have completed Exercise 7.13**

7.8 Accounting of Information Disclosures

An accounting of the releases is also necessary in order to comply with regulations. As noted earlier, most releases require a written authorization, but to comply with HITECH, *all* releases must be accounted for, whether the disclosure is to internal staff members or to external requestors.

Run a Report of Information Disclosures for a Particular Patient

In this scenario, the office manager needs to run a report of information disclosures (or, in this case, access) of the chart of a patient, Corinne T. Hess, whose chart ID is 1592. She is particularly looking for disclosures (accesses) to Ambulatory Summary for today.

Follow these steps to complete the exercise on your own once you have watched the demonstration and tried the steps with helpful prompts in practice mode. Use the information provided in the scenario to complete the information.

1. Click Report Selection . . . F7.
2. Click System.
3. Click Audit Log Report.
4. Click the Patient ID: field.
5. Type "1592".
6. Click the CCDA Doc Type: drop-down.
7. Click Ambulatory Summary.
8. Click Immediate View.
9. Click Close.

✓ You have completed Exercise 7.14

7.9 Information Exchange

Communicating with other healthcare providers is another requirement of Meaningful Use. It is known as **health information exchange (HIE)**. An advantage of utilizing an EHR is that patient care improves through the sharing of patient information at the point of care. With this functionality, care providers can access the findings of other physicians or test results immediately. Of course, this sharing is done through a secure environment, and there are regulations that address telecommunications and networking security as well. Secure email is one way that information can be shared between providers, the National Health Information Network (NHIN) Exchange is another, and there are state and private HIE programs as well. The State HIE Cooperative Agreement Program operates through the use of ONC funding, and its purpose is to coordinate local HIEs or serve as the HIE for a given area.

Health information exchange (HIE) The movement or sharing of information between healthcare entities in a secure manner and in keeping with nationally recognized standards.

for your information **fyi**

Using a search engine, take the time to find your state's HIE on the Internet; each HIE has its own site and includes valuable information for care providers and staff.

 Go to http://connect.mheducation.com to complete this exercise.

 EXERCISE 7.15

Exchange of Information for Continuity of Care

In this scenario, Ian Mikeals is a pediatric asthma patient of Dr. Ingram. Dr. Ingram is referring Ian to a pediatric asthma specialist.

Follow these steps to complete the exercise on your own once you've watched the demonstration and tried the steps with helpful prompts in practice mode.

1. Click Document Import.
2. Click Data Submission.
3. Click Referral Summary (XDS-MS).

(continued)

4. Click the Reason for Referral field.
5. Type "Asthma".
6. Click Preview.
7. Click Print.
8. Click Close.

 You have completed Exercise 7.15

Exchange of Information outside the Organization

Social media Interactive communication sites via the Internet. Examples are Facebook, YouTube, Instagram, Snapchat, and Twitter.

Blog Ongoing conversations about a topic that take place online via the Internet.

There is another type of information exchange that has nothing to do with continuity of care, business purposes, or insurance purposes. It involves communicating *about* care via **social media**. Social media include Facebook, YouTube, Twitter, **blogs** (ongoing conversations about a topic that take place online), and the like. These outlets are used by patients to share their experience with a healthcare organization or to recount their journey through an illness; they can also be used by the organizations themselves as a means of marketing or public relations. Take a look at the Facebook page of Children's Hospital, Boston, for example, by going to http://www.facebook.com/ and searching for the hospital. Here you will find videos, testimonials, facts and figures about its patient population, and links to other related sites, as well as support groups and blogs, awards the organization has won, and a link to its social media policy, which is short and to the point and, in summary, states that although all comments are welcome, they should not be offensive, should be on-topic, and should not violate the privacy of patients or their families.

There is some risk in allowing patients to provide comments, since not all of them will be positive, but by the same token, patient feedback is a vehicle to promote the institution, its accomplishments, and its services. The appropriate use of social media also provides a service to the community by including needed information about the organization as well as links to related sites such as public health, educational sites, and support groups.

Employees of an organization also use social media (Facebook, Twitter, and LinkedIn, for example) and may contribute to blogs about their organization. Since what they say and how they say it can sometimes be misconstrued, it is imperative that healthcare organizations develop a policy to address the use of social media, and such a policy should include this information:

- Circumstances under which an employee may access any social media site during work hours
- Penalties or potential disciplinary action for failure to comply with the organization's social media policy
- Requirements:
  - Employees should maintain a positive tone in their posts, and be respectful of the organization and its staff when posting on an organization-sponsored site.
  - The PHI of patients should *never* be posted (directly or implied).
  - The identity of any patients (directly or implied) should *never* be posted.

- No copyrighted materials should be posted.
- No information about the organization may be posted, as this is the responsibility of the marketing or public relations department.

The use of social media to share information about a particular person is gaining popularity. Use is set up and maintained by someone authorized by the patient, with the objective of keeping family and friends updated on the patient's condition. One such site is Caring Bridge (to locate Caring Bridge's home page, type "CaringBridge" into a search engine). What the patient or family cares to share on this site is under their control, but healthcare professionals who are or were involved in the patient's care need to be careful. A posting that you intend to be caring and helpful may be misinterpreted and perceived as intrusive by the family, so before posting, you should think twice about what you want to say and how you say it!

7.10 Compliance Plans

Think of all the regulations that affect healthcare—HIPAA, ARRA, and HITECH, not to mention Medicare, Medicaid, and managed care plan requirements; it is a daunting task to ensure compliance with all of them. Having a formal compliance plan is key to surviving the regulatory maze. Think of a compliance plan as your office's or facility's policies that ensure regulations are followed, and use it as a check-sheet to ensure that staff and care providers in your office or facility are following your own policies, which in turn ensure the following of rules and regulations. A compliance plan should include

- A named compliance officer—a staff member who monitors new regulations, monitors existing ones, and is the "go-to" person, should an incident occur that is not in compliance
- Written policies that cover, at a minimum,
  - Routine daily operations (registration, scheduling, human resources, etc.)
  - File backup
  - Computer access (both physical access and access to software and databases)
  - Release of patient information
  - Breach of confidentiality, including unauthorized disclosure
  - Security breaches, internal and external
  - Coding and billing (including anti-fraud and -abuse practices)

Policies should be kept in a location accessible to all office staff. All policies should also include the disciplinary process, should policies not be followed, intentionally or unintentionally.

An example of a Policy Statement regarding computer access and use of passwords may read

Access to computer software, databases, and equipment shall be restricted to employees (including care providers) of Greensburg Medical Center. The extent to which access and rights are given is based on position description in order to carry out their job duties. Employees (including care providers) are required to keep their log-in user ID and password confidential; sharing with others is grounds for immediate disciplinary action, up to and including dismissal.

Reporting of compliance with meaningful use is also required; specific compliance strategies to conform with meaningful use will be covered later in this text.

The use of formal internal audits, which should be performed on every staff member (including care providers) on a periodic basis, not only allows the administrative staff to be proactive in finding and correcting problems but also serves as a reminder and an educational tool for staff.

7.11 Safeguarding Your System and Disaster Recovery Planning

Protecting computer hardware and software is as important as protecting the information within the systems. Computer crime, unauthorized access to information, and natural disasters are all security concerns that must be addressed within any healthcare organization that processes or stores digital data.

Written policies, as noted in Section 7.10, are deterrents at a very basic level—in particular, regarding controlling access. Restricting access in offices or areas where computers are present to employees only, turning computer screens away from public view, and shredding printed documents that include patient information are all examples. Encryption of data is necessary to deter unauthorized access to what is documented. Tracking the computer accesses of all employees on a periodic basis helps ensure that access is only on a need-to-know basis. Carefully screening job applicants and verifying previous employment are additional important screening mechanisms, since people are the greatest threat to computer security.

Backing up data on a daily basis is crucial. Backup can be made to online secondary storage, hard disk, optical disk, magnetic tape, and/or flash memory. A key component of backup is that the backed-up files should be stored at an off-site location. Should a fire or flood occur in your office, and the backup files be also damaged by the flood, they will do little good.

Over the past few years, worldwide disasters have shown the need for having a **disaster recovery plan**. The plan must be written and staff must know what to do in the event of a disaster that affects the computer systems within the facility (Williams and Sawyer).

At a minimum, the plan should include

Disaster recovery plan A written document that details an inventory of hardware and software, backup procedure, including location of backup files, the system used to alert users of the disaster, required security training for personnel, and procedure for restoring backup files.

- An accounting of all functions that are performed electronically within the office
- A listing of all computer hardware, software, and data related to each of those functions
- The specific location of the backup files and the format used for the backup
- Step-by-step procedures for restoring the backed-up data
- An alert system to notify personnel of the disaster
- Required security training for all personnel

Unfortunately, many facilities lack a disaster recovery plan and may not realize its importance until a data loss, security breach, or other disaster occurs. Not only should facilities have a plan, they should actually carry out the plan periodically as any other disaster plan would be practiced.

The importance of keeping *all* computerized functions safe, confidential, and secure cannot be overstated.

APPLYING YOUR SKILLS

Write a timeline and summary of the regulations that govern the collection, storage, and release of health information kept in an electronic format. Keeping in mind paper records versus electronic records, why was there a need for more stringent rules?

chapter 7 **summary**

LEARNING OUTCOME	CONCEPTS FOR REVIEW
7.1 Identify the HIPAA privacy and security standards.	– HIPAA passed in 1996
	– Contains privacy and security rules, among others
	– HITECH made HIPAA rules more stringent and gave government authorities the power to enforce the privacy and security rules.
	– Omnibus Final Rule to HITECH went into effect March 2013 with compliance required in September 2013.
	– Enhancements were made to patient privacy and patient rights, strengthened enforcement of the law, and allowed more control over business associates.
	– Fines for privacy breaches were increased.
	– Providers using an EHR must provide patients with electronic copies of their records when requested.
	– Patients paying by cash may instruct the provider not to bill their insurance and not to divulge any information regarding the treatment to the insurance company.
	– The intent is to ensure protected health information (PHI) is private and secure.
	– Covered entities include any healthcare facilities, health plans, clearinghouses, or other businesses that handle PHI.
	– Only minimum necessary information may be released.
	– Standards include
	• Define directory information
	• Use of authorization to release PHI
	• Enforce minimum necessary information release
	– Password configuration and protection
	– Appointment of a privacy and/or security officer
	– System configured to minimize number of log-in attempts
	– Protection from viruses and malware
	– Use of security audits to monitor access
	– Policy to address remote access to the system
	– Policy on use and protection of hardware, particularly wireless devices
	– Written policy and procedures on breach notification
	– Staff education
7.2 Evaluate an EHR system for HIPAA compliance.	– Password protection
	– Use of unique identifier for each user
	– Access to PHI only for those who have a need to know
	– Accounting of all disclosures (internal and external)
	– Security policy that addresses backup of data, storage, and restoration of backed-up data
	– Ability to audit by user or by patient who has accessed a record, and which area(s) of the record were viewed, edited, or deleted
	– Use of code sets—ICD-10-CM/PCS, CPT, and HCPCS—to store and transmit information

LEARNING OUTCOME	CONCEPTS FOR REVIEW
7.3 Describe the role of certification in EHR implementation.	– HIMSS—Health Information and Management Systems Society – AHIMA—American Health Information Management Association – CMS and the Office of the National Coordinator for Health Information Technology (ONC) – Independent agencies
7.4 Apply procedures to set up security measures in Prime Suite.	– Add new clinical users – Assign password to new clinical users – Set up a care provider's user rights – Assign user rights to a healthcare professional (medical assistant) – Assign user rights to an office manager – Create a group – Set general system-wide security requirements – Run an audit trail report
7.5 Follow proper procedures to access sensitive or restricted-access records.	– Sensitive information may or may not be clinical in nature but is embarrassing in nature; therefore, the record is flagged. – Restricted-access records are marked as such so that only select providers or staff may access them.
7.6 Apply procedures to ensure data integrity.	– Integrity of data can be ensured only if it is complete, accurate, consistent, and timely and has not been altered, destroyed, or accessed by unauthorized individuals. – Strict organization-wide policies that are adhered to must be in place. – Amendments and deletions to entries must be obvious, and the original format must remain. – Amend a chart entry – Hide a chart entry – Recover a hidden chart entry
7.7 Apply procedures to release health information using Prime Suite.	– Release of information is necessary for a multitude of reasons, including continuity of care. – Authorization to release information may be required and must be addressed in written organization policies. – Must account for all disclosures to comply with HITECH – Compose correspondence and release immunization record using Prime Suite
7.8 Account for data disclosures using Prime Suite.	– Internal and external disclosures of PHI must be accounted for. – Run a report of information disclosures from a patient's chart

(continued)

LEARNING OUTCOME	CONCEPTS FOR REVIEW
7.9 Exchange information with outside healthcare providers for continuity of care using Prime Suite.	– Meaningful use standards require exchange of information between providers for smooth continuation of care. – Sharing of electronic information must be through secure means. – Exchange information for continuity of care using Prime Suite
7.10 Outline the content of compliance plans.	– Healthcare organizations must have written compliance plans that address how the organization ensures compliance with all regulations governing operation of the organization as well as privacy, security, meaningful use, and general health information regulations. – Written policies must be kept and available to all staff at all times.
7.11 Appraise the importance of disaster recovery planning.	– Contingency plan is equivalent to a back-up plan, should the system fail or a natural or other disaster occur. – All potential security concerns should be addressed with a detailed back-up plan. – Importance of written disaster recovery plan

chapter review

MATCHING QUESTIONS

Match the terms on the left with the definitions on the right.

——— 1. **[LO 7.4]** breach of confidentiality

——— 2. **[LO 7.1]** confidentiality

——— 3. **[LO 7.1]** hardware

——— 4. **[LO 7.4]** audit trail

——— 5. **[LO 7.1]** computer virus

——— 6. **[LO 7.1]** covered entity

——— 7. **[LO 7.1]** password

——— 8. **[LO 7.11]** disaster recovery plan

——— 9. **[LO 7.1]** directory information

——— 10. **[LO 7.1]** encryption

a. person or group who has legal right to access protected health information by virtue of being a healthcare provider, clearinghouse, or health insurance plan

b. private, secure code that allows a user access to computer systems and software

c. security measure in which words are scrambled and can only be read if the receiving computer has the code to read the message

d. listing of patient information, such as hospital room number

e. documentation for addressing critical issues in the event of a crisis

f. permanent record of the changes made to various documents; available even after files are deleted

g. break or failure of security measures that results in information being compromised

h. devices such as laptops, PDAs, and desktop computers that are at risk for theft

i. keeping information about a patient to oneself

j. deviant program, stored on a computer floppy disk, hard drive, or CD, that can destroy or corrupt data

MULTIPLE-CHOICE QUESTIONS

Select the letter that best completes the statement or answers the question:

1. **[LO 7.7]** In the event of a breach, who may be held responsible?
   a. providers
   b. office staff
   c. the facility
   d. all of these

Enhance your learning by completing these exercises and more at http://**connect.mheducation.com**!

2. **[LO 7.1]** Which of the following would be considered a covered entity?
   a. healthcare provider
   b. friend
   c. significant other
   d. teacher

3. **[LO 7.4]** Of the following, which factor contributes to the user rights allowed a user?
   a. annual job performance
   b. job description
   c. level of education
   d. number of patients seen

4. **[LO 7.11]** It is critical that back-up files be stored
   a. in paper form.
   b. off-site.
   c. on-site.
   d. with the originals.

5. **[LO 7.8]** HITECH regulations require that _____ information releases are accounted for.
   a. all
   b. external
   c. internal
   d. no

6. **[LO 7.2]** According to HIPAA regulations, healthcare providers must use _____, as opposed to written documentation, to store and transmit information to insurance carriers.
   a. CPT codes
   b. ICD-10 codes
   c. HCPCS codes
   d. all of these

7. **[LO 7.3]** Meaningful use standards require offices to select an EHR that is
   a. certified.
   b. comprehensive.
   c. fast.
   d. simple.

8. **[LO 7.7]** Releasing information without proper authorization is called a/an
   a. breach of confidentiality.
   b. breach of trust.
   c. information breach.
   d. security breach.

9. **[LO 7.6]** When a document is amended or changed in an EHR, the original documentation is
   a. deleted.
   b. hidden.
   c. printed.
   d. visible.

10. **[LO 7.10]** An office's compliance manual should be kept in a/an _____ location.
    a. accessible
    b. external
    c. electronic
    d. protected

11. **[LO 7.9]** The sharing of health information must be done in a _____ environment.
    a. healthcare
    b. private
    c. public
    d. secure

12. **[LO 7.4]** Under a care provider's order, medical assistants and nurses _____ allowed to send an ePrescription or call in a refill prescription to a pharmacy.
    a. are
    b. are not
    c. might be
    d. should not be

13. **[LO 7.1]** To help guard against security breaches, emails containing protected health information should be
    a. deleted.
    b. encrypted.
    c. forbidden.
    d. sent.

14. **[LO 7.3]** The mission of HIMSS is to
    a. develop competencies for health information education programs.
    b. ensure information security.
    c. lead healthcare transformation through the use of health information technology.
    d. train facilities on HIPAA regulations.

SHORT-ANSWER QUESTIONS

1. **[LO 7.2]** According to the ONC website, how does health information technology help care providers better manage patient care?

2. **[LO 7.7]** Define continuity of care.

3. **[LO 7.5]** If all health information is confidential, explain why it may still be necessary to mark some health records as "sensitive" or "restricted."

4. **[LO 7.6]** Why must a user enter her password in order to change a chart entry in Prime Suite?

5. **[LO 7.10]** List at least six pieces of information that must be included in an office's compliance plan.

 Enhance your learning by completing these exercises and more at http://connect.mheducation.com!

6. **[LO 7.11]** List the six pieces of information that form the minimum requirements of a disaster recovery plan.

7. **[LO 7.4]** When new physicians or employees are hired in a physician's practice, the office manager or office administrator typically has the responsibility to set the physician or employee up in the PM and EHR system(s) as part of the security measures. Explain each type of security role in Prime Suite.

8. **[LO 7.3]** What does it mean if an EHR system has been certified by the Office of the National Coordinator?

9. **[LO 7.1]** Explain what a security audit is, and list one example of when a security audit might need to take place.

10. **[LO 7.9]** Explain one advantage of using an EHR for communicating with other healthcare providers, as discussed in the text.

11. **[LO 7.10]** What is the best way to ensure that your office staff are following all the different regulatory bodies governing healthcare?

12. **[LO 7.8]** Why must an office manager account for all information released, including that released internally?

13. **[LO 7.4]** Would a care provider and a medical assistant be assigned the same rights in Prime Suite? Why or why not?

14. **[LO 7.2]** List six things that an office's EHR team should keep in mind when rolling out a new system.

15. **[LO 7.11]** List three methods to safeguard computer hardware and software systems.

16. **[LO 7.1]** Give an example of when directory information would be needed.

APPLYING YOUR KNOWLEDGE

1. **[LOs 7.1 , 7.9]** Discuss two advantages and two disadvantages of using email to send information between providers.

2. **[LOs 7.1, 7.2, 7.4, 7.10, 7.11]** Discuss why many practices require users to change their passwords after a specified period and why they do not allow users to reuse the same passwords over and over again.

3. **[LO 7.3]** Imagine that you are working in a small healthcare practice. Your supervisor has asked you to spearhead the adoption of an EHR program. Follow the link provided in the text to find the website listing certified EHRs. After browsing the site and looking at the sheer number of products listed, discuss some methods your healthcare office could use to choose the best EHR option.

4. **[LOs 7.6, 7.7]** Provide one example each of an internal and an external breach of confidentiality that might occur in a healthcare setting, and list a possible consequence of each breach. (For example, letting a temporary employee access a patient's chart with your username would be an internal breach; a consequence could be that a patient's health information is compromised when the temp accidentally sends the patient's chart information out in an accidental "reply all" email.)

5. **[LOs 7.1, 7.4, 7.6, 7.10, 7.11]** You are in the office lounge getting some water. One of your colleagues is at her desk, working on a laptop. She gets up to join you at the water cooler. As the two of you are talking, another staff member sits down in your colleague's chair and begins using the laptop to check her email. What is wrong with this scenario?

6. **[LOs 7.1, 7.2, 7.4, 7.6, 7.7, 7.9]** Paul Davies presents to County Hospital's ER with an arm injury. He refuses to talk about how he sustained the injury and says he wants his medical records released to his sister, who will be coming to take him home. How would the objectives of an EHR make handling Mr. Davies' case easier?

7. **[LO 7.4]** Stephanie Byrd is a coder at Greensburg Medical Center. Her user ID is sbyrd. She recently got married and wants her user ID changed to slopez, to reflect her married name. Stephanie is told by the office administrator that once a user ID is assigned, it cannot be changed. Why can't the user ID be changed?

8. **[LO 7.1]** A local TV celebrity has been admitted to the local hospital. She states that she wants her admission to remain private and does not want her room number or the fact that she is there at all released to anyone but her sister, Mary Ann Green. The registration specialist in the ER tells her that is not possible and that if anyone goes to the information desk, he or she will be given her room number. If she does not wish to see the visitor, she will have to ask the nurses on the unit to put a "do not disturb" sign on the door of her room. Is this correct? Explain your answer.

chapter references

Abdelhak, M., Grostick, S., Hanken, M.A., and Jacobs, E. (2007). *Health Information: Management of a Strategic Resource* (3rd ed.). Philadelphia: Elsevier.

American Medical Association. (1995–2013). *HIPAA Violations and Enforcement.* Retrieved from https://www.ama-assn.org/practice-management/hipaa-violations-enforcement

Centers for Medicare and Medicaid Services, Office for Civil Rights. *Collection Use and Disclosure Limitation. The HIPAA Privacy Rule in Electronic Health Information Exchange in a Networked Environment.* Retrieved from www.hhs.gov

Certification Commission for Health Information Technology. (2011). Retrieved from http://www.cchit.org/

CNN.com Entertainment. 27 Suspended for Clooney File Peek. Retrieved from http://www.cnn.com/2007/SHOWBIZ/10/10/clooney.records/

Cox, J.W., Turner, K., and Zapotsky, M.C. "Virus Infects MedStar Health System's Computers, Forcing an Online Shutdown." *The Washington Post,* March 28, 2016).

Department of Health and Human Services. (2010, March 10). Proposed Establishment of Certification Programs for Health Information Technology; Proposed Rule. *Federal Register, 75*(46): 11327–11373. Retrieved from http://edocket.access.gpo.gov/2010/2010-4991.htm

Dimick, Chris. (2010, February). Empowered Patient: Preparing for a New Patient Interaction. *Journal of AHIMA, 81*(2): 26–31.

Heubusch, Kevin. (2011, July). Access Report: OCR Tries Subtraction through Addition in Accounting of Disclosure Rule. *Journal of AHIMA, 82*(7): 38–39.

HIMSS. (2016). *About HIMSS.* Retrieved from http://www.himss.org/ASP/aboutHimssHome.asp

McGuireWoods. (2013). *HIPAA Final Omnibus Rule Implements Tiered Penalty Structure for HIPAA Violations.*

Miaoulis, William M. (2010, March). Access, Use, and Disclosure: HITECH's Impact on the HIPAA Touchstones. *Journal of AHIMA, 81*(3): 38–39, 64.

Williams, B.K., and Sawyer, S.C. (2010). *Using Information Technology: A Practical Introduction to Computers & Communications* (9th ed.). New York: McGraw-Hill Companies.

chapter **eight**

Management of Information and Communication

Learning Outcomes

At the end of this chapter, the student should be able to

8.1 Use software as an internal communication tool.

8.2 Differentiate the steps used to import documents using scanning technology.

8.3 Build master files and templates using Prime Suite.

8.4 Create custom screens within Prime Suite.

8.5 Develop a Task List within Prime Suite.

8.6 Set up system flags within Prime Suite.

Key Terms

Default values
Flags
Internet
Intranet
Live

Master file
Optical character recognition (OCR)
Resolution
Scanner
Templates

The Big Picture

What You Need to Know and Why You Need to Know It

So far in this text, we have mainly looked at the collection of data, which in turn become information about a patient. In this chapter, we will look at communicating that information. The information collected in a healthcare environment is shared with external sources such as other healthcare providers, public health agencies, Medicare, Medicaid, insurance companies, and professional organizations. The information included may be in the form of a summary of a patient's record; a report that answers a question, such as the local public health office asking how many cases of flu-related illnesses were seen during a given time period; or a piece of correspondence from one care provider to another. Additionally, the communication may be internal—within the facility. With PM and EHR software, communicating internally through the use of an internal email system is efficient. Information is key to almost everything we do, personally and professionally, so having the information we need at our fingertips and communicating that information accurately and in a timely fashion are key to a well-run organization. Taking it a step further, patients who receive timely, accurate information and who experience good communication within the practice will have more confidence in the practice as a whole.

8.1 | Internal Communications

Internet A series of networks that allow instant access to information from around the world.

Intranet A secure environment or private internal network that is available only to a select group (e.g., the staff within an organization).

The **Internet** is a series of networks that allow instant access to information from around the world. Some Internet sites are private, requiring a user ID and password to gain access, and some are public sites that can be viewed by anyone. Within an organization, however, an **intranet** exists. An intranet is a secure environment or private internal network that is available only to a select group, such as the staff within the organization. Examples of what might be shared on an intranet site include

Facility's mission and value statements	Directory of staff and care providers	Compliance officer's name and contact information
Policies and procedures	FAQs	Forms, publications, newsletters
Organization charts	Office meeting minutes	Calendar of events
Link to the IT department	Calendar of upcoming events	Internal webmail links

The intranet is a one-stop-shop for staff and providers of a practice or other healthcare organization to gain access to all the information they need to stay informed, as well as a way to send and receive messages among colleagues. Of course, someone (usually a webmaster) has to keep the information up to date; otherwise, the outdated information is not information at all, and there is no benefit to having an intranet. When staff starts noticing that the site is not being kept current, they will stop accessing it and sharing information. If your current employer has an intranet, take some time to navigate it—look there for the information listed in this section as well as other useful information.

The use of internal messaging improves communication within an office. It is particularly helpful for avoiding the "no one ever told me" syndrome. When internal email is used to communicate work-related information, and is not cluttered with personal communications, it is even more valuable. Many organizations have policies regarding use of the office email account, and though they may not mandate that it cannot be used as a personal means of communication, such use is most likely frowned upon and may lead to more stringent policies. Some offices use a priority rating on their work-related emails. This is particularly helpful to the care providers in sifting out what needs to be done immediately versus what can wait for a later time. High-priority messages include patient care matters, those of medium priority include changes in meeting dates or time-sensitive information, and low-priority messages might be information such as that lunch is ready in the lounge. When establishing rules for the priority system, everyone should at least be clear on what *is* or *is not* considered high priority. Remember that if everything is marked as urgent, or high priority, then there is no way to differentiate the item that should truly take priority.

connect Go to http://connect.mheducation.com to complete this exercise.   **EXERCISE** **8.1**

Send an Electronic Message Using Prime Suite Messaging

In this exercise, we will look at carrying out an internal communication using Prime Suite. In the exercise that follows, Dr. Ingram is to attend an EMR meeting, but the date and time have been changed to Thursday at 3:30 p.m. In this instance, the message would be sent only to Dr. Ingram; if the message were for all of the care providers, then it would be sent using a group rather than typing in one name.

This function is accessible from the desktop screen.

Follow these steps to complete the exercise on your own once you have watched the demonstration and tried the steps with helpful prompts in practice mode. Use the information provided in the scenario to complete the information.

1. Click the envelope icon.
2. Click Compose Message.
3. Type "jingram" in the To: field.
4. Click James Ingram (ingram).
5. Type "EMR Meeting" in the Subject: field.
6. Click the Priority: drop-down.
7. Click Medium.
8. Type the salutation "Dr. Ingram," in the message field.
9. Press "Return".
10. Type "Just as a reminder, the EMR meeting this week has been moved to Thursday at 3:30 p.m." in the message field.
11. Click Send.
12. Click Close.

✓ **You have completed Exercise 8.1**

Communication involves many forms other than email messages. Reports, test results, and verifications of insurance coverage, just to name a few, are communicated many times throughout the day. These reports may be sent to the practice in digital or hard-copy format but, in the end, must be merged with the appropriate patient's electronic medical record.

For example, Dr. Ingram sent Max Shaw to Memorial Hospital for a chest x-ray. The x-ray is completed and the report of the radiologist's findings is sent electronically to Greensburg Medical Center. It then needs to be merged with (attached to) the patient's chart; the flow of this is depicted in Figure 8.1.

Not all documents can be sent electronically, however. Let's say a patient, David Malone, had his chest x-ray at Duffields Hospital, which does not yet have electronic capability. Instead, the report of the x-ray findings is in hard-copy form only. It can be faxed, mailed, or picked up from the hospital by a staff member. Since the goal of Greensburg Medical Center is a paperless office with a unit record for all patients, a hard-copy image needs to be manually scanned into the EHR once it arrives at the office (Figure 8.2).

When a hard-copy document needs to be scanned, the healthcare professional simply feeds the document through the scanner (or lays the document flat on a screen) (Figure 8.3), follows the prompts that appear on the computer screen, and finally merges (attaches) the document with the proper patient's electronic record within Prime Suite. The process of scanning is much like the process of making a photocopy. Just as a hard-copy document can be misfiled, so can a scanned image. Before a scanned image is attached to a patient's health record, the healthcare professional verifies that the correct patient and the correct visit are selected. Also, the type of document (correspondence, authorization, history, or physical exam, for example) may be bar-coded so that the document is easily retrievable electronically. It is also important to remember that, although it is necessary to include relevant medical documentation in patients' electronic health records, scanned

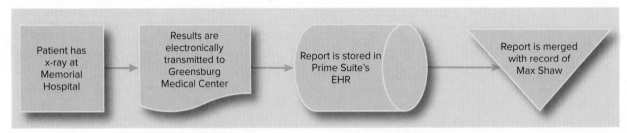

Figure 8.1 **Flow of Report from Hospital to Merging with Appropriate Record in Prime Suite**

Figure 8.2 **Flow of Faxed Report from Hospital to Prime Suite**

documents take up "space," or memory, so avoid scanning unnecessary documents.

Scanners digitize documents into a format that is readable by a computer. The scanning of documents utilizes **optical character recognition (OCR)** technology to convert the document into a format that is computer readable. It is important to ensure that scanned images are as good as the originals. This is known as **resolution**, in which the higher the resolution, the better the quality of the image. There are other scanning functions that you may be aware of and may not even realize it—in a grocery store, for instance, the cashier passes the bar code from a can of green beans across a small light source, scanning the bar code so that the computer reads it as a 15.5-ounce can of green beans with a price of $1.25. In that case, the optical reader reads a bar code rather than words. This process not only results in a price for the item but also is part of an inventory control system—the persons responsible for re-order now know that there is one less can of beans on the shelf.

Figure 8.3 **Scanner Used to Import a Document** © Ryan McVay/Getty RF

Scanner A piece of equipment that digitizes documents into a format that is readable by a computer.

Optical character recognition (OCR) Technology that converts a document into a format that is computer readable—that is, into an electronic file.

Resolution The quality of a scanned image as it will appear in the record. The higher the resolution, the crisper the image.

Master file Dataset that provides structure and is the building block for parts of chart notes within an EHR.

Templates Preformatted documents built into practice management and electronic health record systems.

8.3 Master Files and Templates

Care providers and all other healthcare professionals are extremely busy. Their first concern is the patient, not documentation, but documentation is essential to patient care. So to make documenting easier and faster, **master files** (datasets that provide structure and are the building blocks for parts of the chart notes) and **templates** (preformatted documents built into practice management (PM) and electronic health record (EHR) systems) are used. The use of master files and templates are used often in an electronic health record system, for instance when documenting a history and physical exam. Figure 8.4 is an example of a master file for selecting conditions in a patient's past medical history.

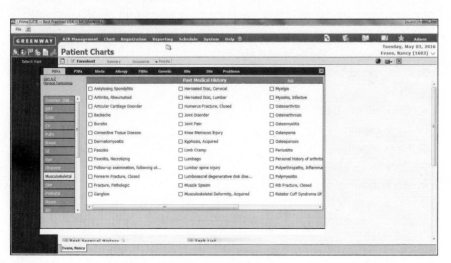

Figure 8.4 **Past Medical History Master File**

Live The point at which computer software or systems are put into real-time use within a practice or hospital.

At Greensburg Medical Center, before the EHR went **live**, staff members built these master files with input from care providers. Master files list common conditions and diagnoses that patients at Greensburg Medical Center have had. Diagnoses can be added to an individual's record, or to the master file itself. Other master files in Prime Suite include PE (physical exam), ROS (review of systems), orders, diagnosis favorites, and HPI (history of present illness).

Building templates within the system is an administrative task that is done prior to going live, but they can be edited as necessary. Templates are preformatted documents that allow screenshots to be built, letters to be written, and progress notes to appear out of individual selections from master files. Care providers may prefer their documentation to look a certain way, so a practice that has five care providers may have five templates for written progress notes. Templates can also be used to facilitate return to work or school notes, draft letters to patients, document lab results, and a assist with a number of other functions.

EXERCISE **8.2**   Go to http://connect.mheducation.com to complete this exercise.

Build a Master File in Prime Suite

To build a master file in Prime Suite, the Desktop will be accessed and then Review of Systems Admin will be selected from the Chart menu. In the exercise that follows, we will build the master file for Review of Systems (ROS). The end product will be indicative of what this care provider wants as the **default values** (the values that automatically appear in a field on the ROS screen and appear each time he sees a patient). For instance, the care provider wants the default value for weight loss to be a negative response; in other words, if a patient is asked if she has experienced unexplained weight loss, most of the time the answer will be no; therefore, this response will show as (–) weight loss on the ROS screen.

Default value A value that automatically appears in a field each time it appears on a screen (e.g., the current date in a date field, the local area code in a home phone number field).

Setting up these default values is done from the System Set-Up module on the Chart menu.

Follow these steps to complete the exercise on your own once you have watched the demonstration and tried the steps with helpful prompts in practice mode.

1. Click Review of Systems Admin.
2. Click Constitutional.
3. Click fatigue.
4. Click weight loss.
5. Click Genitourinary.
6. Click urgency.
7. Click frequency.
8. Click dysuria.
9. Click Save icon.

✔ **You have completed Exercise 8.2**

Care providers, registration staff, medical assistants, nurses, therapists, billers, and coders all use the information in the PM and EHR software. But not all of the users "see" things the same way. The way subsets of information display in relation to one another on a computer screen is often most effective when the user is satisfied with how the information appears. Many PM and EHR software packages include flexibility to allow the customization of screen configurations, and Prime Suite is no exception. Care providers, and healthcare professionals in general, will be more accepting of an EHR if they know they have some say in the appearance of the information and can customize it to meet the needs of the facility.

    Go to http://connect.mheducation.com to complete this exercise. **PM** **EHR** **HIM** **EXERCISE** **8.3**

Customize a Facesheet Screen

We will now look at a couple of exercises in which customization is possible. The first task is to customize a Facesheet screen. In this scenario, the healthcare professional is going to customize a Facesheet. He starts by entering the User Settings Admin within the System Set-up module that is in the Chart menu. Watch as he chooses the elements that will show on the Facesheet and then how he changes the order in which they appear.

Follow these steps to complete the exercise on your own once you have watched the demonstration and tried the steps with helpful prompts in practice mode.

1. Click User Settings Admin.
2. Click the Facesheet & History tab.
3. Click History Sections.
4. Click Facesheet Sections.
5. Click Save icon.
6. Click Patient Charts.
7. Click Customize Facesheet.
8. Click Reason for Visit.
9. Click Allergy List.
10. Click Clinical Alerts.
11. Click Confidential.
12. Click Flowsheets.
13. Click Medication List.
14. Click Orders Tracking History.
15. Click Past Surgical History.
16. Click Problem List.
17. Click Task List.
18. Click Visit History.
19. Click Vital Signs.
20. Click anywhere to the left of the Customize Facesheet menu to close it.
21. Drag Medication List and drop on Confidential.

In addition to the Facesheet, the desktop can also be customized to the individual user's preferences.

 You have completed Exercise 8.3

Customize a Clinical Desktop

Watch as this user sets up the Desktop (the first screen that appears when a user logs on) to meet her needs and preferences.

Follow these steps to complete the exercise on your own once you have watched the demonstration and tried the steps with helpful prompts in practice mode.

1. Click Customize Desktop.
2. Click Patient List.
3. Click Use Clinician Desktop.
4. Click Show Task List.
5. Click the Section First radio button.
6. Click the display drop-down.
7. Click Patient List.
8. Click Save.

✔ **You have completed Exercise 8.4**

8.5   Using Software to Organize Your Work—Task Lists

With all the requirements we deal with in healthcare, having help with organizational skills is certainly an advantage! In Prime Suite, there is a functionality called Task List or Tasks, whereby a care provider or other healthcare professional assigns tasks to another staff member or to an entire group. For instance, Dianna Pike, a care provider, wants a particular report to be run by the office administrator, Jon Viria. The request is simply put into Jon's Task List so that he is aware that he has a task to complete. Or a task that needs to be completed by an entire group, such as the health information department staff—for instance, the completion of a computerized in-service—can be assigned to the group rather than to each individual, saving the office administrator much time and ensuring that everyone gets the *same* message.

Some examples of tasks include

- Calling patients to change appointments due to the change in a provider's vacation dates
- Registering for an upcoming seminar
- Calling a patient regarding the need for a follow-up laboratory test
- Making reservations for the office holiday party
- Ordering supplies or equipment

As you can see, the tasks may not be clinical in nature; they can be anything that needs to be done by an individual or individuals in the practice.

Create a Task for the Receptionist

In the scenario that follows, a task is set up for Jane Baxter to schedule a training session on ePrescribing. The message is "Jane, will you please contact Greenway and arrange a training session covering ePrescribe? I would like to have this done between June 1 and July 31. Thanks!" (without the quotation marks). (In addition, use one space after the question mark after "ePrescribe" and one space after the period after "31.")

This function also allows the user to select the priority of the task—high, medium, or low. Practice policy may dictate what circumstances dictate each, and whether prioritization is used at all.

Follow these steps to complete the exercise on your own once you have watched the demonstration and tried the steps with helpful prompts in practice mode. Use the information provided in the scenario to complete the information.

1. Click Tasks.
2. Click Add New Task.
3. Click Type:.
4. Click General Task.
5. Click Send To:.
6. Click Baxter, Jane (jbaxter).
7. Click OK.
8. Click Subject:.
9. Type "eRX training".
10. Click the Due Date: field.
11. Click 25.
12. Click the Status: drop-down.
13. Click New.
14. Click Add Comment:.
15. Type the required message in the Comment field.
16. Click OK.
17. Click Save & Return.
18. Click Close.

☑ **You have completed Exercise 8.5**

8.6 Using Software as a Reminder

If you work in healthcare, you have a lot to remember, as you have already seen. It would be next to impossible to remember every situation about every patient. Using the functionality of PM or EHR software, including Prime Suite, makes keeping on top of everything easier, though, by including alerts, or reminders, in a patient's chart, through a series of flag alerts (reminders) or icons, each of which has a particular meaning.

Flags can be added in the system and be used for all patients. Examples of common flags include these:

- Patient frequently cancels appointments
- Phone number on file is no longer in service

Flag A message that appears on a screen in written form or as an icon to serve as a reminder to staff and care providers.

- Confidentiality messages (such as do not leave message on home phone)
- Co-pay required (and can include amount)
- Patient is noncompliant
- Account in collections
- Do not charge late fee
- Payment plan set up
- Allergic to penicillin (can have several different medications)
- Environmental allergy to _____
- Sensitive information contained in chart
- Clinical alerts
  - Bone density scan due
  - Diabetic patient
  - Requires patient education
  - Pap smear due

A flag can be set up in the system for just about anything the office sees a need for. A word of caution, though: Do not set up so many flags that it is difficult to remember their meaning or that the alert becomes the rule rather than the exception and therefore is ignored.

EXERCISE 8.6

Go to http://connect.mheducation.com to complete this exercise.

Assign a Flag to a Patient's Chart

In this exercise, you will set up a system flag for a patient. In this case, Jessie Hamilton is allergic to latex, so the healthcare professional will add that flag to Jessie's chart.

Follow these steps to complete the exercise on your own once you have watched the demonstration and tried the steps with helpful prompts in practice mode. Use the information provided in the scenario to complete the information.

1. Click Search for Patient.
2. Type "Hamilton" in the *Last Name field.
3. Click Search.
4. Click Jessie.
5. Click Select.
6. Click View/Edit Patient Flag.
7. Click Allergic to Latex.
8. Click Save.

As you can see, computerization of the practice management and health record functions has many other benefits to care providers and staff than just maintenance of the information they collect. The use of software streamlines the processes and increases efficiency.

 You have completed Exercise 8.6

APPLYING YOUR SKILLS

Virginia Park called Dr. Hilliard today. He was looking at her medical history in her EHR, then sent an email to his nurse from within the history section of Prime Suite. The body of the email read

"Jane, Ms. Park has called five times with the same questions. I'm tired of her calling me. Please take care of this—I have better things to do than to deal with a hypochondriac."

Could this become an issue for Dr. Hilliard? Defend your answer.

chapter 8 **summary**

LEARNING OUTCOME	CONCEPTS FOR REVIEW
8.1 Use software as an internal communication tool.	– Difference between Internet and intranet. – Examples of information commonly shared on an intranet – Send a message using Prime Suite.
8.2 Differentiate the steps used to import documents using scanning technology.	– Reports within a chart are a type of communication. – Documents may be imported from within Prime Suite or from an external source. – Scanning a document involves a process of feeding (or laying flat) the document in the scanner, then attaching the document to the appropriate patient's chart. – Scanning digitizes documentation into readable format. – Optical character recognition (OCR) allows scanned images to be edited.
8.3 Build master files and templates using Prime Suite.	– Master file—list of possible choices such as a list of allergies, list of conditions, or list of surgeries – Templates allow for building an end product such as a progress note, a piece of correspondence, or a screen view. – Build a master file for an ROS.
8.4 Create custom screens within Prime Suite.	– Allow flexibility and personalization for individual users. – Design a Facesheet view for a user.
8.5 Develop a Task List within Prime Suite.	– Tasks are reminders that a job has been assigned. – Can be made by any user. – Can be a task set for a single user or a group. – Assign a task to a user in Prime Suite.
8.6 Set up system flags within Prime Suite.	– Flags are alerts, or reminders. – Use them sparingly; otherwise, they no longer point out the exception to the rule but rather become the rule. – Set up a flag on a patient's record in Prime Suite.

chapter review

MATCHING QUESTIONS

Match the terms on the left with the definitions on the right.

_____ 1. **[LO 8.6]** flag

_____ 2. **[LO 8.3]** default value

_____ 3. **[LO 8.3]** master file

_____ 4. **[LO 8.3]** templates

_____ 5. **[LO 8.1]** intranet

_____ 6. **[LO 8.3]** live

_____ 7. **[LO 8.2]** scanner

_____ 8. **[LO 8.2]** optical character recognition (OCR)

a. secure internal environment available only to a select group

b. device that digitizes documents into a format readable by computers

c. alert, or reminder, that appears in a patient's chart

d. dataset that provides structure and is the building block for parts of the chart notes

e. technology that converts a document into a computer readable format

f. using something in real time

g. preassigned value that automatically appears in a field

h. preformatted documents built into an EHR or PM system

MULTIPLE-CHOICE QUESTIONS

Select the letter that best completes the statement or answers the question:

1. **[LO 8.1]** The Internet is _____ and an intranet is _____.
   a. public; private
   b. private; public
   c. private; private
   d. public; public

2. **[LO 8.2]** A hard-copy document is attached to a patient's electronic chart by
   a. copying.
   b. emailing.
   c. scanning.
   d. shredding.

3. **[LO 8.3]** Using templates makes it easier for care providers to focus on their first priority, which is
   a. documentation.
   b. patient care.
   c. office staff.
   d. training.

Enhance your learning by completing these exercises and more at http://connect.mheducation.com!

4. **[LO 8.4]** Prime Suite allows each user to _____ certain features to their liking.
   a. access
   b. customize
   c. delete
   d. revise

5. **[LO 8.1]** A facility needs to make sure that the information on its intranet does not become
   a. outdated.
   b. overused.
   c. private.
   d. secure.

6. **[LO 8.6]** It is _____ to have too many flags set up in Prime Suite.
   a. impossible
   b. possible
   c. necessary
   d. recommended

7. **[LO 8.3]** The Review of Systems menu choices in Prime Suite are an example of a/an
   a. index.
   b. master file.
   c. real-time menu.
   d. template.

8. **[LO 8.5]** A healthcare professional may assign work to another user with Prime Suite's _____ functionality.
   a. Assignment
   b. Groups
   c. Tasks
   d. Workload

9. **[LO 8.6]** Jane Howard often misses appointments; an alert is set to appear on her record; this alert is known as a/an _____ in Prime Suite.
   a. flag
   b. avatar
   c. decal
   d. symbol

10. **[LO 8.4]** Which of the following Prime Suite functions may be customized by a user?
    a. Access Rights
    b. Insurance Policies
    c. Patient Information
    d. Screen Layout

SHORT-ANSWER QUESTIONS

1. **[LO 8.1]** List four topics that might be found on an organization's intranet.

2. **[LO 8.3]** Can a medical office have more than one template for a referral letter? Explain.

3. **[LO 8.1]** What will happen if an office's intranet is not kept current? Be specific.

4. **[LO 8.3]** List four advantages of using master files and templates in a healthcare office.

5. **[LO 8.6]** List at least eight common flags used in Prime Suite.

6. **[LO 8.6]** Why might it be good to have a "Sensitive information contained in chart" alert pop up when users access specific patient charts?

7. **[LO 8.5]** Explain how using the Task List function in Prime Suite helps organize work.

8. **[LO 8.4]** Why might healthcare professionals be more accepting of an EHR if they are able to customize it in some way?

APPLYING YOUR KNOWLEDGE

1. **[LO 8.4]** How might a care provider "see" the information display in Prime Suite in the same way a patient registration staff member does?

2. **[LOs 8.1, 8.2, 8.6]** As office manager, what are some ways for you to ensure that staff members remember to attach hard-copy documents to the patient charts they are working on?

3. **[LO 8.3]** Discuss two advantages and any potential disadvantages to using templates for communication documents.

4. **[LOs 8.5, 8.6]** You are the office manager for a small practice. Since your office recently implemented an EHR system, you would like to have a staff training session to set forth guidelines and best practices for using system flags. Explain how you would use Prime Suite to assist you in your task, and come up with four talking points about the proper use of flags and alerts.

5. **[LOs 8.3, 8.4]** Dr. Stewart hired a new associate, Dr. Reynolds, about six months ago. Dr. Reynolds has been trying without success to use Prime Suite efficiently. Though he likes the template method of documenting, he has found that much of what he prefers to document is not part of the existing templates, and he has to type freehand a lot of that data. He feels he is not paying as much attention to his patients as he should during visits because he is typing, and he is concerned that his E&M code levels are lower than they should be. He comes to you, the office manager, to vent his frustrations. What, if anything, can be done to make his use of Prime Suite more effective and efficient? Would any of this have an impact on Dr. Reynolds' E&M code levels?

 Enhance your learning by completing these exercises and more at http://**connect.mheducation.com**!

chapter references

Content related to Greenway Health™, Greenway Prime Suite™, or other related products retrieved from http://www.greenwayhealth.com (or earlier iterations of the website) from 2011–2016.

Williams, B.K., and Sawyer, S.C. (2011). *Using Information Technology: A Practical Introduction to Computers & Communications* (9th ed.). New York: McGraw-Hill Companies.

chapter **nine**

Decision and Compliance Support: Utilizing the Database

Learning Outcomes

At the end of this chapter, the student should be able to

9.1 Describe the uses of the dashboard in Prime Suite to meet Meaningful Use standards.

9.2 Explain how data and information are used in decision support.

9.3 Set up system reports using Prime Suite.

9.4 Set up custom reports using Prime Suite.

9.5 Illustrate uses for an index.

9.6 Describe uses for a registry.

9.7 Explain how data gathered in Prime Suite are used in the credentialing process.

Key Terms

Aggregate
Benchmarking
Centers for Medicare and Medicaid Services (CMS)
Certified Electronic Health Record Technology (CEHRT)
Core objectives
Credentialing
Custom report
Dashboard
Detail report
Drug formulary

Healthcare Integrity and Protection Data Bank (HIPDB)
Index
In-network
Meaningful Use
Menu objectives
National Practitioner Data Bank (NPDB)
Physician Quality Reporting Initiative (PQRI)
Query
Registry
Summary report
Variable

What You Need to Know and Why You Need to Know It

Running reports, supplying information to government agencies, and ensuring compliance with Meaningful Use, licensing agencies, Medicare/Medicaid rules, managed care plans, and accrediting agencies are all responsibilities of administrative personnel. This person may be an MA who is an office manager, a health information professional, or a healthcare administrator. Participation in the Meaningful Use incentive program, or a similar program, will require submission of data that show compliance with specific standards in order to receive incentive grants and avoid penalties. In this chapter, we will cover Prime Suite functionality that allows us to prove compliance with Meaningful Use, licensing agencies, insurance providers, and state and federal reporting requirements.

9.1 Using the Dashboard in Prime Suite to Meet Meaningful Use Standards

In order for eligible professionals and hospitals to receive stimulus money, as part of HITECH legislation they must successfully show meaningful use of electronic health data. In other words, eligible professionals and hospitals that implement (or upgrade) certified electronic health record systems and comply with the core and menu objectives (covered below) will be eligible for monetary grants and avoid penalties for noncompliance.

Meaningful Use was developed to ensure that the use of EHRs by healthcare providers will improve quality, safety, and efficiency, as well as reducing health disparities within healthcare. Specifically, Meaningful Use has been developed with the following health outcomes policy priorities in mind:

- Improving quality, safety, and efficiency and reducing health disparities
- Engaging patients and families in their own health
- Improving the coordination of care
- Improving population and public health
- Ensuring adequate privacy and security protection for personal health information

The **Centers for Medicare and Medicaid Services (CMS)** administers the Meaningful Use program and has developed a plan for implementing three stages within five years. Stage 1 of the evolution of Meaningful Use focused on data capturing and sharing and was implemented in 2011. The 15 Stage 1 **core objectives** to show Meaningful Use of electronic health records are listed in Table 9.1. Stage 2 of Meaningful Use is currently in progress, and Stage 3, which will focus on demonstrating improved outcomes, is being finalized for implementation by 2018.

For hospitals, the core objectives include all of those listed in the table *except* ePrescribing.

The 2011 **menu objectives** for Medicare include those listed in Table 9.2. Of the 10 listed, 5 needed to be met, 1 of which must include a population/public health measure.

Menu objectives are additional functions that allow for greater use of EHR functionality—for instance, running statistical reports, registries, or

Meaningful Use The use of certified electronic health record technology with the purpose of improving quality, safety, and efficiency, as well as reducing health disparities within healthcare.

Centers for Medicare and Medicaid Services (CMS) An agency of the Department of Health and Human Services, responsible for administering the Medicare and Medicaid programs.

Core objectives Basic functions or collection of data that should be completed on a patient's visit or hospitalization.

Menu objectives Additional functions that allow for greater use of EHR functionality.

TABLE 9.1	**Medicare Core Objectives, 2011, Stage 1**

Core Objective	Explanation
Use of computerized physician order entry (CPOE)	Medication orders made by care providers are done electronically rather than in writing in a paper record.
Drug–drug and drug–allergy checks	An alert system exists, based on the medications and allergies entered for a patient, for potential drug-to-drug or drug-to-allergy effects.
ePrescribing	Care providers place prescriptions electronically rather than by paper.
Recording of patient demographic information	The following demographics must be collected on all records: – Preferred language – Gender – Race – Ethnicity – Date of birth
Recording of a problem list	A list of all current and active diagnoses for which the patient is being treated must be maintained.
Recording of a medication list	A list of all current and active medications being taken by the patient—if the patient is on no medications, the record must reflect that as well.
Recording of a medication allergy list	A list of medication(s) to which the patient is allergic
Recording of vital signs	On each visit, the following must be recorded: – Height – Weight – Blood pressure – Body Mass Index (BMI) – Maintenance of a growth chart (for children 2–20 years, including BMI)
Recording of smoking status	For patients 13 years of age and older, smoking status must be recorded.
Clinical decision support functionality	At least one clinical decision support rule must be implemented. Example: A patient with a fasting blood sugar above 120 mg/dL may trigger an alert for diabetes mellitus, type 2.
Reporting clinical quality measures	Each provider must specify the Reporting Numerators, Denominators, and Exclusions for each quality measure reported.
Ability to exchange key clinical information between/among care providers	The capability to share among care providers such information as problem list, medication list, allergies, and diagnostic test results

(continued)

Core Objective	Explanation
Ability to provide an electronic copy of health information	Patients must be provided with electronic health information upon request, including test results, problem list, medication list, and medication allergies.
Ability to provide clinical summaries	For each office visit, a clinical summary should be provided to each patient.
Privacy and security provisions	The software in use meets or exceeds standards set forth by the ONC Meaningful Use standards and includes technical specifications that ensure the privacy and confidentiality of information found in the database.

Source: Centers for Medicare and Medicaid Services. Medicare & Medicaid EHR Incentive Program: Meaningful Use Stage 1 Requirements. Retrieved from https://www.cms.gov/EHRIncentivePrograms/Downloads/MU_Stage1_ReqOverview.pdf

TABLE 9.2   **Medicare Menu Objectives, 2011, Stage 1**

Drug formulary A list of provider-preferred generic and brand-name drugs covered under various insurance plans.

Menu Objective	Explanation
Drug-Formulary Checks	The office or hospital has access to at least one internal or external **drug formulary** (a list of provider-preferred generic and brand-name drugs covered under various insurance plans).
Lab Test Results Documented in the EHR	Results of laboratory tests ordered must be entered into the patient's EHR rather than being filed in paper format; results may be entered electronically through electronic data interchange, scanned into the record via manual scanning methods, or manually keyed in to the record from the paper results.
Keeping of Patient Lists	The ability to generate a list of patients with a specific condition in order to satisfy quality improvement initiatives, reduce disparities, for research, or for outreach to patients with that diagnosis
Patient Reminders Generated	The ability to send reminder letters (or electronic reminders) for preventive and/or follow-up care
Timely Electronic Access	The ability to provide patients with their electronic record within four business days of the information being available in electronic form
Patient Education	Access to educational resources using EHR technology and providing the resources to patients, if appropriate
Medication Reconciliation	Documentation of medications the patient is taking as prescribed by other care providers

Menu Objective	Explanation
Summary of Care	The care provider submits a summary of care to physicians or another healthcare facility that is assessing the patient or taking over the care of the patient.
Immunization Registries	The capability to submit electronic data to immunization registries or other immunization information systems in accordance with applicable law
Syndromatic Surveillance	The capability to submit electronic data to public health agencies in accordance with applicable law

Source: Centers for Medicare and Medicaid Services. Medicare & Medicaid EHR Incentive Program: Meaningful Use Stage 1 Requirements. Retrieved from https://www.cms.gov/EHRIncentivePrograms/Downloads/MU_Stage1_ReqOverview.pdf

lists; checking for drug interactions; and providing patients with educational materials about their illness.

See Figure 9.1 for a Clinical Visit Summary given to a patient at the conclusion of the visit, which would satisfy the Summary of Care objective.

Hospitals had to incorporate 5 of the 10 menu objectives listed in Table 9.2 to be eligible for incentive grants in 2011.

Medicaid-eligible providers (physicians, dentists, nurse midwives, nurse practitioners, or physicians' assistants in rural health clinics), with some restrictions based on percentage of patients who are covered by Medicaid, will qualify for the full stimulus amount in the first year if a practice shows it has adopted, upgraded, or implemented EHR.

Eligible professionals (EPs) and hospitals (including critical access hospitals, or CAHs) must meet Stage 1 Meaningful Use of electronic health data before progressing to Stage 2. Though the final rule for Stage 2 was effective on September 4, 2012, implementation of Stage 2 requirements has been extended through 2016, and Stage 3 begins in 2018 for providers who have completed at least two years in Stage 2.

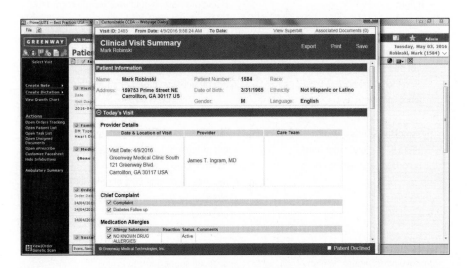

Figure 9.1   Clinical Visit Summary

Table 9.3 illustrates the EP Core Objectives for Stage 2 as excerpted from the CMS Stage 1 vs. Stage 2 Comparison Table. All 17 are required to meet Stage 2 Meaningful Use.

TABLE 9.3	Eligible Professional (EP) Core Objectives: Stage 2 Meaningful Use
Stage 2 Explanation	**Comparison to Stage 1**
CPOE to be used for medication, laboratory, and radiology orders directly entered by any licensed healthcare professional who can enter orders into the medical record per state, local, and professional guidelines	Stage 1 addressed medications only, and at least 30% of unique patients had to have medication(s) ordered using CPOE Stage 2 requires more than 60% of medication, 30% of laboratory, and 30% of radiology orders created by the EP during the EHR reporting period be recorded using CPOE
Generate and transmit permissible prescriptions electronically (eRx)	Stage 1 required that more than 40% of permissible prescriptions written by an EP were transmitted electronically Stage 2 requires more than 50% of all permissible prescriptions written by the EP to be compared to at least one drug formulary and transmitted electronically using Certified EHR Technology
EHR must show evidence that the following demographics are included in the EHR of each patient: • Gender • Preferred language • Race • Ethnicity • Date of birth	Stage 1 required more than 50% of unique patients' EHR to show evidence of collection of the demographics collected in structured format Stage 2 requires more than 80% of unique patients to have the demographics collected in structured format
The following vital signs must be recorded: • Height • Weight • Blood pressure • Calculate and display BMI • Plot and display growth charts for children 2–20 years, including BMI	Stage 1 required more than 50% of all unique patients age 2 and over to show evidence of blood pressure, height, and weight recorded as structured data Stage 2 requires more than 80% of unique patients to have blood pressure (for patients age 3 and over only) and height and weight (for all ages) recorded as structured data
The smoking status of patients 13 years of age and older must be recorded as structured data.	Stage 1 required more than 50% of patients 13 years old or older to have smoking status recorded as structured data Stage 2 requires more than 80% of patients 13 years old or older to have smoking status recorded as structured data
Use clinical decision support to improve performance on high priority health conditions.	Stage 1 required the EP to implement one clinical decision support rule

Stage 2 Explanation	Comparison to Stage 1
	Stage 2 requires 1. Five clinical decision support interventions related to four or more clinical quality measures, if applicable, be implemented at a relevant point in patient care for the entire EHR reporting period 2. The EP or hospital EHR has functionality for drug–drug and drug–allergy interaction checks be in place for the entire EHR reporting period.
Provide patients the ability to view online, download, and transmit their health information within four business days of the information being available to the provider.	Stage 1 required that more than 50% of all patients who request an electronic copy of their health information be provided it within three business days Stage 2 requires more than 50% of patients seen during the EHR reporting period be provided timely (available to the patient within four business days after the information is available to the provider) online access to their health information And more than 5% of all patients seen during the EHR reporting period (or their authorized representative) be able to view, download, or transmit to a third party their health information
Provide clinical summaries for patients for each office visit.	Stage 1 required that clinical summaries were provided to patients for more than 50% of all office visits within three business days Stage 2 requires that clinical summaries be provided to patients within one business day for more than 50% of office visits
Protect electronic health information created or maintained by the Certified EHR Technology through the implementation of appropriate technical capabilities.	Stage 1 required EPs to conduct or review a security risk analysis and implement security updates as necessary and correct identified security deficiencies as part of its risk management process Stage 2 requires an EP to conduct or review a security risk analysis, including addressing the encryption/security of data at rest, and implement security updates as necessary and correct identified security deficiencies as part of its risk management process
Incorporate clinical lab test results into Certified EHR Technology as structured data.	Stage 1 required more than 40% of all clinical lab test results ordered by the EP during the EHR reporting period whose results were either in a positive/negative or numeric format be included in the EHR as structured data Stage 2 requires more than 55% of all clinical lab test results ordered during the EHR reporting period whose results are either in a positive/negative or numeric format be included in the EHR as structured data

(continued)

Stage 2 Explanation	Comparison to Stage 1
Generate lists of patients by specific conditions to use for quality improvement, reduction of disparities, research, or outreach.	Stage 1 required an EP to generate at least one report listing patients of the provider with a specific condition The Stage 1 requirement remained the same in Stage 2.
Use clinically relevant information to identify patients who should receive reminders for preventive/follow-up care.	Stage 1 required more than 20% of all unique patients 65 years or older or 5 years old or younger to be sent an appropriate reminder during the EHR reporting period Stage 2 requires the use of EHR technology to identify and provide reminders for preventive/follow-up care for more than 10% of patients with two or more office visits in the last 2 years
Use Certified EHR Technology to identify patient-specific education resources and provide those resources to the patient if appropriate.	Stage 1 required more than 10% of all patients seen by the EP be provided patient-specific education resources Stage 2 requires patient-specific education resources identified by **Certified Electronic Health Record Technology (CEHRT)** be provided to patients for more than 10% of all unique patients with office visits seen by the EP during the EHR reporting period
The EP who receives a patient from another setting of care or provider of care or believes an encounter is relevant should perform medication reconciliation	Stage 1 required that the EP perform medication reconciliation for more than 50% of transitions of care in which the patient is transitioned into the care of the EP The Stage 1 requirement remained the same in Stage 2.
The EP who transitions a patient to another setting of care or provider of care or refers a patient to another provider of care should provide a summary of care record for each transition of care or referral.	Stage 1 required that the EP who transitioned or referred the patient to another setting of care or provider of care provide a summary of care record for more than 50% of transitions of care and referrals Stage 2 requires 1. The EP who transitions or refers a patient to another setting of care or provider of care to provide a summary of care record for more than 50% of transitions of care and referrals 2. The EP who transitions or refers a patient to another setting of care or provider of care to provide a summary of care record either (a) electronically transmitted to a recipient using CEHRT or (b) where the recipient receives the summary of care record via exchange facilitated by an organization that is a NwHIN Exchange participant or is validated through an ONC-established governance mechanism to facilitate exchange for 10% of transitions and referrals

Certified Electronic Health Record Technology (CEHRT) A complement to Meaningful Use Stage 2; certification by the Office of the National Coordinator (ONC) of EHR software that meets certain standards.

Stage 2 Explanation	Comparison to Stage 1
	3. The EP who transitions or refers a patient to another setting of care or provider of care must either (a) conduct one or more successful electronic exchanges of a summary of care record with a recipient using technology that was designed by a different EHR developer than the sender's or (b) conduct one or more successful tests with the CMS-designated test EHR during the EHR reporting period
Capability to submit electronic data to immunization registries or immunization information systems and actual submission except where prohibited and in accordance with applicable law and practice	Stage 1 required the performance of at least one test of Certified EHR Technology's capacity to submit electronic data to immunization registries Stage 2 requires successful ongoing submission of electronic immunization data from Certified EHR Technology to an immunization registry or immunization information system for the entire EHR reporting period
Use secure electronic messaging to communicate with patients on relevant health information.	This objective did not exist in Stage 1. Stage 2 requires the capability for a secure message to be sent using the electronic messaging function of CEHRT by more than 5% of unique patients seen during the EHR reporting period

Source: Centers for Medicare and Medicaid Services. (2012, August). *Stage 1 vs. Stage 2 Comparison Table for Eligible Professionals.* Retrieved from https://www.cms.gov/Regulations-and-Guidance/Legislation/EHRIncentivePrograms/Downloads/Stage1vsStage2CompTablesforEP.pdf

The following Stage 1 core objectives were incorporated elsewhere in Stage 2, and therefore, there was no need to list them as separate objectives:

- Implement drug–drug and drug–allergy interaction checks.
- Maintain an up-to-date problem list of current and active diagnoses.
- Maintain an active medication list.
- Maintain an active medication allergy list.
- Report clinical quality measures (CQMs) to CMS or the states.
- Have the capability to exchange key clinical information (e.g., problem list, medication list, medication allergies, diagnostic test results) among providers of care and patient-authorized entities electronically.
- Implement drug-formulary checks.
- Provide patients with timely electronic access to their health information (including lab results, problem list, medication lists, medication allergies) within four business days of the information being available to the EP.

Hospitals (including CAHs) have similar core objectives, as listed above for eligible professionals. The requirement to generate and transmit permissible prescriptions electronically is a menu objective rather than a core objective in hospitals. Also, the requirement to receive reminders for preventive/follow-up care does not apply to hospitals. The demographics objectives for hospitals include those listed for eligible professionals and include date and preliminary cause of death in the event of mortality in the eligible hospital or critical access hospital. Eligible hospitals are required to submit electronic syndromic surveillance data to public health agencies and actual submission except where prohibited and in accordance with applicable law and practice. Also in core objectives, eligible hospitals must have the electronic means to automatically track medications from order to administration using assistive technologies in conjunction with an electronic medication administration record (eMAR). In the paper system, that was known as a medication administration record (MAR).

Table 9.4 recaps the menu objectives for Stage 2 as they apply to eligible professionals. EPs are required to comply with three of the six menu objectives to qualify for Meaningful Use.

TABLE 9.4	Eligible Professional (EP) Menu Objectives: Stage 2 Meaningful Use	
Stage 2 Explanation	**Comparison to Stage 1**	
Have the capability to submit electronic syndromic surveillance data to public health agencies and actual submission except where prohibited and in accordance with applicable law and practice.	Stage 1	required at least one test of Certified EHR Technology's capacity to provide electronic syndromic surveillance data to public health agencies
	Stage 2	requires successful ongoing submission of electronic syndromic surveillance data from Certified EHR Technology to a public health agency for the entire EHR reporting period
Record electronic notes in patient records.	Stage 1	did not include this menu objective
	Stage 2	requires an EP to enter at least one electronic progress note created, edited, and signed for more than 30% of unique patients
Imaging results consisting of the image itself and any explanation or other accompanying information are accessible through CEHRT.	Stage 1	did not include this menu objective
	Stage 2	requires more than 10% of all scans and tests whose result is an image ordered by the EP for patients seen during the EHR reporting period be incorporated into or accessible through Certified EHR Technology
Record patient family health history as structured data.	Stage 1	did not include this menu objective
	Stage 2	requires more than 20% of all unique patients seen by the EP during the EHR reporting period to have a structured data entry for one or more first-degree relatives or an indication that family health history has been reviewed
Have the capability to identify and report cancer cases to a state cancer registry, except where prohibited, and in accordance with applicable law and practice.	Stage 1	did not include this menu objective
	Stage 2	requires successful ongoing submission of cancer case information from Certified EHR Technology to a cancer registry for the entire EHR reporting period
Have the capability to identify and report specific cases to a specialized registry (other than a cancer registry), except where prohibited, and in accordance with applicable law and practice.	Stage 1	did not include this menu objective
	Stage 2	requires successful ongoing submission of specific case information from Certified EHR Technology to a specialized registry for the entire EHR reporting period

Source: Centers for Medicare and Medicaid Services. (2012, August). *Stage 1 vs. Stage 2 Comparison Table for Eligible Professionals.* Retrieved from https://www.cms.gov/Regulations-and-Guidance/Legislation/EHRIncentivePrograms/Downloads/Stage1vsStage2CompTablesforEP.pdf

Eligible hospitals (including CAHs) desiring to meet Stage 2 menu objectives must also meet three of six possible objectives, which include the following:

- Record whether a patient 65 years old or older has an advance directive.
- Record electronic notes in patient records.
- Imaging results consisting of the image itself and any explanation or other accompanying information are accessible through CEHRT.
- Record patient family health history as structured data.
- Generate and transmit permissible discharge prescriptions electronically (eRx).
- Provide structured electronic lab results to ambulatory providers and transmit permissible discharge prescriptions electronically (eRx).

As you read through the core and menu objectives, notice how often "structured data" is mentioned. These data elements must be chosen from libraries within the EHR system rather than in free text within the EHR notes.

Not only was more functionality added in Stage 2, but the measure thresholds were increased as well.

In Stage 2, the ability to share patient information with other providers and healthcare facilities is a major emphasis; after all, a prime reason for using electronic health records is the improvement of patient care and outcomes by sharing patient information between and among providers, hospitals, and other healthcare facilities. A 2012 study conducted by CapSite, a healthcare technology research firm, revealed that 71% of hospitals in the United States plan to join an HIE (CapSite, September 2012), and a 2013 study conducted by the same research firm found that 46% of U.S. physician groups plan to join an HIE (CapSite, June 2013).

Having the ability to view Meaningful Use **dashboards** is an important component of all EHR programs, as it allows a practice or an organization to compare actual performance to the required performance to ensure compliance. An example of a dashboard is depicted in Figure 9.2. Note that the

Dashboard A visual comparison of actual performance to required performance.

Figure 9.2 **Example of Meaningful Use Dashboard**

color-coding will help users identify areas of strength or weakness when viewing the dashboard.

9.2 Data and Information Used in Decision Support

According to the Health Information Management and Systems Society, "Clinical Decision Support (CDS) is defined broadly as a clinical system, application, or process that helps health professionals make clinical decisions to enhance patient care. Clinical knowledge of interest could range from simple facts and relationships to best practices for managing patients with specific disease states, new medical knowledge from clinical research, and other types of information" (HIMSS, 2013).

CDS includes reminders and alerts, diagnostic and therapeutic guidance, links to expert resources (CDC, Mayo Clinic, and clinical trials, for example), and results of best practices. Many EHR vendors link directly to one of these expert sites. The trigger that a clinical alert or support should be displayed comes from the data that has already been captured in the patient's record. This is where the data dictionary and structured data that we covered in an earlier chapter apply. In the exercise that follows, the trigger for the alert flag will be the patient's age (calculated by the system), the CPT codes for colonoscopy, and whether or not one of those codes has been assigned to any visit for a patient over the past five years (derived from calculating five years prior to the date of the visit). Decision support, or clinical decision support, is a functionality of an EHR whose value cannot be overestimated. Use of CDS tools improves patient safety, decreases duplication of procedures, reduces the performance of unnecessary testing, and as a result reduces the cost of healthcare, while improving patient outcomes, efficiency of care, and provision of clinically relevant, evidence-based care. Clinical decision support tools are built into most EHRs, including Prime Suite, and they are instrumental in improving patient compliance and assisting physicians in providing quality care.

Recall that Meaningful Use requires that at least five clinical decision support interventions related to four or more clinical quality measures be implemented during the entire reporting period. An alert that pops up to ask a patient if he or she has had a colonoscopy does not meet the requirement unless that alert appears based on certain information found in the EHR about *that* patient compared to evidence-based criteria that have been embedded in the EHR software. For instance, an alert for colonoscopy would appear when a patient is 50 years of age and older, and/or there is an entry in the patient's problem list showing a history of rectal bleeding, or a family history of colon cancer is documented in the history section of his chart, and no CPT procedure codes for colonoscopy have appeared in the patient's visit history in the past five years.

By setting parameters (age, diagnosis, length of time since the last procedure was performed, etc.) for specific objectives and wellness initiatives, such as with a colonoscopy, a mammogram, or cholesterol testing, EHR systems have the ability to audit patients' charts to identify if they are due or overdue for screening or testing. This ensures that providers can order tests, procedures, immunizations, and screenings when they are needed. Doing so provides opportunities for patients to remain proactive in their own healthcare and can even lead to early detection of disease, which will result in improved patient outcomes and a lower overall cost of healthcare.

Of course, if a care provider has this functionality available through the practice's EHR software and does not use it, then it is not beneficial to the patient, to the care provider, or to the practice, or to satisfy Meaningful Use standards. There are still care providers who view CDS systems as "cookbook medicine"—those who find it too time consuming or who are annoyed by the pop-up reminders. One incentive to encourage the use of a CDS is pay-for-performance programs available in certain managed care plans. In other words, if the practice's fiscal position is improved by using CDS technology, then the care providers are more accepting of CDS systems.

connect Go to http://connect.mheducation.com to complete this exercise.

EXERCISE 9.1

Build a Clinical Alert, Part A

In this scenario, we are going to build a clinical alert in Prime Suite. This is a lengthy process for the alert we have chosen, so this will be done in two parts—Exercise 9.1 (Part A) and Exercise 9.2 (Part B).

We are going to build a clinical alert for all patients who are 50 years of age or older who have not had a colonoscopy in the past five years. To do this, we will use CPT codes for colonoscopy, of which there are eight. There are many CPT codes for colonoscopy because the codes differ based on the reason for doing the procedure as well as the extent of the procedure. (You will enter these codes in the order code fields in numeric order during the exercise.) The colonoscopy codes are

45378	45382
45379	45383
45380	45384
45381	45385

These are called "filters," which will select (or exclude) patients from the database who do (or in this case do not) meet certain criteria. In this particular alert we will **query** the database for patients who are 50 years of age or older and who do not have one of the colonoscopy codes listed above attached to any of their visits for the past five years; once the alert is set up, their electronic record will then have the red ribbon icon attached to show that a colonoscopy is needed. To query means that we are going to search, or "ask," the database for records that meet (or do not meet) the criteria noted in the filters. In our example, we are querying the database for patients who are 50 years of age or older and who *do not* have one of the eight colonoscopy codes listed above attached to any of their visits over the past five years.

Follow these steps to complete the exercise on your own once you have watched the demonstration and tried the steps with helpful prompts in practice mode. Use the information provided in the scenario to complete the information.

1. Click Clinical Alerts.
2. Click in the Clinical Alert Description field.
3. Type "Patient due for colonoscopy".
4. Click Clinical Alert Filters.

Query Searching a database for patients who meet certain criteria.

(continued)

5. In the "Include patients that meet All of the following criteria:" section, click the Field Name drop-down menu.

6. Click Patient: Age.

7. Click the Operator drop-down menu.

8. Click is greater than or equal to.

9. Click the Match Value field.

10. Type "50".

11. In the "Exclude the patients that HAVE or DO meet ANY of the following criteria:" section, click the Field Name drop-down menu.

12. Click Order: Order Code.

13. Click the Operator drop-down menu.

14. Click matches any value in list.

15. Click Create Match List.

16. Type "45378" in the Order: Order Code field.

17. Click Add.

18. Type "45379".

19. Click Add.

20. Type "45380".

21. Click Add.

22. Type "45381".

23. Click Add.

24. Type "45382".

25. Click Add.

26. Type "45383".

27. Click Add.

28. Type "45384".

29. Click Add.

30. Type "45385".

31. Click Add.

32. Click OK.

☑ **You have completed Exercise 9.1**

EXERCISE **9.2**   Go to http://connect.mheducation.com to complete this exercise.

Build a Clinical Alert, Part B

In Part B we will continue adding filters, and you will need the following information:

The URL needed for the Clinical Alert is http://www.cdc.gov/cancer/colorectal/basic_info/screening/guidelines.htm. This practice has chosen to use the Centers for Disease Control and Prevention (CDC) as the organization from which they base their expert advice.

This alert will be named "Colonoscopy Needed" (without the quotes).

Follow these steps to complete the exercise on your own once you have watched the demonstration and tried the steps with helpful prompts in practice mode. Use the information provided in the scenario to complete the information.

1. Click the first blank Field Name drop-down menu.
2. Click Order: Order Date.
3. Click the Operator drop-down menu.
4. Click in the past.
5. Click the number sign #.
6. Click 5.
7. Click year(s).
8. Click OK in dialog box.
9. Click OK.
10. Click Clinical Alert Flag.
11. Click Colonoscopy Alert.
12. Click OK.
13. Click the Clinical Alert URL field.
14. Enter the clinical alert URL.
15. Click Save.
16. Type "Colonoscopy Needed" in the Enter Alert Name field.
17. Click Save.
18. Click Garza, Alfredo Jose.

✓ **You have completed Exercise 9.2**

9.3 Use of Report-Writer for System Reports

Prime Suite and other PM/EMR software offer a multitude of standard reports that are set to run at certain times (end of month, for example) or on demand, as the information is needed. Some of the standard reports available in Prime Suite are

- Payment analysis
- Procedure code analysis
- Provider revenue summary
- Patient balances
- Referring provider
- Appointment analysis report

The standard reports listed above and others in the reports library are necessary for efficient running of the office. Not keeping a close watch over revenue or balances and constantly battling scheduling conflicts are not good business practices. Surprises in any of these areas can negatively impact the bottom line and cause unhappy staff, providers, and patients.

Running standard reports is as easy as a click of a button. It is always important to know the date ranges you want to include and, if it is a report you run on a routine basis, you should always use the same parameters for consistency. In other words, if you run a report routinely that includes all of the care providers, do not make the mistake of running it next time with just a few of the providers; otherwise, you are not comparing apples to apples! Figure 9.3 shows the A/R Management Report Selection screen.

Figure 9.3 **Report Selection Screen**

This is the screen from which you would choose to run a Procedure Code Analysis Report, for example. This is a report that shows all procedures, and the volume of each, that are performed in the office. They are listed by CPT code. If you work for a dermatologist, the CPT code 42400, biopsy of salivary gland, should not appear on your Procedure Code Analysis Report, for example. If it does, then someone has made a coding error, since dermatologists typically do not excise salivary glands. If this does happen, then the affected account should be found and the code corrected. Another use for this type of report is cost justification. If one of the providers wants to purchase a newer model of a particular piece of equipment, and it will cost approximately $200,000, the managing partners in the practice most likely will not approve the purchase if only a small number of procedures it will be used for are performed each year. When making large purchasing decisions, all practices should consider the return on investment (ROI) of the item(s), meaning when they can expect to make their money back. A $200,000 piece of equipment is not likely to turn a profit, or even pay for itself, if not enough procedures are performed on it. Running the CPT report would be able to provide this information to the practice for the decision-making process.

Major decisions, especially those that involve funding, should always be analyzed, and standard reports are a good starting point for the analysis. The findings from these reports give information—either baseline findings or changes over time. If information in these reports is not analyzed, decisions will be made arbitrarily rather than based on facts. Additionally, reports can be used to identify trends, which help practices forecast for the future.

Standard clinical reports are used as well. Examples include a listing of all active patients in the practice with a particular diagnosis, or a listing of all patients with an alert flag of smoker. You may want to run this type of report to answer a survey, where just the number of active smokers is requested. In this case, a **summary report** that includes only the total number (**aggregate**) of active smokers for a specific time period would be included rather than

Summary report A statistical report that includes totals rather than data for individual patients. Examples include a report of total patients seen during a particular time by gender; a report of the total number of patients seen in the office with E&M code 99214.

Aggregate The sum total; for instance, the sum total of patients between the ages of 60 and 100 in a practice as opposed to a separate listing for each patient between the ages of 60 and 100.

their name, address, and so on. Reports that do include patient identifying information and list each case individually are known as **detail reports**.

Figure 9.4 depicts a Provider Revenue Summary report in Prime Suite.

Detail report Any report that includes patient identifying information and lists each case individually rather than as total number of cases.

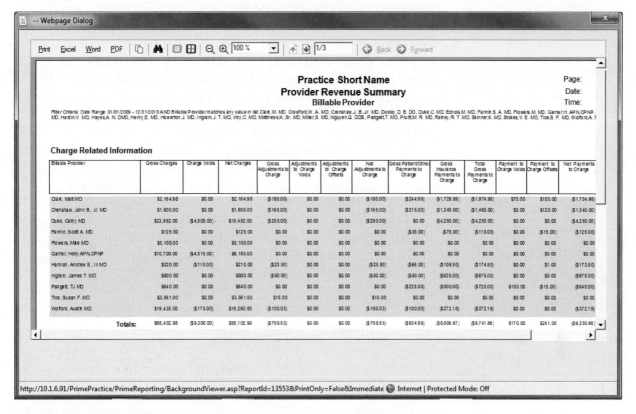

Figure 9.4   Provider Revenue Summary

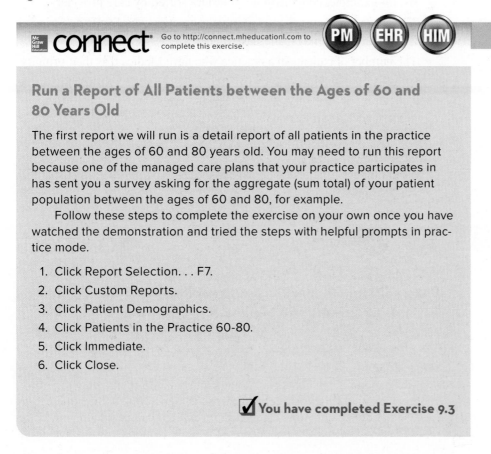

Go to http://connect.mheducationl.com to complete this exercise.

PM   EHR   HIM   **EXERCISE   9.3**

Run a Report of All Patients between the Ages of 60 and 80 Years Old

The first report we will run is a detail report of all patients in the practice between the ages of 60 and 80 years old. You may need to run this report because one of the managed care plans that your practice participates in has sent you a survey asking for the aggregate (sum total) of your patient population between the ages of 60 and 80, for example.

Follow these steps to complete the exercise on your own once you have watched the demonstration and tried the steps with helpful prompts in practice mode.

1. Click Report Selection. . . F7.
2. Click Custom Reports.
3. Click Patient Demographics.
4. Click Patients in the Practice 60-80.
5. Click Immediate.
6. Click Close.

☑ **You have completed Exercise 9.3**

Custom report Report that is designed by the office or hospital rather than coming as part of a software package (standard report).

Variable In relation to a statistical report, the factor that varies from one patient to the next. Examples include age, ZIP code, and diagnoses.

A **custom report** can be built to include **variables**. Variables are the factors that vary from one patient to the next (e.g., age, ZIP code, diagnosis code, procedure code). We select the variables in these reports that we want our patients to meet or not meet. In Exercise 9.3 there was only one variable—the patient's age—which had to be between 60 and 80 years. If we had wanted to narrow our search to patients between 60 and 80 years old who live in ZIP code 21122, then we would have had to run a custom report in order to capture only those patients who live in the locality with a ZIP code of 21122 and are between 60 and 80 years old.

We often run these custom reports to answer inquiries from managed care agencies, federal or state departments of health, public health agencies, or accrediting agencies. We may even do so for a newspaper reporter or a student who just wants aggregate data about a particular diagnosis in order to write an article or a research paper. A cardiology practice may take part in a study with other cardiology practices in town and will run a custom report to compare its patient demographics to those of the other practices. When statistics concerning one practice or hospital are compared to the statistics of other practices or hospitals, this is referred to as **benchmarking**, which is the comparison of one set of statistics to the overall statistics (using the same variables). As always, remember HIPAA! While we can run reports and share generic information, we are not able to share specific or identifiable personal information, such as linking their names with the data, about patients without their consent.

Other custom report examples include

Benchmarking Comparison of one set of statistics to the overall statistics when the same variables are used for each.

- The number of patients treated in the practice with a particular diagnosis, for example, congestive heart failure sorted by care provider
- The number of patients treated in your practice who live in a particular ZIP code, are smokers, and have diabetes
- The number of patients in a practice who have Medicaid as their primary source of payment and are between the ages of 30 and 60 years
- The number of patients in a practice who have not had a specific screening test, such as all female patients over the age of 40 who have not had a mammogram within one year, which would allow the provider to send letters so these patients will know they are overdue for testing
- The number of patients who have allergies to penicillin, are Hispanic, and live in ZIP code 12345

EXERCISE **9.4** **PM** **EHR** **HIM** Go to http://connect.mheducation.com to complete this exercise. **McGraw Hill Education** **connect**

Build a Custom Report to See What Providers Are Referring Patients to Greensburg Medical Center

In this custom report we are going to create a report that will show us which providers patients are referred from, as well as which providers Greensburg Medical Center providers are referring to. The terms *referring* and *referral* are both used and mean the same thing, but it is important to understand your relationship with other medical practices in the area, both on the receiving and the sending ends of a referral. One reason a patient may be referred to another provider is because the patient needs to see a specialist such as a cardiologist or dermatologist. If your office is family practice, then you would be referring *to* the specialist. The specialist's office would be accepting the referral. Another reason for referral may be a patient who was seen in an urgent care or emergency department; the patient would most likely be referred for follow-up to a family practitioner or an internist, or a specialist, depending on the reason for the visit. An organization may want to see where patients are being referred from so it can do some marketing in that area, or even to see about creating a partnership with the referring organization to ensure continuity of care for patients; thus, the organization would need to run a referral report to locate the names of physicians or practices that are referring to your practice.

Follow these steps to complete the exercise on your own once you have watched the demonstration and tried the steps with helpful prompts in practice mode.

1. Click Report Designer.
2. Click Referral Management.
3. Click Import.
4. Click Registration.
5. Click Referral Management.
6. Click Reports.
7. Click Referral Tracking Report (v2).
8. Click Start Import.
9. Click the text box in the Custom Reports--Webpage Dialog window.
10. Type "Referring Provider Report".
11. Click OK.
12. Click Referral Management.
13. Click Referring Provider Report.
14. Click Filter.
15. Click Current Report Filters.
16. Click the Field Name drop-down menu.
17. Click Referral: Referral From Provider Name.
18. Click the Operator drop-down menu.
19. Click matches any value in list.
20. Click Create Match List.
21. Click Bones, George MD.
22. Click Woodard, Tyler T. MD.
23. Click OK.
24. Click OK.
25. Click Properties.
26. Click the Name: field.
27. Type "Referral From Provider Report".
28. Click the Description: field.
29. Type "Referring Provider Report from External Providers".
30. Click Save.
31. Click Save.
32. Click Report Selection . . . F7.
33. Click Custom Reports.
34. Click Referral Management.
35. Click Referral From Provider Report.
36. Click Immediate.

 You have completed Exercise 9.4

Build a Custom Report to Add a Flag to Multiple Records at One Time

In this custom report, we will show how easy it is to add a flag to many records at one time. In our scenario, we will add an exclamation point icon to the charts of all patients 13 years of age and older who do not have a smoking status on the registration page. Collection of this data is a Meaningful Use requirement.

Follow these steps to complete the exercise on your own once you have watched the demonstration and tried the steps with helpful prompts in practice mode.

1. Click Clinical Alerts.
2. Click the Clinical Alert Description field.
3. Type "Smoking Status Documentation".
4. Click Clinical Alert Filters.
5. Click the Field Name drop-down menu.
6. Click Patient: Age.
7. Click the Operator drop-down menu.
8. Click is greater than or equal to.
9. Click the Match Value field.
10. Type "13".
11. On the lower half of the screen, click the Field Name drop-down menu.
12. Click History: SHx.
13. Click the Operator drop-down menu.
14. Click is equal to.
15. Click the Match Value field.
16. Type "unknown".
17. Click OK.
18. Click Clinical Alert Flag.
19. Click Smoking Status Unknown.
20. Click OK.
21. Click Save.
22. Type "Smoking Status Documentation".
23. Click Save.

The records of all patients 13 years of age and older who do not have a smoking status indicated will now have the smoking indicator icon attached to their record.

☑ **You have completed Exercise 9.5**

Index A listing—for instance, a Diagnosis Index is a report that is sorted by diagnosis code and includes the total number of patients seen with that disease for a given period of time; a Master Patient Index (MPI) is a listing of all patients who have ever been seen in a hospital or a practice.

9.5   Uses of Indexes

An **index** is a listing. Indexes, also known as indices, are generally used to find basic information; a Disease Index is run and is sorted by ICD-10-CM diagnosis code and under each code lists each patient by name and health record number (dates of admission/discharge, attending physician, discharge disposition may also be included). Hospitals run the Disease Index to get a grasp of the types of patients being seen in the facility. This is also a good way to check for inaccuracies in coding. Another example is a listing of all patients who are assigned to each care provider individually. In inpatient and outpatient settings, the Disease, Operation (procedure), and Physicians' Indexes are commonly run reports.

Managed care insurance plans often want to see the Physicians' Index or Disease Index to get a profile of the type of patients treated by a practice before considering it for **in-network** status (meaning that there is a contract between a managed care plan and the provider to offer services to members of the managed care plan at a prenegotiated rate, called capitation). Another reason to see this index is to provide proof that a physician has cared for a certain number of patients when he or she is seeking board certification, as in the case of a board-certified urologist or board-certified obstetrician. Disease Indexes are also used for case finding for such entities as the cancer registry, trauma registry, birth defect registries, and so on. Registries will be discussed in the next section.

A common index in a hospital setting is the Master Patient Index (MPI) (the listing of all patients seen in a hospital), which includes basic identifying information. Running the entire MPI may be done to look for missing information, to look for duplicate patients, or to look for names entered outside the practice's defined specifications (that is, making sure that names are formatted according to data dictionary specifications).

In-network Care providers who contract with a managed care plan to offer services to members of the managed care plan at a prenegotiated rate.

9.6 Uses of Registries

Whereas an index is a listing of information, a **registry** is also a listing, but it is in chronological order. Examples in a hospital are admission and discharge registries, since they are run on a daily basis and include the names of all patients admitted and all patients discharged on a certain date. Another example is a birth registry—it is kept by date and time of birth, but it is sorted by the name of the newborn and includes the name of the mother, the time of birth, and the name of the attending physician. And death registries, which are kept by date and time of death, include the patient's name, the cause of death, and the signature of the person pronouncing the death, among other data elements.

Registry A listing that is filed in chronological order based on when something occurred. Examples include a birth registry, a death registry, a cancer registry, and a trauma registry.

Cancer registries are required by law. These are registries of all patients diagnosed or treated for cancer. The registry of these patients is then sent to the state cancer registry, where statewide statistics are compiled regarding the incidence of each type of cancer as well as survival rates by type of cancer in that state. The state registry is responsible for reporting to the Centers for Disease Control and Prevention (CDC). Hospitals, physicians' offices, outpatient radiation therapy facilities, and ambulatory care centers may keep and report a registry of cancer patients on a yearly basis. Take the time to look for the most commonly diagnosed cancers in the United States, found at http://www.cdc.gov/cancer/dcpc/data/types.htm. Cancer registries will be covered in more detail in another course.

Trauma registries are one of the newer registries, created in the early 1990s; as the name implies, this is a registry of all patients diagnosed or treated with traumatic injuries, including fractures, burns, open wounds, and the like. The 2015 Annual Report of the American College of Surgeons'

National Trauma Databank can be found at https://www.facs.org/quality-programs/trauma/ntdb/docpub. It is interesting to page through the report; you will see the enormous amount of data reported by hospitals throughout the country. In Table 15 on page 39 of the report, you will see a breakdown by mechanism of injury (fall, fire/flame, suffocation, transport vehicles, motor vehicle accidents, etc.). From there, the data gets more specific—for instance, incidence of falls by age or incidents by region of the country (Table 41, page 99). As you can see, the southern part of the country has the highest incidence of traumatic incidents, at 38.64%. The Northeast has the lowest, at 16.96%. State and local health and safety officials can then use this information to analyze reasons for a higher-than-average incidence (in the case of the South) or a lower-than-average incidence (as is the case in the Northeast).

Immunization registries are of particular importance to public health. Some private physicians' offices keep a registry of immunizations by patient; however, not all medical practices keep this registry; it may just be a public health department that does so. Some states require reporting of immunizations by law. For instance, a West Virginia state law requires all providers to report all immunizations they administer to children under age 18 within two weeks of administering the immunization.

Other registries include birth defect, diabetes, implant (any material implanted into the body), transplant, and HIV/AIDS registries. The requirements for these vary from state to state, as well as by managed care plan or other third-party requirements, and for quality reporting purposes.

Prime Suite, like most other EHR systems, makes the process of running an index or a registry very fast. Its accuracy depends on whether the entry of the data was correct in the first place! This is another reason accuracy and attention to detail are so important. Remember that data obtained from any software program will only be as good and accurate as the person who inputs it.

The Centers for Medicare & Medicaid Services (CMS) receives registry information directly from Prime Suite. This information satisfies the **Physician Quality Reporting Initiative (PQRI)** measures. Participation in PQRI is voluntary and is a pay-for-performance incentive program. Participating care providers submit data on any of the 100 designated quality measures, which include diabetes, hypertension, stroke, and glaucoma, just to name a few. The full list is accessible at https://www.cms.gov/apps/ama/license.asp?file=/PQRS/downloads/PQRS_2016_Measure_List_01072016.xlsx. PQRS preceded the Accountable Care Organizations, discussed in the chapter on financial management.

Physician Quality Reporting Initiative (PQRI) A voluntary pay-for-performance incentive program. Participating care providers submit data on any of the 100 designated quality measures and receive monetary incentives for doing so.

Prime Suite includes an option to receive an alert at the point of care if the information entered for a patient qualifies for one or more of the PQRI Measure Groups.

There are times when hospitals, medical practices, or other healthcare entities contribute to outside registries. Of note is the **National Practitioner Data Bank (NPDB)**, which came about as part of the Health Care Quality Improvement Act of 1986. This is a database of malpractice payments, revocation of privileges, licensure denial or suspension, denial of medical staff privileges, and the like. Reporting any of these adverse actions to the NPDB is required by law. Hospitals or offices considering granting privileges to or hiring of care providers, state boards of medical examiners or

National Practitioner Data Bank (NPDB) Required by law, a database of malpractice payouts, revocation of privileges, licensure denial or suspension, denial of medical staff privileges, and similar actions.

licensing boards, state boards of medicine, or the care providers themselves can query the data bank when necessary. Healthcare entities that are considering granting privileges to a physician must query the NPDB during the hiring/privileging process.

Hospitals, care providers, and all other healthcare organizations must report adverse actions related to fraud and abuse to the **Healthcare Integrity and Protection Data Bank (HIPDB)**. Reporting to either the NPDB or the HIPDB can be done on one site rather than attempting to determine which specific data bank to report incidences to. More information about both of these can be found at http://www.npdb-hipdb.com/.

Healthcare Integrity and Protection Data Bank (HIPDB) A database of adverse actions related to fraud and abuse.

9.7 The Credentialing Process

Credentialing does not involve a database, nor does the process necessarily require the use of a database. It is mentioned here because information is captured and maintained for reporting purposes when a healthcare professional files for renewal of a medical license, applies for board certification (and continuing board certification), applies for hospital privileges (or maintaining such privileges), and reports to managed care entities.

Credentialing The process of ensuring a care provider has the proper qualifications (education, experience, malpractice coverage) to practice medicine.

Credentialing is the process of ensuring a care provider has the proper qualifications to practice medicine. In other words, if a physician claims to be a cardiac surgeon, then the practice or hospital must verify that he has the educational background and experience (medical residency) necessary to perform surgeries typically carried out by a cardiac surgeon. It must verify that he has shown verification that he is a qualified medical professional in that specialty. Also, it means that he is in compliance with specific policies (called bylaws) for that organization, and that he has purchased sufficient malpractice insurance coverage. Some insurance carriers will not reimburse providers who perform medical care for which they are not qualified. Further, some will not invite physicians to be participating providers in an insurance plan unless they are board-certified. Board certification involves successfully completing a test that is directly related to the specialty area, and which goes above and beyond state medical licensure. Physicians must be Medicare-credentialed in order to submit claims to Medicare for payment. When a medical practice hires a new care provider, information regarding education, experience, state license number, DEA number, NPI number, proof of malpractice insurance, and documentation of any pending or settled claims against the care provider are all on file, usually within the PM software. And, as noted earlier, the NPDB and HIPDB must also be queried prior to granting privileges, hiring, or including him as a participating provider by insurance carriers.

APPLYING YOUR SKILLS

In the chapter on reimbursement, we discussed a new outcome-based pay-for-performance reimbursement method, the Accountable Care Organization (ACO). How will the concepts in this chapter apply to care professionals and hospitals who are part of an ACO?

chapter 9 **Summary**

LEARNING OUTCOME	CONCEPTS FOR REVIEW
9.1 Describe the uses of the dashboard in Prime Suite to meet Meaningful Use standards.	– List Meaningful Use Stage 1 and 2 core objectives for providers and hospitals. – List Meaningful Use Stage 1 and 2 menu objectives for providers and hospitals. – View a dashboard in Prime Suite to assess performance.
9.2 Explain how data and information are used in decision support.	– Define clinical decision support. – Use improves patient safety, decreases duplication, reduces unnecessary testing, reduces cost of healthcare. – Use improves patient outcomes, improves efficiency. – Some care providers are not accepting of CDS technology.
9.3 Set up system reports using Prime Suite.	– Standard reports are commonly used by most medical practices. – Standard reports are system built. – Administrative as well as clinical standard reports are available. – Differentiate between summary and detail reports.
9.4 Set up custom reports using Prime Suite.	– Custom reports are run based on specific parameters or variables. – Custom reports are used when standard reports do not provide the level of detail necessary.
9.5 Illustrate uses for an index.	– An index is a list. – Typically used to find all patients who meet certain criteria – Examples: Master Patient Index, Disease Index, Procedure Index, Physician Index
9.6 Describe uses for a registry.	– A listing of information in chronological order – Examples: birth registry, cancer registry, trauma registry, PQRI Measures registry – Submissions required by National Practitioner Data Bank (NPDB) – Submissions required by Healthcare Integrity and Protection Data Bank (HIPDB)

9.7 Explain how data gathered in Prime Suite are used in the credentialing process.	– Verification that care provider holds certain credentials
	– Included in the credentials are
	  • education (undergrad as well as medical school)
	  • residency(ies) dates and institution(s)
	  • pending or settled malpractice cases
	  • proof of purchase of malpractice insurance

chapter review

MATCHING QUESTIONS

Match the terms on the left with the definitions on the right.

_____ 1. **[LO 9.1]** dashboard

_____ 2. **[LO 9.5]** in-network

_____ 3. **[LO 9.1]** Meaningful Use

_____ 4. **[LO 9.6]** CMS

_____ 5. **[LO 9.5]** registry

_____ 6. **[LO 9.5]** index

_____ 7. **[LO 9.2]** decision support

_____ 8. **[LO 9.1]** CEHRT

_____ 9. **[LO 9.3]** summary report

_____ 10. **[LO 9.1]** core objectives

_____ 11. **[LO 9.6]** PQRI measures group

_____ 12. **[LO 9.1]** drug formulary

_____ 13. **[LO 9.7]** credentialing

_____ 14. **[LO 9.1]** Meaningful Use Stage 2

_____ 15. **[LO 9.3]** detail report

a. requires more than 80% of unique patients have the demographics collected in structured format

b. consolidated clinical data that removes any patient information in the printout

c. tool built into most EHRs that provides staff with results of research and best practices to enhance patient care

d. software used to capture health information that meets standards set by the Office of the National Coordinator

e. subgroup of common or similar conditions pulled from registry data

f. consolidated clinical data that includes specific, demographic, or patient identifying information in the printout

g. verification process that ensures a care provider is legally authorized through education and experience to practice medicine

h. care provider or practice that contracts with insurance companies to provide care to its subscribers at a reduced rate

i. feature of Prime Suite that allows a provider to visually track its fulfillment of core objectives

j. requirements that must be met for a professional to receive Medicare stimulus money to purchase or upgrade an EHR

k. benchmark tasks that demonstrate Meaningful Use of electronic health information

l. agency to which quality reporting measures are reported

m. list of specified information, such as all patients covered by one care provider

n. list of provider-preferred generic and brand-name drugs covered under various insurance plans

o. chronological list used in calculating statistics and record-keeping

 Enhance your learning by completing these exercises and more at http://**connect**.mheducation.com!

MULTIPLE-CHOICE QUESTIONS

Select the letter that best completes the statement or answers the question:

1. **[LO 9.7]** A credentialing requirement is
   a. being hired by a professional organization.
   b. gaining additional medical degrees.
   c. having malpractice insurance.
   d. knowing procedures outside one's specialty.

2. **[LO 9.1]** In the CPOE standard, Stage 1 addressed only
   a. laboratory orders.
   b. medication orders.
   c. radiology orders.
   d. transfer orders.

3. **[LO 9.2]** When an alert is created, specifying a detail such as "search for patients 30 years or older" is an example of using a/an
   a. decision.
   b. filter.
   c. outlier.
   d. trend.

4. **[LO 9.5]** A healthcare professional will typically use an index to locate _____ information.
   a. basic
   b. encrypted
   c. statistical
   d. virtual

5. **[LO 9.1]** Healthcare facilities have _____ year[s] after the adoption of an EHR to prove Meaningful Use.
   a. 1
   b. 2
   c. 3
   d. 4

6. **[LO 9.3]** Prime Suite's reports can be used to
   a. justify the cost of new equipment.
   b. perform quality checks.
   c. track care provider data.
   d. all of these.

7. **[LO 9.2]** Meaningful Use requires that a practice not only implement at least one clinical support rule but also
   a. reduce alerts.
   b. reduce costs.
   c. track compliance.
   d. use evidence.

8. **[LO 9.4]** Custom reports have at least _____ variable(s) that is/are not available through a standard report.
   a. one
   b. two
   c. three
   d. four

9. **[LO 9.6]** You are reviewing a report that shows the patients born at Memorial Hospital from January 1, 2016, through December 31, 2016. The report is sorted by date and includes patient name, name of mother, time of birth, and name of obstetrician. Which type of report are you reviewing?
   a. dashboard
   b. index
   c. registry
   d. summary

10. **[LO 9.3]** Prime Suite's Referring Provider report is an example of a _____ report.
    a. clinical
    b. custom
    c. special
    d. standard

11. **[LO 9.5]** Care providers who contract with insurance carriers typically agree to a _____ rate of reimbursement for those services.
    a. higher
    b. lower
    c. special
    d. standard

12. **[LO 9.6]** Currently, participation in the Physician Quality Reporting Initiative is
    a. discouraged.
    b. mandatory.
    c. standard.
    d. voluntary.

SHORT-ANSWER QUESTIONS

1. **[LO 9.1]** What does it mean for a healthcare setting to report clinical quality measures?

2. **[LO 9.5]** Why might a hospital need to periodically run an entire Master Patient Index?

3. **[LO 9.3]** Contrast a summary report and a detail report.

4. **[LO 9.1]** Discuss the consequences (if any) if a provider does not achieve her core menu/objective percentages.

5. **[LO 9.2]** Explain the purpose of using filters when running a report.

6. **[LO 9.7]** What information is included in a provider's credentials?

7. **[LO 9.4]** If you needed to run a report of all the patients in your practice who were diagnosed with asthma, were African American, and were under the age of 15, what type of report would you be running? Explain your answer.

8. **[LO 9.3]** What is a Procedure Code Analysis Report?

9. **[LO 9.2]** List the benefits of clinical decision support.

10. **[LO 9.6]** List three things a registry might be used for.

11. **[LO 9.1]** Discuss the difference between the Stage 1 and Stage 2 Meaningful Use requirements for providing patients the ability to view or transmit their health information.

APPLYING YOUR KNOWLEDGE

1. **[LO 9.1]** Why might hospitals be exempt from the e-Prescribing core objective?

2. **[LOs 9.1, 9.3, 9.4, 9.5, 9.6]** As a healthcare professional, part of your job is answering patient questions. One day, a patient comes in, very concerned. When you ask what's wrong, she says, "I read about this term called *syndromatic surveillance,* and it really worries me! I don't want the government keeping tabs on me when I'm sick!" What would you say to her to alleviate her fears?

3. **[LO 9.6]** Why are registries kept in chronological order?

4. **[LO 9.2]** How could Prime Suite assist a practice in the fight against cancer?

5. **[LOs 9.2, 9.3, 9.4, 9.6]** Imagine that the state you reside in recently passed a measure requiring that a report of all immunizations administered at your practice be submitted to the state office of public health. How would you go about fulfilling this request while maintaining patient confidentiality? How could your office use the data to improve patient care?

6. **[LO 9.7]** Dr. Smith is a new provider in your office. Currently, he does not have board certification. Is it imperative that he obtain this credential? Why or why not?

7. **[LO 9.1]** Discuss why the Stage 2 Meaningful Use requirements are more stringent than those for Stage 1.

chapter references

Capsite: *2012 Ambulatory EHR & PM Study.* (2012, September). Retrieved from http://capsite.com/assets/Uploads/2012-Ambulatory-EHR-PM-StudyTOC.pdf

Capsite: *2012 Health Information Exchange Study.* (2012, September). Retrieved from http://capsite.com/assets/Uploads/2012-Health-Information-Exchange-StudyTOC2.pdf

Capsite: *Fifth Annual Ambulatory PM and EHR Study.* (2013, June). Retrieved from http://capsite.com/assets/Uploads/2013-Ambulatory-EHR-Study-TOC6.pdf

Centers for Medicare and Medicaid Services. (2012, August). *Stage 1 vs. Stage 2 Comparison Table for Eligible Hospitals and CAHs.* Retrieved from https://www.cms.gov/regulations-and-guidance/legislation/ehrincentiveprograms/downloads/stage1vsstage2comptablesforhospitals.pdf

Centers for Medicare and Medicaid Services. (2016, October). *2016 Program Requirements.* Retrieved from https://www.cms.gov/Regulations-and-Guidance/Legislation/EHRIncentivePrograms/2016ProgramRequirements.html

HIMSS. (2016). *Clinical Decision Support.* Retrieved from http://www.himss.org/ASP/topics_clinicalDecision.asp

U.S. Department of Health and Human Services. (2016). *The DataBank.* Retrieved from http://www.npdb-hipdb.hrsa.gov/

Content related to Greenway Health™, Greenway Prime Suite™, or other related products retrieved from http://www.greenwayhealth.com (or earlier iterations of the website) from 2011–2016.

Chapter **ten**

Looking Ahead— the Future of Health Information and Informatics

Learning Outcomes

At the end of this chapter, the student should be able to

10.1 Compare health information management to health informatics.

10.2 Discuss barriers to the adoption of electronic health records.

10.3 Describe ancillary technologies or models that are improving the care of patients through information technology.

10.4 Illustrate three mobile devices that will make the collection and sharing of health information more timely and efficient.

10.5 Describe how virtual private networks (VPNs) and cloud computing are advancing the use of EHRs.

Key Terms

Cloud computing
Decryption
Evidence-based medicine
Health informatics
Health information exchange (HIE)
Health information management (HIM)
Local area network (LAN)
Patient-Centered Medical Home (PCMH)
Patient portal

Personal digital assistant (PDA)
Personal health record (PHR)
Smartphone
Tablet computer
Telehealth
Telemedicine
Virtual private network (VPN)
Wide area network (WAN)
Wi-Fi

What You Need to Know and Why You Need to Know It

Technology is part of the healthcare world, whether you are a clinician or hold an administrative role. It was mentioned earlier that healthcare as a whole has been reluctant to embrace the digital age. That is not so when it comes to computerization of medical technology such as diagnostic and treatment procedures, however. Newer technologies are less invasive, require shorter recovery time, require less (or no) hospitalization, and are safer overall than previous procedures. Though we are far ahead in the use of medical technology for diagnostic and treatment purposes, we lag far behind other industries where computerization of *information* is concerned. In this chapter we will explore some of the more common methods to access electronic records and will discuss newer (at least to healthcare) technologies that are in limited use but gaining in momentum. As a healthcare professional, it is imperative that you stay abreast of emerging technologies. Even if you do not initially hold a position where you are involved in selection or implementation, you will definitely *use* technology in all the positions you will hold throughout your career. And since you have chosen healthcare as a profession, you have also chosen to become a lifelong learner—do not get too comfortable with how something is done today, as it will surely change in the blink of an eye!

10.1 Health Information versus Health Informatics

The American Health Information Management Association (AHIMA) Committee on Professional Development states the vision of **health information management (HIM)** as follows:

> *Health information management is the body of knowledge and practice that ensures the availability of health information to facilitate real-time healthcare delivery and critical health related decision-making for multiple purposes across diverse organizations, settings, and disciplines. (AHIMA)*

Health information management (HIM) A profession that encompasses services in planning, collecting, aggregating, analyzing, and disseminating individual patient and aggregate clinical data (in paper or electronic format).

The health information management professional's role in the provision of quality healthcare is to ensure the availability of complete, accurate, timely health information and the collection of data necessary to make healthcare decisions, whether related to either a particular patient or to the population as a whole.

Whereas health information management pertains to both paper and automated capture, retrieval, storage, and use of health information, **health informatics** is the management of automated health information in particular. Health information professionals whose work is geared more toward informatics focus on the structure of data, interoperability, the design of input and output tools, security controls, the development of data dictionaries, workflow configuration in an automated environment, and the classification systems and terminologies used in a computerized healthcare system.

Health informatics The management of automated health information; the technological side of managing health information—the design, development, structure, implementation, integration, and management of the technical aspects of electronic (automated) health record-keeping.

In short, health informatics is the technological side of managing health information—the design, development, structure, implementation, integration, and management of the technical aspects of electronic record-keeping. HIM professionals have historically ensured accurate, complete, readily available health information for use by care providers, administrators, researchers, public health officials, and insurers. Their focus is the content of the record, the integration of systems, and the ability to share electronic information.

They manage health information regardless of the media on which it is kept. The HIM professional and the IT professional within a facility have always worked very closely together to ensure that standards are met and information is available yet private and secure. In health informatics, there is a melding of the two disciplines—IT expertise with HIM expertise—and both may be embodied in the same person.

For years, health information management programs at all levels have included coursework in information-related software, as well as electronic record-keeping, in their curricula. Colleges and universities include in-depth coverage of the electronic health record in their medical assisting, medical billing and coding, medical office management, and healthcare administration programs. Providing these core concepts is instrumental to preparing students in these allied health disciplines for their careers in healthcare.

In a physician's office, as well as other outpatient facilities, there may not be degreed health information professionals per se, but there is an individual in the facility who should know the requirements of a legal electronic health record, documentation requirements, and privacy and security regulations. Software service providers also have support staff who actively participate in the installation and training of a PM or EHR system, as well as know the most up-to-date IT security requirements for the storage, retrieval, and sharing of sensitive patient data. They advise practices on using the software efficiently and effectively to ensure the security and privacy of the information collected, as well as to ensure that documentation requirements are being met. If the practice does not have a full- or part-time technology position staffed, the office will contract with either a consultant or the software service provider's team.

Check Your Understanding

1. Between health information management and health informatics, which discipline is most closely associated with IT and which with information itself?

2. How can a practice management software service provider assist an office or a facility that does not have a degreed HIM professional on staff?

10.2 Initial Adoptions of Electronic Health Records

We started our journey through the electronic health record system by pointing out that there was a great deal of resistance to giving up paper records; this subject is worth revisiting, as you may encounter other healthcare workers who have been a part of the transition to EHRs and may still demonstrate some resistance to using them.

For years, care providers have been documenting the health records of patients by writing orders, progress notes, and chart notes or by dictating History & Physicals (H&Ps), discharge summaries, operative reports, consultation reports, and correspondence. They were used to it, as that was how it had always been done. Providers would have known that if a laboratory test result was needed during a patient's visit, they needed only to flip to the laboratory tab of the patient's folder and it would be there (well, hopefully it would be). Additionally, paper and folders are inexpensive, relatively speaking, so this was perceived as the ideal way to create, maintain, and store patient records. If it was impossible to complete the record at the time the patient was seen, the record was sent to the health information department for completion at a later time, or if a patient was seen in the office and the provider needed to dictate the chart note, it was easy enough to take the record back to her private office to complete later. Many care providers saw this paper system as being easier, and it may have seemed more efficient; however, the quality of the documentation that was written or dictated days (or even weeks) after the care was provided could be considered questionable. Handwritten paper records were often illegible, and if dictation and transcription were used, there was lag time before the typed report could be filed in the record. Additionally, from a security perspective, a paper record could easily have been picked up by someone with no need to have or see it and, if a paper record was lost, hours of staff time would have been spent searching for it.

Implementing and maintaining an electronic record is expensive, that is true. But the argument for patient safety, higher-quality medical care, point of care documentation, faster results of diagnostic tests, and the ability to both share information with other care providers when necessary and access a patient's chart from any location (not to mention access clinical decision support) should outweigh the "high cost" argument. Financial incentives through HITECH were the initial driving forces for many practices that had decided to convert to a paperless (or almost paperless) system. Beginning in 2011, hospitals and physicians' practices that adopted and proved meaningful use of EHRs started receiving incentive payment. Shortly afterwards, physicians were expected to begin the transition of compliance, and there was neither an incentive nor a penalty. In 2015, those who held out and had not implemented EHR, likely thinking that it would go away, began to receive penalties and fines for noncompliance.

Converting from a paper system to an electronic system was considered a lengthy, sometimes chaotic process. It no doubt caused a loss of productivity for both staff and care providers. When office procedures that seemed efficient in the manual form became computerized, errors in conversion were expected, some steps in the process may have been overlooked, and many of those involved became frustrated. However, planning, heeding the advice of the software service provider's installation team, and accepting the fact that the conversion, training of staff, and use of the system were expected to be a difficult and lengthy transition made the process more tolerable. In any healthcare facility or practice using EHR, it took a great deal of time and effort to convert to and use the electronic systems, but the same can be said for any change in procedure in any profession. Use of EHRs is now an industry expectation, and it has proven to provide better functionality, an increase in patient safety, and improved continuity of care.

Check Your Understanding

1. Healthcare facilities with greater than ten employees that do not adopt electronic record technology began facing penalties in the year _____.

2. What was the initial driving force behind facilities adopting EHRs?

Patient Portals

Patients today are more interested and involved in their own healthcare. They are taking a more active role and, thanks to the Internet, arrive at their appointments knowing what their care provider may ask and why, as well as what treatment options exist. They have a list of questions ready for the care provider, which allows for a more productive visit. **Patient portals** are another means for better, more meaningful communication with a care provider, and they are a functionality of EHRs that satisfies Meaningful Use regulation. A patient portal is a method of accessing portions of one's own office health record. These portals are secure and can be accessed only with a user ID and password. Through it, patients can

- Email the practice with questions or concerns regarding care
- Make appointments
- Complete history forms and authorizations online
- Request prescription refills
- Get results of tests
- Access the contents of one's own health record

More information is available about the Greenway Health patient portal at http://www.greenwayhealth.com/solution/patient-portal-messaging/.

By using the secure portal, the office staff spends less time answering phone calls, calling patients back (or playing phone tag), and entering data in the record; patients are more satisfied because their questions are answered more promptly, and they feel that they are more in control of their care. You may not realize that your care provider offers patient portals; if the office is automated, and an EHR is in use, ask about it!

Many insurance plans have similar options for their subscribers, including communicating with a nurse or care provider to answer questions about symptoms, treatment options, coverage, and the like. Take a few moments to look at the website for your own health insurance—does it have patient portal capability? If so, what functionalities are provided? How can you use this to engage in your own healthcare?

Personal Health Records (PHRs)

A **personal health record (PHR)**, which is maintained and kept by the patient, is a record of his or her past and current health information, including drug allergies or reactions, immunization dates, past and present medical conditions, surgical procedures, family history, list of current medications, and insurance information. The PHR is not a legal record because it is just that—personal; there are no safeguards to ensure that it is complete, it is not written by a medical professional, much of it may have been compiled from memory, and it does not meet the legal requirement of "being compiled during the normal course of business." However, it is a valuable tool when a patient seeks medical care, particularly if emergency care is required or if there has been a change in care providers. The PHR is only as good as the information in it—all of the information should be up-to-date and accurate. It also needs to be available when needed. If patients expect their PHR to be

Patient portal A method of accessing portions of one's own health information from the care provider's or hospital's electronic health record.

Personal health record (PHR) A record, kept by the patient, that contains a person's health history, immunization status, current and past medications, allergies, and instructions given by a care provider; it often includes patient education materials as well.

a useful document, family members should know where it is kept, and it should be taken to office visits or to the emergency department when such visits occur and updated with any new or changed information. Patients may keep the PHR in a paper format or online (or may print it from the online portal). There are many options for doing so, including the PHR websites of many major insurance carriers and the AHIMA PHR website, found at http://www.myphr.com/. Other free online PHRs include https://www.healthvault.com/and https://www.mychartlink.com/mychart/, just to name a couple. The AHIMA website provides a full list. PHRs are not a new technology, but their use is becoming increasingly widespread.

Telemedicine

Telehealth and **telemedicine** are of great benefit to patients who do not have the means to travel to a doctor's appointment or who live in remote, medically under-served areas. Telehealth is more associated with preventive care. With the use of audiovisual equipment, the patient and the care provider or healthcare professional can connect through teleconferencing technology, allowing each to see and hear the other. Through telemedicine technology, a patient's blood pressure, heart rate, respiratory rate, EKG tracing, or medical imaging can be monitored remotely. Should the care provider find something that is not within normal limits, the patient would then need to seek on-site care or have emergency care dispatched. The imaging technology of Picture Archiving and Communications Systems (PACS), whereby radiologic images are viewed remotely, is one of the original uses of telemedicine.

Telehealth Associated with preventive care, telehealth is the use of audiovisual equipment through which the patient and the care provider or healthcare professional can connect remotely.

Telemedicine The use of technology to remotely monitor a patient's vital signs and perform tests such as an EKG, or forward radiologic images.

Using telemedicine offers cost savings to both the insurance carrier and the patient; patients who would not otherwise be able to make visits to their care providers now have better access to care, which in turn improves outcomes and generally is more convenient for patients, particularly those who do not have transportation or who live a distance away from their care provider.

The Institute of Medicine's report Telemedicine: A Guide to Assessing Telecommunications for Health Care can be downloaded online by searching by the title.

Many Veterans Affairs Medical Centers provide telemedicine or telehealth to assist in the care of veterans. The Department of Veterans Affairs telehealth website can be found at http://www.telehealth.va.gov/index.asp.

Patient-Centered Medical Home (PCMH)

Patient-Centered Medical Home (PCMH) is a model that was developed to care for patients with chronic conditions by the American Academy of Family Practitioners. The premise encourages and facilitates the patient's (and family's) involvement in his or her own care. It is mentioned in this chapter because it ties in with the concept of a patient-centric health model. The PCMH also encourages a primary care physician approach to patient care. This is also the premise of many managed care insurance plans that require a "gatekeeper" to reduce redundancy and overutilization of testing and services and to provide overall more efficient and effective healthcare.

Patient-Centered Medical Home (PCMH) A model that was developed to care for patients with chronic conditions by the American Academy of Family Practitioners, to encourage and facilitate a patient's (and family's) involvement in his or her own care.

The use of health information technology is paramount to the PCMH model because the use of quality measures, including registries, referral tracking, results tracking, medication alerts, performance measures, evidence-based medicine, updated problem lists and current medication lists, are all part of the PCMH model—all of the elements that are requirements of Meaningful Use as well.

Evidence-Based Medicine

Evidence-based medicine
Diagnostic and treatment protocols that are based on proven research and documented best practices.

Meaningful Use of data requires decision support capability as part of the EHR. This is also known as **evidence-based medicine** because the diagnostic and treatment protocols are based on proven research and best practices from physicians' experiences with patients and their responses to treatment. Through evidence-based medicine, a patient's plan of care is based on current, proven practice. Alerts, or reminders, automatically appear in a patient's chart based on data captured about that patient. An example is a female patient who has just passed her fortieth birthday. The FDA Office of Women's Health recommends a screening mammogram be performed at the age of 40 and every one to two years thereafter (FDA). Current EHR software makes it possible for physicians to be alerted to the latest diagnostic and treatment recommendations and modalities, which in turn improves efficiency, patient care, and clinical outcomes. An office, for example, can set parameters within the EHR software that meet the industry standards for wellness screening, such as that all female patients over the age of 40 have an annual mammogram. Once these parameters are set, the EHR can perform wellness screening searches to determine which patients are overdue for testing and screening, which gives the practice an opportunity to order the tests or screening. Better compliance with these initiatives results in earlier diagnosis and treatment of diseases and conditions. It is clear why the use of evidence-based medicine is part of the Meaningful Use regulations.

Check Your Understanding

1. What are the diagnostic and treatment protocols of evidence-based medicine based on?

2. Is a patient's personal health record a legal document? Explain your answer.

3. For a patient being monitored using telemedicine, what would happen if an abnormal reading were found?

4. How might a PCMH make a patient's experience more positive?

10.4 Making the World of Health Informatics User-Friendly and Convenient

In order for an electronic health record system to be successful, the care providers need to be satisfied with the product. They typically look for portability, mobility, flexibility, and convenience—all the qualities of the products used in the 21st century and all requirements of the healthcare team if they are to work efficiently.

Portable devices allow for flexibility and mobility. They are advantageous because they are convenient (the provider does not have to find a computer to use); they are cost effective (the provider can use an inexpensive device and there is no need to rework because notes and procedure codes are entered at the point of care, which reduces the number of lost or missing charges); they improve accuracy (the care provider does not have to jot down notes that must be transferred into the record later); and, in general, they create overall satisfaction, since the information needed to care for patients is available at any time from any location. A connection to the EHR may be through a **local area network (LAN)** or a **wide area network (WAN)**. LANs link computers and related devices that are physically close to one another, such as within a building; WANs connect computer networks together that are not physically close (Figure 10.1). And, of course, access can be via the Internet. The types of portable devices used include **personal digital assistants (PDAs)**; they are small enough to fit in one's hand yet allow access to LANs, WANs, and the Internet; they may also have phone capability. **Smartphones** are telephones that also allow Internet browsing, as well as audio, video, and camera functionality; and **tablet computers** are larger than PDAs or smartphones yet smaller than laptop computers—they, too, provide access to LANs, WANs, and the Internet. Though PDAs and tablets are used, smartphones have much of the same functionality, and many users prefer carrying one device rather than two or more. As with all healthcare technology, consideration of HIPAA requirements should be given to ensure the privacy and safety of protected health information (PHI) accessed via devices such as these.

Local area network (LAN) Links computers and related devices that are physically close to one another such as within a building.

Wide area network (WAN) Connects computer networks together that are not physically close.

Personal digital assistant (PDA) A mobile device that is small enough to fit in one's hand, yet allows access to local area networks (LANs), wide area networks (WANs), and the Internet; may also have telephone capability.

Smartphone Telephone that allows Internet browsing, audio, video, and camera functionality.

Tablet computer Computer that is larger than a PDA or smartphone yet smaller than a laptop computer; allows access to local area networks (LANs), wide area networks (WANs), and the Internet.

Figure 10.1   Depiction of a Wide Area Network (WAN)

Source: Williams, B.K., and Sawyer, S.C. (2011). *Using Information Technology: A Practical Introduction to Computers & Communications* (9th ed.). New York: McGraw-Hill Companies. Reprinted by permission.

Check Your Understanding

1. What are smartphones?
2. Describe three instances when access to an EHR on a mobile device would improve a care provider's efficiency or save time.

10.5 Virtual Private Networks—Advancing the Use of EHRs Remotely Yet Securely

Wi-Fi Data exchange via high radio frequency.

Virtual private network (VPN) Software that encrypts (codes) the data being sent as well as interprets the data being received.

Decryption Interpretation of data being received in encrypted (scrambled) form.

To use mobile functionality, a wireless connection is necessary. This is known as **Wi-Fi**, which sends data via high radio frequency. Of course, utilizing mobile technology does require high levels of security. The use of a **virtual private network (VPN)** is one way to ensure the security of the information flowing between the mobile device and the EHR. A VPN uses the Internet as its path, but built into the VPN is software that encrypts (codes) the data being sent and interprets the data being received (**decryption**). A VPN also verifies the identity of the user through his or her user ID and password, and it allows access only to users who have been granted permission to sign on to the network. A VPN is also used for employees who telecommute (work from home) and are dialing into the facility's computer system from a home computer or laptop. A VPN provides a secure environment for users to share information with other users at remote locations. In addition to the VPN, a firewall is another security method (Figure 10.2).

Figure 10.2 Placement of a Firewall between Computers, Servers, and the Internet

Source: C. Holcombe and J. Holcombe (2012). *Survey of Operating Systems* (3rd ed.). New York: McGraw-Hill Companies. Reprinted by permission.

Firewalls prevent unauthorized access into or out of the network through use of both hardware and software devices that filter activity over the network. Based on predefined rules, the firewall acts as a barrier—activity that passes the rules may continue into or out of the network; activity that does not pass the rules may not.

These security measures are necessary to exchange information on a small scale within or among related medical practices or hospitals, as well as between the **health information exchanges (HIEs)** that are the vision of the Office of the National Coordinator (ONC).

Cloud Computing

In recent years, there has been a rise in the number of systems that do not reside on a physical server owned, maintained, and operated by a hospital or medical practice. Rather, the data is housed in a cloud environment, which is a commercially maintained site on the Internet. In **cloud computing**, the cloud service provider, rather than an Internet service provider, is in control, and a cloud environment has unlimited processing and storage capacity. In a private cloud configuration, the storage space is solely for a single organization. It is scalable; the facility or office uses just the amount of storage space it needs and then expands its storage space as needed, thus, paying only for the space they are using (Dinh). If there should be an equipment failure or damage of some sort, the database is not affected. Think of email services such as Gmail® (Google) or Yahoo!® or document storage services such as Google Docs, Evernote, or Dropbox; if a person loses his or her laptop or if a desktop computer is destroyed in a fire, emails and documents are not lost, since the data is stored on Google's or Yahoo!'s server. The security of the data is ensured. There is no hardware cost (for servers) associated with data stored in the cloud, and the system is mobile, allowing care providers to utilize mobile devices to access records and receive important, time-sensitive notifications at any time.

Cloud computing means that data is still Internet-centric, so privacy and security of the data is a concern. Compliance with HIPAA regulations must be considered before choosing a cloud service provider.

Pulling It All Together

The intent of this worktext has been to introduce students to the automation of health information, with emphasis on those who have chosen to study health information management, medical assisting, and medical billing and coding. Having chosen one of these professions, you will work closely with automated systems. Many of you will be lucky enough to be involved in choosing a system from the very first steps, others will use the systems on a daily basis, and yet others will climb the ladder into implementation, training, and development of computer programs and systems that will enhance the automated exchange of information.

Medicine and healthcare are not static; changes occur daily. Those changes need to be communicated, implemented, and tracked to determine their impact on patient care. As a healthcare professional, you will not be observing from

Health information exchange (HIE) The movement or sharing of information between healthcare entities in a secure manner and in keeping with nationally recognized standards.

Cloud computing The housing of data in a cloud environment, which is a commercially maintained site on the Internet.

the sidelines; instead, you will be an active participant in improving quality healthcare through the availability of complete, accurate, and secure health information.

Check Your Understanding

1. How does a VPN verify a user's identity?
2. What role does encryption play in using VPNs?
3. Explain what is meant by the scalability of cloud computing.

APPLYING YOUR SKILLS

As a healthcare consumer, name 5 to 10 experiences you have had or have witnessed in which any aspect of healthcare was electronic rather than manual.

chapter 10 **summary**

LEARNING OUTCOME	CONCEPTS FOR REVIEW
10.1 Compare health information management to health informatics.	– Define health information management. – Define health informatics. – Role of HIM professional in each
10.2 Discuss barriers to the adoption of electronic health records.	– Written records and dictation have been the norm. – Paper and dictation are fairly inexpensive. – Lengthy process to convert to electronic records – Training time is extensive. – Loss of productivity – High frustration level
10.3 Describe ancillary technologies or models that are improving the care of patients through information technology.	– Patient portals—means of communication between patients and medical practice – Personal health record—patient keeps own record of history, immunizations, allergies, surgeries, past conditions, and family history – Telemedicine—allows patient to be "seen" without leaving the home – Patient-Centered Medical Home (PCMH)—primary care physician is leader of a team that cares for the patient; patient is more involved than in traditional approach; use of technology inherent in the process – Evidence-based medicine—technology "researches" best practices and decision support to assure that patient is receiving most up-to-date diagnostic and treatment options
10.4 Illustrate three mobile devices that will make the collection and sharing of health information more timely and efficient.	– Use of EHR can be more convenient by making it mobile; use of personal digital assistants (PDAs), smartphones, and tablet computers allow for portability. – Wireless (Wi-Fi) connections are required to use portable devices.
10.5 Describe how virtual private networks (VPNs) and cloud computing are advancing the use of EHRs.	– Though portability is necessary, so is security. – Virtual private networks encrypt and interpret information that is sent and received via wireless networks. – Use of firewalls as a security device – Cloud computing: commercially maintained storage site on the Internet – Unlimited storage and processing capability – Scalable (pay for as much or as little storage as used) – Private cloud is for use by one organization. – Database not affected by equipment failure, power outages, or physical damage

chapter review

MATCHING QUESTIONS

Match the terms on the left with the definitions on the right.

_____ 1. **[LO 10.5]** decryption

_____ 2. **[LO 10.1]** health information management

_____ 3. **[LO 10.3]** patient portal

_____ 4. **[LO 10.3]** evidence-based medicine

_____ 5. **[LO 10.3]** personal health record

_____ 6. **[LO 10.3]** telemedicine

_____ 7. **[LO 10.5]** VPN

_____ 8. **[LO 10.5]** Wi-Fi

_____ 9. **[LO 10.1]** health informatics

_____ 10. **[LO 10.5]** cloud computing

_____ 11. **[LO 10.4]** wide area network (WAN)

_____ 12. **[LO 10.3]** Picture Archiving and Communications S ystems

a. clinical decision support based on research and best practices

b. allow radiologists to remotely view and interpret x-rays

c. link computers within the same company that are not located in close proximity

d. uncoding coded data to make it readable

e. high radio frequency wireless connection used by smartphones, PDAs, and other electronic devices

f. unlimited storage and processing capability

g. secure method of accessing individual health records and information through an EHR

h. secure Internet environment that encrypts data and allows remote access to health information

i. medical history maintained and kept by an individual patient

j. monitoring or exchange of health information remotely

k. improving healthcare through working with data and ensuring that the best information is available for decision making

l. science that deals with health information, its structure, acquisition, and uses

MULTIPLE-CHOICE QUESTIONS

Select the letter that best completes the statement or answers the question:

1. **[LO 10.1]** Health informatics is basically the _____ part of managing health information.
   a. critical
   b. structural
   c. technological
   d. usable

2. **[LO 10.4]** One benefit of accessing the EHR through mobile devices is a reduction in
   a. cost.
   b. errors.
   c. satisfaction.
   d. both cost and errors.

3. **[LO 10.2]** Incentives are being offered to EHR adopters through _____ legislation.
   a. CCHIP
   b. HIPAA
   c. HITECH
   d. ONC

4. **[LO 10.3]** Care providers use _____ as a way to support their decisions and diagnoses.
   a. current medical trends
   b. evidence-based medicine
   c. Meaningful Use
   d. patient-centric care

5. **[LO 10.1]** Which of the following stakeholders are served by the health information management profession?
   a. patient care organizations
   b. payers
   c. research agencies
   d. all of these

6. **[LO 10.2]** Which of the following is a way to make the transition to EHRs easier?
   a. Allow staff members to be frustrated and anxious about the change.
   b. Follow the advice and suggestions of the EHR service provider's installation team.
   c. Provide immediate training so that ramp-up is quicker.
   d. Save money for EHR costs by eliminating staff.

7. **[LO 10.3]** A PCMH focuses on _____ communication between patients and providers.
   a. decreased
   b. increased
   c. random
   d. structured

8. **[LO 10.1]** Of the following, which is an accurate statement?
   a. Eligible providers taking advantage of HITECH funds must have a credentialed or degreed health information professional on staff.
   b. In the event the eligible provider is unable to hire a credentialed or degreed health information professional on staff, he or she must use the services of a paid health information consultant.
   c. Though not required, the expertise of a health information professional on staff, as a consultant or as offered by the service provider, is helpful.
   d. The EHR software is already written to handle any health information–related issues; therefore, no additional input or services from a health information professional are necessary.

 connect Enhance your learning by completing these exercises and more at http://connect.mheducation.com!

9. **[LO 10.4]** There must be a(n) _____ available in order for providers to use portable devices to access health information.
    a. computer terminal
    b. Internet hookup
    c. wireless connection
    d. wireless mouse

10. **[LO 10.3]** Who is responsible for maintaining a personal health record?
    a. HIM professional
    b. patient
    c. provider
    d. medical staff

11. **[LO 10.2]** Penalties for facilities not adopting electronic health records began in
    a. 2014.
    b. 2015.
    c. 2016.
    d. 2017.

12. **[LO 10.3]** Videoconferencing and remote vital sign monitoring are part of
    a. patient-centric care.
    b. a patient portal.
    c. telemedicine.
    d. virtual health networks.

13. **[LO 10.5]** What does VPN stand for?
    a. verifying provider network
    b. verified protocol network
    c. virtual private network
    d. virtual provider network

14. **[LO 10.3]** Recent advances in healthcare rely increasingly on
    a. change.
    b. precedent.
    c. technology.
    d. tradition.

SHORT-ANSWER QUESTIONS

1. **[LO 10.1]** Explain the difference between health information and health informatics.

2. **[LO 10.3]** What are some advantages to a healthcare facility's use of the patient portal function?

3. **[LO 10.4]** What is a mobile device?

4. **[LO 10.5]** How does a VPN ensure data integrity and security?

5. **[LO 10.2]** Explain why many care providers view a paper-based system as easier than an electronic one.

6. **[LO 10.1]** What does an HIM professional do?

7. **[LO 10.2]** How can healthcare facilities make the adoption of EHRs as easy and painless as possible?

8. **[LO 10.4]** How do mobile applications reduce costs and errors?

9. **[LO 10.3]** Describe a Patient-Centered Medical Home (PCMH).

10. **[LO 10.5]** Explain what Wi-Fi is.

APPLYING YOUR KNOWLEDGE

1. **[LO 10.3]** After reading about the patient portal in your text, can you think of any potential disadvantages of patients using the patient portal system within the EHR? Justify your answer.

2. **[LO 10.2]** What is your opinion on the use of incentives to encourage healthcare facilities to adopt EHRs? Explain your answer.

3. **[LOs 10.4, 10.5]** You are a healthcare professional who has the ability to work from home on certain days. How would you go about accessing the work you needed to do on a given day from your home?

4. **[LOs 10.1, 10.2, 10.3, 10.4, 10.5]** Your healthcare office is beginning to discuss adopting an EHR system, mobile accessibility, and other new capabilities such as telemedicine. Your supervisor has asked you to come up with some brief talking points for the staff discussing the new technologies, their advantages, and ways in which each staff member will be affected by the new systems. Come up with a short outline for your presentation.

5. **[LO 10.5]** Justify why a physician's practice or hospital may choose cloud computing over on-site servers. Are there any drawbacks to using a cloud environment instead of traditional servers? Explain.

chapter references

Abdelhak, M., Grostick, S., Hanken, M.A., and Jacobs, E. (2007). *Health Information: Management of a Strategic Resource.* Philadelphia: Saunders.

American Health Information Management Association (AHIMA). (2003). Body of Knowledge, A Vision of the e-HIM Future: A Report from the AHIMA e-HIM Task Force. Supplement to the *Journal of AHIMA.*

American Telemedicine Association. Telemedicine Defined. Retrieved from www.americantelemed.org/

Association for Medical Ethics. (2011). *History of Evidence-Based Medicine, 98.*

Cantrell, S. (2010). Reference and Information Services in the 21st Century: An Introduction, 2nd ed. *Journal of the Medical Library Association, 98*(3): 264–265. doi: 10.3163/1536-5050.98.3.019

Dinh, Angela K. "Cloud Computing 101." *Journal of AHIMA 82*(4) (April 2011): 36–37.

FDA Office of Women's Health. (2011). *Mammograms.* Retrieved from http://www.fda.gov/

Institute of Medicine. (1996). *Telemedicine: A Guide to Assessing Telecommunications for Health Care.* Retrieved from http://www.nap.edu/openbook.php?record_id=5296&page=R1

LaTour, K.M., and Eichenwald-Maki, S. (2010). *Health Information Management: Concepts, Principles and Practice, AHIMA Press.*

Menachemi, N., Powers, T.L., and Brooks, R.G. (2011). Physician and Practice Characteristics Associated with Longitudinal Increases in Electronic Health Records Adoption. *Essentials of the U.S. Health Care-System, 56*(3): 183–197. Retrieved from EBSCO*host.*

Shi, L., and Sing, D.A. (2010). *Essentials of the U.S. Health Care System* (2nd ed.). Sudbury, MA: Jones and Bartlett Publishers.

Additional Practice

What You Need to Know and Why You Need to Know It

In previous chapters of the book, you had the chance to complete guided exercises using step-by-step directions. In this chapter, you will have the opportunity to apply the knowledge you have learned to a scenario that will take you through the entire medical documentation and billing process. Using source documents and references to earlier chapters, you will use your critical thinking skills to complete the simulated exercises related to this scenario.

Here is the scenario:

> Harper Anna Jacobi has called in to Greensburg Medical Center to make an appointment. She says that she is a new patient and would like to see Dr. Ingram, as she has heard he is a great doctor. Harper states she would like to get in as soon as possible because she is miserable, with a sore throat, fever, and urinary symptoms.

You will use the following Source Documents, located at the end of the chapter, to help you complete several of the exercises:

- Source Document A: Patient Registration Form
- Source Document B: Insurance Card
- Source Document C: Patient Intake Sheet
- Source Document D: Office Visit Notes
- Source Document E: Remittance Advice (RA)

EXERCISE 11.1

Go to http://connect.mheducation.com to complete this exercise. Mc Graw Hill Education **connect®**

Register the Patient (Refer to Chapter 3 for assistance.)

The information the healthcare professional enters in Exercise 11.1 is taken while on the initial phone call with the patient. Basic information such as full name, date of birth, address, and telephone numbers are entered into Prime Suite. The healthcare professional will email some paperwork to Harper before she arrives for her appointment. For our purposes we will say she filled out the **Patient Registration Form** (Source Document A) and had her friend drop it off the same day she called in.

Register the patient using the information found on Source Document A. In addition, please note that the patient indicated that email is her preferred communication during the initial phone call.

✔️ **You have completed Exercise 11.1**

EXERCISE 11.2

Go to http://connect.mheducation.com to complete this exercise. Mc Graw Hill Education **connect®**

Capture Insurance Information of the Patient (Refer to Chapter 3 for assistance.)

Harper included her insurance information on the lower half of the Registration Form.

Capture the insurance information from the Patient Registration form and enter it into Prime Suite. The expiration date of the insurance is 6/20/2016.

✔️ **You have completed Exercise 11.2**

EXERCISE 11.3

Go to http://connect.mheducation.com to complete this exercise. Mc Graw Hill Education **connect®**

Schedule an Appointment (Refer to Chapter 3 for assistance.)

While on the initial phone call with the healthcare professional, Harper also made an appointment.

Schedule an appointment for Harper at the Greensburg Medical Center with Dr. Ingram on June 20, 2016, for an ROV-New Patient Exam at 9:30 a.m. Enter the chief complaint using the **Office Visit Notes** (Source Document D).

✔️ **You have completed Exercise 11.3**

Go to http://connect.mheducationl.com to complete this exercise.

EXERCISE 11.4

Check In the Patient Who Has Arrived (Refer to Chapter 3 for assistance.)

The scenario moves ahead and Harper has now arrived for her appointment. Check Harper into Prime Suite.

☑ **You have completed Exercise 11.4**

 Go to http://connect.mheducationl.com to complete this exercise.

EXERCISE 11.5

Post the Co-payment to the Account (Refer to Chapter 6 for assistance.)

Post the co-pay to Harper's account in Prime Suite. Refer to the **Insurance Card** (Source Document B) for the co-pay amount. She paid her co-pay with check number 5879. You will need to type "Check #5879" in the additional info field as part of the exercise.

☑ **You have completed Exercise 11.5**

connect Go to http://connect.mheducationl.com to complete this exercise.

EXERCISE 11.6

Enter the Patient's Past Medical History (Refer to Chapter 4 for assistance.)

The healthcare professional has come out to the waiting room to take Harper back to an exam room. While in the exam room, more information is gathered from the patient regarding past medical history, current medications, and allergies. Finally, a set of vitals is taken and entered in Harper's chart. A flag is also put on the chart to alert anyone on the healthcare team.

Enter the patient's Past Medical History using the **Patient Intake Sheet** (Source Document C) and bullet points below.

- Chronic Bronchitis Details: Date Onset 1998. In the notes area in Prime Suite, type "Symptoms started when she was 10 years old".
- Social Drinker. In the notes area in Prime Suite, type "Social monthly drinker".
- Substance Abuse is the category where you find caffeine use. In the notes area in Prime Suite, type "2 cups of coffee per day".
- For the Education level, choose College graduate.

☑ **You have completed Exercise 11.6**

EXERCISE **11.7** Go to http://connect.mheducation.com to complete this exercise.

Enter the Patient's List of Current Medications (Refer to Chapter 4 for assistance.)

Enter Harper's current medications into Prime Suite using the information on the Patient Intake Sheet, as well as the additional information below:

- Enter the medication in the Outside Prescribed Medication area.
- The patient takes 1 oral tablet of the medication.
- The Dispense Amount is #90.
- The prescription has 4 refills.

☑ **You have completed Exercise 11.7**

EXERCISE **11.8** Go to http://connect.mheducation.com to complete this exercise.

Enter the Patient's Known Drug Allergies (Refer to Chapter 4 for assistance.)

Enter Harper's known drug allergies into Prime Suite using the Patient Intake sheet.

☑ **You have completed Exercise 11.8**

EXERCISE **11.9** Go to http://connect.mheducation.com to complete this exercise.

Enter the Patient's Vital Signs (Refer to Chapter 4 for assistance.)

Enter Harper's vital signs into Prime Suite using Office Visit Notes.

☑ **You have completed Exercise 11.9**

EXERCISE **11.10**   Go to http://connect.mheducation.com to complete this exercise.

Assign a Flag to the Patient's Chart (Refer to Chapter 8 for assistance.)

Assign the "HIPAA Form Signed" flag to Harper's chart in Prime Suite.

☑ **You have completed Exercise 11.10**

Enter Diagnosis and Procedure Codes (Refer to Chapter 6 for assistance.)

Dr. Ingram spent 20 minutes with Harper, ran a couple of lab tests (strep screen and urinalysis), and has determined she has strep throat and a UTI.

In this exercise, enter the diagnosis and procedure codes for Harper's visit into Prime Suite. Following is some information needed to complete the exercise:

- For the ROS: Enter information found on Source Document D.
- For the Assessment: Type "Strep throat" in the Add New field.
- Click on Streptococcal sore throat.
- Click the Add New field again and type in "Urinary tract infection".
- Then, choose modifiers "acute cystitis" and "without hematuria".
- For the Plan: Add Orders for Rapid Strep (CPT code 87880) and Automated dipstick urinalysis (CPT code 81001) with microscopy, and map each to its diagnosis code.
- For the E&M: Use CPT code 99202.
- ***Remember to Save and Sign.

 You have completed Exercise 11.11

Using ePrescribe (Refer to Chapter 5 for assistance.)

Create a prescription in Prime Suite using the ePrescribe function for Harper. Refer to the Office Visit Notes for the prescription details.

 You have completed Exercise 11.12

Create a Task for the Receptionist (Refer to Chapter 8 for assistance.)

Harper needs a note to return to work. Compose a return to work letter for her to take with her before she leaves the office. The healthcare professional sends a task to the receptionist to create the note for Harper and tells Harper to stop by the front desk to pick it up on her way out.

Send a task through Prime Suite to Alisha Acy with the Subject "Note for Work" for Harper Jacobi with High Priority so Alisha sees it right away. Put a due date of 6/20/2016. In the comment area, type "Please write a note for Harper Jacobi to return to work on Wednesday June 22, 2016 per Dr. Ingram."

 You have completed Exercise 11.13

Go to http://connect.mheducation.com to complete this exercise. **connect**

Compose a Correspondence Letter (Refer to Chapter 7 for assistance.)

Compose a correspondence letter for return to work for Harper Jacobi, entering the information for dates under care from 6/20/2016 to 6/20/2016, and and returning to work on 6/22/2016 with no restrictions and no other instructions.

☑ **You have completed Exercise 11.14**

Go to http://connect.mheducation.com to complete this exercise. **connect**

Investigate an Unpaid Insurance Claim (Refer to Chapter 6 for assistance.)

Harper called the billing office because she received her Explanation of Benefits (EOB) and noticed the insurance company did not pay anything on her claim. The EOB has an explanation of "Not eligible for benefits."

Usually, when an EOB states "Not eligible for benefits," it means the policy is expired or that the policy or group number may have been entered wrong. You want to verify this with Harper, so you go to her insurance information and ask her what her policy number is on her card. She tells you it is HAJ5679045. This is not what is entered in the computer. Fix the error on her policy number in Prime Suite.

☑ **You have completed Exercise 11.15**

Go to http://connect.mheducation.com to complete this exercise.

Post an Insurance Payment to an Account (Refer to Chapter 6 for assistance.)

Three weeks later, after resubmitting the claim, your office received an RA from Harper's insurance company. This includes the payments and adjustments as well as the patient responsibility for the date of service 6/20/2016.

Post the insurance payment to Harper's account in Prime Suite. Refer to **Remittance Advice (RA)** (Source Document E) for information needed for this exercise. The patient ID is 1611.

☑ **You have completed Exercise 11.16**

Go to http://connect.mheducationl.com to complete this exercise.

Send an Electronic Message Using Prime Suite Messaging (Refer to Chapter 8 for assistance.)

Dr. Ingram is very active in the community and does many charitable fundraisers. One of the big events he does each year is to compete in the annual city triathlon, for which the proceeds go to help those in need. Dr. Ingram is sending a message to a few employees to challenge them to compete in this year's event. If any of them beat him in the race, he will buy everybody in the clinic lunch on Monday.

Send an electronic message using Prime Suite Messaging. Here are some details you will need:

- Send the message to Albert Hart, Brenda Galfano, Charles Renal, Ema Dean, and John Crenshaw.
- Subject should be "Up for a challenge?"
- Body of message should be "A challenge from Dr. Ingram Beat me at the tri, and I will buy! Dr. Ingram will buy lunch for the entire clinic if any of you beat him at the triathlon this year. All money donated goes to a good cause to help those in need. Have some fun and get lunch . . . maybe!"

✓ **You have completed Exercise 11.17**

Go to http://connect.mheducationl.com to complete this exercise.

Add a New Clinical User and Assign a Password (Refer to Chapter 7 for assistance.)

The healthcare professional has been on the job for a year and a half. Her supervisor feels that she is ready for some more administrative duties, so she is shown how to add a new user to Prime Suite. A new MA and a new care provider are starting today, so the healthcare professional sets up and assigns Prime Suite access rights to the new employees. The healthcare professional also sets up general security for password maintenance.

Add the new medical assistant, and assign a password and user rights in Prime Suite. Here is some information you will need:

- New medical assistant: Cecelia Strong
- DOB: 12/28/1989
- Password: *******
- User rights:
  - Default for Chart Registration
  - Check the boxes for Add patients or Persons to the System, View Patient or Person Registration Information, Modify Patient or Person Registration Information, Check-In Patients, View and Modify Chart Patient Flags, and View Clinical Alerts Flags. The SSN is 456-78-9101.

✓ **You have completed Exercise 11.18**

Set Up a Care Provider (Refer to Chapter 7 for assistance.)

Set up the new care provider in Prime Suite. Here is some information you will need:

- New provider: Ariana Gladstone, MD
- NPI: 1234567892
- State License: 789456
- DEA: GA1234567
- This care provider is On Staff and Billable.
- User ID: agladstone

☑ **You have completed Exercise 11.19**

Build a Master File in Prime Suite (Refer to Chapter 8 for assistance.)

The new provider wants specific criteria set up because her specialty is cardiology. This will allow her to enter data faster, as well as spend more time examining patients.

Build a master file for ROS in Prime Suite. Here is some information you will need:

- Click on Review of Systems admin.
- Choose Cardiovascular.
- Then choose (-) for chest pain, light-headedness, irregular heartbeats, and rapid heart rate.

☑ **You have completed Exercise 11.20**

Set General Security (Refer to Chapter 7 for assistance.)

Set General Security for password maintenance in Prime Suite. Here is some information you will need for System Configuration:

- Minimum Password Chars=8
- Days Password is Valid=60
- Inactivity limit=20
- Days prevent password reuse=180
- Banner="Have a great day!"

☑ **You have completed Exercise 11.21**

connect Go to http://connect.mheducationl.com to complete this exercise.

Create a Custom Report (Refer to Chapter 9 for assistance.)

One part of the healthcare professional's new duties is to build a report that identifies patients whose primary language is not English. The practice wants to see if it would be beneficial to have Spanish-speaking interpreters on staff rather than go through an agency and contract with interpreters.

Create a customer report in Prime Suite: Report for Primary Language is NOT English. Here is some information you will need:

- Go to Custom Reports.
- Choose Patient Demographics.
- Choose Patient Demographic Summary.
- In Current report filters, choose
  - Field Name: Patient: Primary Language
  - Operator Field: is not equal to
  - Match Value: type "English"
- Save report name "Patient Language Not English"
  - Description: Patients with primary language other than English
- Run the report.

☑ You have completed Exercise 11.22

Chapter 11 Source Documents

Greensburg Medical Center
REGISTRATION FORM
(Please Print)

Today's date: *June 18, 2016*	Care Provider: **Dr. Ingram**

PATIENT INFORMATION

Patient's last name:	First:	Middle:	☐ Mr. ☐ Mrs.	☐ Miss ☒ Ms.	Marital status (circle one)
Jacobi	*Harper*	*Anna*			(Single) / Mar / Div / Sep / Wid

Is this your legal name?	If not, what is your legal name?	(Former name):	Birth date:	Age:	Sex:
☒ Yes ☐ No			*05/15/1988*	*27*	☐ M ☒ F

Street address:	Social Security no.:	Home phone:	Cell phone:
117 Catawba Lane	*555-77-2222*	*770-555-5545*	*770-555-3528*

P. O. Box:	City:	State:	ZIP Code:
	Carrollton	*GA*	*30117*

Occupation:	Employer:	Employer phone no.:
Product Developer	*Greenway Medical Technologies*	*770-555-6666*

E-mail address: *hajacobi@greenwayhealth.com*

Race: *declined*	Ethnicity: *White – non Hispanic*	Primary language: *English*	Religion: *Protestant*

Other family members seen here: *none*

INSURANCE INFORMATION

(Presentation of Insurance Card is required at time of each visit)

Person responsible for bill:	Date of birth:	Address:	Home phone:	Cell phone:
Harper Anna Jacobi	*05/15/1988*	*117 Catawba Lane, Carrollton, GA 30117*	*770-555-5545*	*770-555-3528*

Is this person a patient here?	☐ Yes ☒ No

Occupation:	Employer:	Employer address:	Employer phone no.:
Product Developer	*Greenway Medical Technologies*	*4450 Greenway Blvd., Carrollton, GA 30117*	*770-555-6666*

Is this patient covered by insurance?	☒ Yes ☐ No

Please indicate primary insurance	☒ McGraw-Hill Healthmark Insurance	☐ BlueCross/ Blue Shield	☐ [Insurance]	☐ [Insurance]	☐ [Insurance]

☐ [Insurance]	☐ Workers' Compensation	☐ Medicare	☐ Medicaid *(Please provide card)*	☐ Other

Subscriber's name:	Subscriber's S.S. no.:	Date of birth:	Group no.:	Policy no.:	Co-payment:
Harper Anna Jacobi	*555-77-2222*	*05/15/1988*	*6500*	*HAJ5679015*	$ *20.00*

Patient's relationship to subscriber:	☒ Self	☐ Spouse	☐ Child	☐ Other	Effective Date: *01/06/2014*

Name of secondary insurance (if applicable): *None*	Subscriber's name:	Group no.:	Policy no.:

Patient's relationship to subscriber:	☒ Self	☐ Spouse	☐ Child	☐ Other

IN CASE OF EMERGENCY

Name of local friend or relative (not living at same address):	Relationship to patient:	Home phone no.:	Work phone no.:
		( )	( )

The above information is true to the best of my knowledge. I authorize my insurance benefits be paid directly to the physician. I understand that I am financially responsible for any balance. I also authorize [Name of Practice] or insurance company to release any information required to process my claims.

Harper Jacobi	*06/18/2016*
Patient/Guardian signature	Date

Source Document A Patient Registration Form

McGraw-Hill Healthmark.

Subscriber Name:

HARPER ANNA JACOBI

Identification Number:

HAJ5679045

Group Number: 6500	Office Copay $20
Coverage Date: 01/06/2014	Emergency Copay $100
	RX Generic Copay $25
SINGLE	RX Brand Copay $50
	RxID: 062788
	RxNFP: 6874

PPO℞

Source Document B   Insurance Card

Date:	6/20/2016	Provider: *Dr. Ingram*

Patient Name: *Harper Anna Jacobi*	DOB: *05/15/1988*	MRN: *1611*

Personal Health Information

Allergies (List all allergies and reactions)

Codeine, difficulty breathing and swelling of lips, tongue and throat. Reaction date 9/10/2001.

Medications (all prescription and over-the-counter)

Multivitamin once a day

Family Medical History (list age and health history)

Mother: *59 years old, diabetes Type II at 28 years*

Father: *62 years old, no medical problems*

Sister(s): *none*

Brother(s): *26 years old, asthma started at age 5*

Other:

Past Medical History	Yes	No	If yes, when?
Asthma		✓	
Bronchitis	✓		1998
Cancer		✓	
Diabetes		✓	
Gout		✓	
Heart Disease		✓	
Hernia		✓	
High Blood Pressure		✓	
High Cholesterol		✓	
HIV Positive		✓	
Kidney Disease		✓	
Liver Disease		✓	
Migraines		✓	
Pneumonia		✓	
Thyroid Problems		✓	
Other *seasonal allergies/hay fever*			
Other			
Surgeries (list below)			
Appendectomy		*2004*	

Social History (Check all that apply)

Tobacco Use: (Choose one)

Current – every day? _____

Current – occasional? _____ How often? _____

Former smoker? _____

Never smoked? ✓

Alcohol Use:

Non Drinker? _____

Social Drinker? *occasional* How often? *Monthly*

Heavy Drinker? _____ How often? _____

Caffeine Use: Yes ✓ No_ Type? *2 cups of coffee per day*

Marital Status:

Single ✓ Married _____

Divorced _____ Other _____

Education:

High school _____ College ✓ Post-graduate _____

Occupation: *Product Developer*

Language

Preferred language *English*

Current Medical Problems	Yes	No	Details
Unexplained weight loss		✓	
Headaches		✓	
Pain	✓		*sore throat*
Dental problems		✓	
Arthritis		✓	
Diarrhea/Constipation		✓	
Urinary problems	✓		*burning*
Menstrual problems		✓	
Fatigue		✓	
Problems with eating		✓	
Problems with memory		✓	
Chronic coughs/colds		✓	
Back problems		✓	
Other			

Source Document C   Patient Intake Sheet

Greensburg Medical Center
Office Visit Notes

Date:	6/20/2016 Provider: Dr. Ingram

Patient Name: Harper Anna Jacobi DOB: 05/15/1988	MRN: 1611

CC:	C/o sore throat and "burning with urination"
PI:	Pt states that she developed a sore throat about three days ago and has difficulty swallowing. She states that she may have had a fever, but has not taken her temperature. She has been treating her symptoms with OTC pain relievers, allergy medications, and throat spray with very little relief. Patient also states that she developed a burning sensation with urination about a week ago. She has experienced increased frequency and urgency, slight lower abdominal pain, and pressure with urination. She has been drinking cranberry juice and has increased her water intake with no improvement in symptoms.
ROS:	ROS Normal and pt reports no signs of blood in urination, no flank or back pain, no nausea/vomiting or chills/sweats, no recent changes in weight. Abnormals: + difficulty swallowing and throat pain ⊕ painful urination, frequency, urgency, and lower abd pain.
Vitals:	T: 99.8°F R: 26 P: 84 bpm BP: 112/74 mm HG Ⓡ arm, sitting Ht: 65 in Wt: 143#
Exam:	27 y/o female in no apparent acute distress, well nourished, well developed, alert, cooperative Exam: bilateral lymph nodes in the neck, throat is clear with slight tonsillar redness and swelling, abdomen soft, nontender and without distension. No notable splenic or hepatic enlargement or tenderness. Eyes: PERRLA Ears: External auditory canals and tympanic membrane clear. Nose: No nasal discharge. Lungs: Clear to auscultation and percussion. Cardiac: Regular rhythm, no peripheral edema, cyanosis, or pallor, no bruits.
Meds:	Multivitamin once a day. Allergic to codeine, results in difficulty breathing and swelling.
Tests:	Strep screen, urinalysis with microscopy
Rx:	Ciprofloxaxin 250 mg, administer 5 mL po bid x 7 days
F/U	Take antibiotic until gone, return to clinic if symptoms worsen or as needed, gargle with salt water for symptomatic relief of sore throat. Use Ibuprofen OTC 400 mg every 6 hours as needed for pain.

Source Document D   Office Visit Notes

McGraw-Hill Healthmark®

Greensburg Medical Center

PAGE: 1 OF 1
DATE: 07/22/2016
ID NUMBER: HAJ5679045

PROVIDER: JAMES INGRAM, M.D.

PATIENT: JACOBI, HARPER ANNA   CLAIM: 1659P1611

FROM DATE	THROUGH DATE	PROC CODE	UNIT	AMT BILL	AMT ALLOW	AMT PAID	DED	COPAY	ADJ	COIN	PROV PAID	REASON CODE*
06/20/16	06/20/16	99202	1	75.00	75.00	0.00	8.13	20.00	14.36	32.51	0.00	PR1/PR3
06/20/16	06/20/16	87880	1	25.00	25.00	5.02	4.82	0.00	15.16	0.00	0.00	PR1
06/20/16	06/20/16	81001	1	25.00	25.00	8.07	5.75	0.00	11.18	0.00	0.00	PR1
CLAIM TOTALS				125.00	125.00	13.09	18.70	20.00	40.70	32.51	0.00	

PAYMENT SUMMARY		TOTAL ALL CLAIMS		EFT INFORMATION	
TOTAL AMOUNT PAID	13.09	AMOUNT CHARGED	125.00	NUMBER	59715674
PRIOR CREDIT BALANCE	.00	AMOUNT ALLOWED	125.00	DATE	07/22/16
CURRENT CREDIT DEFERRED	.00	DEDUCTIBLE	18.70	AMOUNT	13.09
PRIOR CREDIT APPLIED	.00	COPAY	20.00		
NEW CREDIT BALANCE	.00	COINSURANCE	32.51		
NET DISPERSED	13.09				

*REASON CODES

PR1 - Deductible   PR3 – Co-pay   V – VOID   ADJ - Adjustment

Source Document E   Remittance Advice (RA)

CMS-1500

HEALTH INSURANCE CLAIM FORM

APPROVED BY NATIONAL UNIFORM CLAIM COMMITTEE (NUCC) 02/12

CARRIER

| | PICA | | | | | | | | PICA | |

1. MEDICARE ☐ (Medicare#) MEDICAID ☐ (Medicaid#) TRICARE ☐ (ID#/DoD#) CHAMPVA ☐ (Member ID#) GROUP HEALTH PLAN ☐ (ID#) FECA BLK LUNG ☐ (ID#) OTHER ☐ (ID#)

1a. INSURED 'S I.D. NUMBER (For Program in Item 1)

2. PATIENT 'S NAME (Last Name, First Name, Middle Initial)

3. PATIENT 'S BIRTH DATE MM DD YY SEX M ☐ F ☐

4. INSURED 'S NAME (Last Name, First Name, Middle Initial)

5. PATIENT 'S ADDRESS (No., Street)

6. PATIENT RELATIONSHIP TO INSURED Self ☐ Spouse ☐ Child ☐ Other ☐

7. INSURED 'S ADDRESS (No., Street)

CITY STATE

8. RESERVED FOR NUCC USE

CITY STATE

ZIP CODE TELEPHONE (Include Area Code) ( )

ZIP CODE TELEPHONE (Include Area Code) ( )

9. OTHER INSURED 'S NAME (Last Name, First Name, Middle Initial)

10. IS PATIENT 'S CONDITION RELATED TO:

11. INSURED 'S POLICY GROUP OR FECA NUMBER

a. OTHER INSURED 'S POLICY OR GROUP NUMBER

a. EMPLOYMENT? (Current or Previous) YES ☐ NO ☐

a. INSURED 'S DATE OF BIRTH MM DD YY SEX M ☐ F ☐

b. RESERVED FOR NUCC USE

b. AUTO ACCIDENT? YES ☐ NO ☐ PLACE (State)

b. OTHER CLAIM ID (Designated by NUCC)

c. RESERVED FOR NUCC USE

c. OTHER ACCIDENT? YES ☐ NO ☐

c. INSURANCE PLAN NAME OR PROGRAM NAME

d. INSURANCE PLAN NAME OR PROGRAM NAME

10d. CLAIM CODES (Designated by NUCC)

d. IS THERE ANOTHER HEALTH BENEFIT PLAN? YES ☐ NO ☐ **If yes**, complete items 9, 9a, and 9d.

PATIENT AND INSURED INFORMATION

READ BACK OF FORM BEFORE COMPLETING & SIGNING THIS FORM.

12. PATIENT 'S OR AUTHORIZED PERSON 'S SIGNATURE I authorize the release of any medical or other information necessary to process this claim. I also request payment of government benefits either to myself or to the party who accepts assignment below.

SIGNED _____ DATE _____

13. INSURED 'S OR AUTHORIZED PERSON 'S SIGNATURE I authorize payment of medical benefits to the undersigned physician or supplier for services described below.

SIGNED _____

14. DATE OF CURRENT ILLNESS, INJURY, or PREGNANCY (LMP) MM DD YY QUAL.

15. OTHER DATE QUAL. MM DD YY

16. DATES PATIENT UNABLE TO WORK IN CURRENT OCCUPATION MM DD YY FROM TO MM DD YY

17. NAME OF REFERRING PROVIDER OR OTHER SOURCE

17a.

17b. NPI

18. HOSPITALIZATION DATES RELATED TO CURRENT SERVICES MM DD YY FROM TO MM DD YY

19. ADDITIONAL CLAIM INFORMATION (Designated by NUCC)

20. OUTSIDE LAB? YES ☐ NO ☐ $ CHARGES

21. DIAGNOSIS OR NATURE OF ILLNESS OR INJURY Relate A-L to service line below (24E) ICD Ind.

A. ____ B. ____ C. ____ D. ____
E. ____ F. ____ G. ____ H. ____
I. ____ J. ____ K. ____ L. ____

22. RESUBMISSION CODE ORIGINAL REF. NO.

23. PRIOR AUTHORIZATION NUMBER

24. A. DATE(S) OF SERVICE						B. PLACE OF SERVICE	C. EMG	D. PROCEDURES, SERVICES, OR SUPPLIES (Explain Unusual Circumstances)		E. DIAGNOSIS POINTER	F. $ CHARGES	G. DAYS OR UNITS	H. EPSDT Family Plan	I. ID. QUAL.	J. RENDERING PROVIDER ID. #
From MM	DD	YY	To MM	DD	YY			CPT/HCPCS	MODIFIER						
1														NPI	
2														NPI	
3														NPI	
4														NPI	
5														NPI	
6														NPI	

PHYSICIAN OR SUPPLIER INFORMATION

25. FEDERAL TAX I.D. NUMBER SSN ☐ EIN ☐

26. PATIENT 'S ACCOUNT NO.

27. ACCEPT ASSIGNMENT? (For govt. claims, see back) YES ☐ NO ☐

28. TOTAL CHARGE $

29. AMOUNT PAID $

30. Rsvd for NUCC Use

31. SIGNATURE OF PHYSICIAN OR SUPPLIER INCLUDING DEGREES OR CREDENTIALS (I certify that the statements on the reverse apply to this bill and are made a part thereof.)

SIGNED _____ DATE _____

32. SERVICE FACILITY LOCATION INFORMATION

a. NPI b.

33. BILLING PROVIDER INFO & PH # ( )

a. NPI b.

NUCC Instruction Manual available at: www.nucc.org *PLEASE PRINT OR TYPE* APPROVED OMB-0938-1197 FORM 1500 (02-12)

UB-04

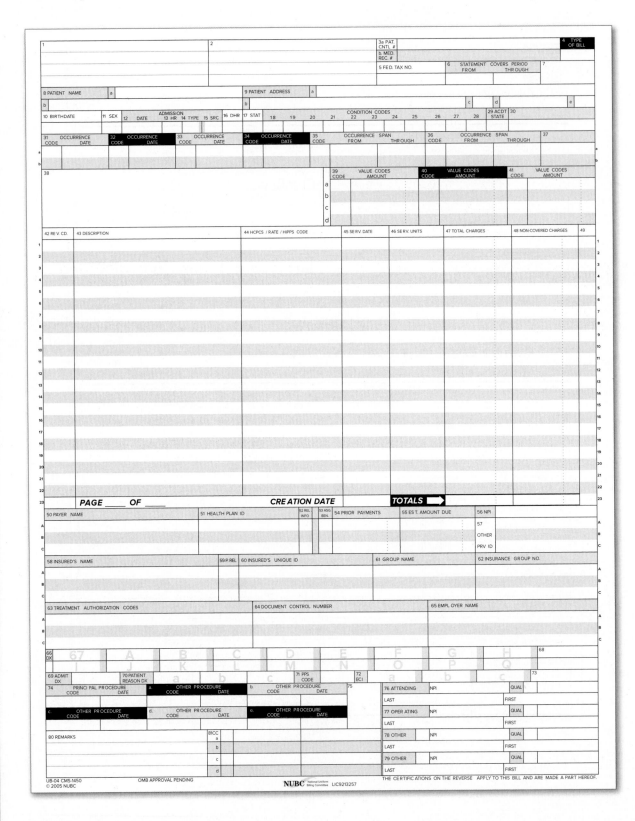

glossary

a

Abuse   Coding and billing that is inconsistent with typical coding and billing practices.

Access report   A report of all persons (within the facility) who have had access to a patient's protected health information.

Accountable Care Organization (ACO)   A reimbursement model where hospitals, physicians, and other healthcare providers form partnerships whereby all are accountable for the quality of care, efficiency of medical services (to contain costs), and patient satisfaction; a pay-for-performance model of healthcare reimbursement.

Accounting of disclosures   Providing the patient, upon request, with a listing of all disclosures of his/her health information, both internally and externally.

Accounts payable   Monies being paid from the medical practice—for instance, to pay for supplies, rent, utilities, payroll, etc.

Accounts receivable   Monies coming into a medical practice—for instance, insurance payments or payments made by patients.

Adjudication   The process of reviewing claims to determine payment.

Administrative data   Identifying information, insurance-related information, authorizations, and business correspondence found in a patient's health record.

Affordable Care Act (ACA)   Signed into law in 2010, the ACA resulted in improved access to affordable healthcare coverage and protection from abusive practices by healthcare insurance companies. Gives consumers more control over their healthcare coverage and ties reimbursement to quality, patient satisfaction, and coordination of care.

Aggregate   The sum total; for instance, the sum total of patients between the ages of 60 and 100 in a practice as opposed to a separate listing for each patient between the ages of 60 and 100.

American Health Information Management Association (AHIMA)   A professional association for the field of health information management.

American Recovery and Reinvestment Act (ARRA)   Signed into law by President Obama on February 17, 2009; this economic "stimulus plan" includes provisions for the Health Information Technology for Economic and Clinical Health (HITECH) Act.

Application   Software that has a special purpose, such as word processing or spreadsheet, or for a particular industry such as practice management or electronic health record software.

Audit trail   A permanent record or accounting of accesses, additions, amendments, or deletions to a health record. Also a report that shows accesses by user to each function of the software.

b

Benchmarking   Comparison of one set of statistics to the overall statistics when the same variables are used for each.

Blog   Ongoing conversations about a topic that take place online via the Internet.

Breach of confidentiality   Releasing information without a required, properly executed authorization or as restricted by law.

c

Care provider   Term used to refer to a physician, physician's assistant, dentist, psychologist, nurse practitioner, or midwife.

Centers for Medicare and Medicaid Services (CMS)   An agency of the Department of Health and Human Services, responsible for administering the Medicare and Medicaid programs.

Certification Commission for Health Information Technology (CCHIT)   A nonprofit, nongovernmental agency whose purpose was to certify electronic health records for functionality, interoperability, and security.

Certified Electronic Health Record Technology (CEHRT)   A complement to Meaningful Use Stage 2; certification by the Office of the National Coordinator (ONC) of EHR software that meets certain standards.

Chief complaint   The reason for which a patient has made an appointment (usually in his/her own words, for instance, "I have a sore throat.").

Clearinghouse   A service that processes data into a standardized billing format and checks for inconsistencies or other errors in the data.

Clinical decision support (CDS)   Allows access to current treatment options for a disease, through electronic or remote methods. Alerts the care provider to possible medication interactions, gives treatment options based on results of clinical trials or research, and alerts the provider that a patient may have a particular diagnosis based on the data found in the patient's electronic record.

Clinical Documentation Architecture (CDA)   Developed by HL7, a document markup standard that specifies the structure and semantics of clinical documents such as discharge summary, operative report, etc.

Cloning (copy and paste)   Used in an electronic environment, copying similar or identical information from a previous encounter of the same or a different patient.

Cloud computing   The housing of data in a cloud environment, which is a commercially maintained site on the Internet.

CMS-1500   The form used by physicians' offices to submit insurance claims.

Co-payment (co-pay)   The amount due from the patient at the time of the office visit; typically a requirement of managed care plans.

Code linkage   On an insurance claim, this is the relationship between each procedure (CPT code) and a diagnosis (ICD-10 code) to demonstrate medical necessity.

Coinsurance   A form of cost-sharing in which the insurance carrier pays a percentage of the claim and the patient pays the remaining percentage. Medicare, for example, has an 80-20 coinsurance, in which Medicare pays 80% and the patient pays 20% of the charges.

Compliance plan   A formal, written document that describes how the hospital or physician's practice ensures rules, regulations, and standards are being adhered to.

Computer virus   A deviant program, stored on a flash drive, hard drive, or CD, that can cause unexpected and often undesirable effects, such as destroying or corrupting data.

Computerized physician order entry (CPOE)   Entering physician orders electronically rather than on paper. The order is transmitted directly to the appropriate department; for instance, an order for an x-ray would go directly to the radiology department, whereas an order for a CBC would go directly to the laboratory.

Confidentiality   The patient's right to expect that his/her health information will not be released to any person or entity without the patient/guardian's written authorization or as required by law or regulation.

Continuity of Care Document (CCD)   A document exchange standard used to share patient summary information, such as in the case of a patient being referred from one healthcare provider to another.

Core objectives   Basic functions or collection of data that should be completed on a patient's visit or hospitalization.

Covered entity   Any healthcare entity that captures or utilizes health information. These include healthcare plans (insurance companies), clearinghouses that process healthcare claims, individual physicians and physician practices, any type of therapist (mental health, physical, speech, occupational), dentists, hospital staffs, ambulatory facilities, nursing homes, home health agencies, pharmacies, and employers.

Credentialing   The process of ensuring a care provider has the proper qualifications (education, experience, malpractice coverage) to practice medicine.

Current Procedural Terminology (CPT)   Coding system used to convert narrative procedures and services into numeric form. CPT is used to code procedures and services in a physician's office; in a hospital setting, it is used for outpatient coding (emergency room, outpatient diagnostic testing, or ambulatory surgery, for example).

Custom report   Report that is designed by the office or hospital rather than coming as part of a software package (standard report).

d

Dashboard   A visual comparison of actual performance to required performance.

Data   A single, raw fact such as a patient's name, height, or weight. Often used interchangeably with information, though they are not synonymous terms.

Data dictionary   A document that specifies the format of each data field as well as a detailed explanation or definition for that field, which allows for consistency of data collection.

Data integrity   Maintaining the accuracy and consistency of data.

Decryption   Interpretation of data being received in encrypted (scrambled) form.

Deductible   The out-of-pocket payment amount that a policyholder must meet before insurance covers the service(s).

Default value   A value that automatically appears in a field each time it appears on a screen (e.g., the current date in a date field, the local area code in a home phone number field).

Demographic (identifying) data   Data that identify the patient. Consist of name, date of birth, sex, race, and Social Security number (may vary by facility policy).

Detail report   Any report that includes patient identifying information and lists each case individually rather than as total number of cases.

Directory information   The fact that a patient is an inpatient (or being treated as an outpatient) as well as his/her location within the facility.

Disaster recovery plan   A written document that details an inventory of hardware and software, backup procedure, including location of backup files, the system used to alert users of the disaster, required security training for personnel, and procedure for restoring backup files.

Discharge summary   A report completed by a care provider that summarizes a patient's stay in the hospital. It generally includes the final diagnoses, a summary of the patient's course in the hospital, any procedures performed, a recap of diagnostic results, and discharge instructions.

Drug formulary   A list of provider-preferred generic and brand-name drugs covered under various insurance plans.

#

Electronic claims submission   Submitting insurance claims via wire to a clearinghouse or directly to the insurance carrier.

Electronic health record (EHR)   Comprehensive record of all health records for a patient, which is able to be shared electronically with other health providers as necessary.

Electronic medical record (EMR)   The legal patient record that is created within any healthcare facility (hospital, nursing home, ambulatory surgery facility, physician's office, etc.). The EMR is the data source for the electronic health record (EHR).

Encounter form   A document (paper or electronic) that is used in medical offices to capture the diagnoses and services or procedures performed and from which the CMS-1500 billing form is completed. Also known as a routing slip or Superbill.

Encryption   A security method in which words are scrambled and can only be read if the receiver has a special code to decipher the scrambled message.

ePrescribing   Electronically transmitting prescriptions from care provider to pharmacy.

Evaluation and Management (E&M)   The CPT codes used to capture the face-to-face time between a patient and the care provider; takes into consideration the extent of the history, the extent of the physical exam, and the level of medical decision making required.

Evidence-based medicine Diagnostic and treatment protocols that are based on proven research and documented best practices.

Explanation of benefits (EOB) An explanation of the charges for services, the amount paid by the insurance company, and the amount due by the subscriber, which is sent to the subscriber (and to the provider, in some instances).

f

Family history (FH) Documentation of conditions and diseases found in immediate family members (e.g., diabetes mellitus, cancer, or heart disease).

Fee schedule The amount charged for services rendered in a physician's office by Current Procedural Terminology (CPT) code.

Firewall A system of hardware and/or software that protects a computer or a network from intruders by filtering activity over the network.

Flag A message that appears on a screen in written form or as an icon to serve as a reminder to staff and care providers.

Fraud Intentional deception, which in healthcare takes advantage of a patient, an insurance company, Medicare, or Medicaid.

h

Hardware The tangible items that are used in automation (e.g., the processing unit, screen, keyboard, mouse, laptops, hand-held devices).

Health informatics The management of automated health information; the technological side of managing health information—the design, development, structure, implementation, integration, and management of the technical aspects of electronic (automated) health record-keeping.

Health information exchange (HIE) The movement or sharing of information between healthcare entities in a secure manner and in keeping with nationally recognized standards.

Health information management (HIM) A profession that encompasses services in planning, collecting, aggregating, analyzing, and disseminating individual patient and aggregate clinical data (in paper or electronic format).

Health Information Technology for Economic and Clinical Health (HITECH) Act A portion of the American Recovery and Reinvestment Act (ARRA) that is meant to increase the use of an electronic health record by hospitals and physicians through a monetary incentive program.

Health Insurance Portability and Accountability Act (HIPAA) Passed in 1996, this act includes regulations that afford people who leave their employment the ability to keep their insurance or obtain new health insurance even if they have a pre-existing medical condition. Also sets standards for storing, maintaining, and sharing electronic health information while ensuring its privacy and security.

Health Level Seven (HL7) A set of standards that makes sharing of data between or among healthcare entities possible.

Healthcare administrator A leadership position within a healthcare facility, including chief executive officer, chief operating officer, chief financial officer, chief information officer, or other higher-level management positions. May also be referred to as healthcare manager or health systems manager.

Healthcare Common Procedure Coding System (HCPCS) Coding system required by Medicare and Medicaid to document services and procedures (Level 1, Current Procedural Terminology, CPT) and equipment, supplies, and transport (HCPCS Level 2).

Healthcare Information and Management Systems Society (HIMSS) An association of health informatics and information professionals formed to promote a better understanding of healthcare informatics and management systems.

Healthcare Integrity and Protection Data Bank (HIPDB) A database of adverse actions related to fraud and abuse.

Healthcare systems administrator A leadership position specifically responsible for the information technology (IT) functions within an organization or facility. May also be known as a chief information officer.

History &Physical (H&P) A report completed by a care provider that includes the reason(s) the patient is being seen or admitted; the history of present illness; the pertinent past medical, surgical, social, and family histories; other current conditions/diseases the patient is being treated for; the report of a physical examination; working diagnoses; and plan of care.

History of present illness (HPI) The patient's description of current complaints such as when the symptoms started, the location of the condition, quality of the symptoms, severity of the symptoms, anything that makes the symptoms better or worse, and additional symptoms the patient is experiencing.

i

In-network Care providers who contract with a managed care plan to offer services to members of the managed care plan at a prenegotiated rate.

Index A listing—for instance, a Diagnosis Index is a report that is sorted by diagnosis code and includes the total number of patients seen with that disease for a given period of time; a Master Patient Index (MPI) is a listing of all patients who have ever been seen in a hospital or a practice.

Information Raw facts that, when viewed as a whole, have meaning. Example: a report of all patients treated in the emergency department of Memorial Medical Center with a primary diagnosis of streptococcal pharyngitis (strep throat), sorted by patients' age.

Information governance As defined by AHIMA, information governance is "the enterprise-wide framework for managing information throughout its lifecycle and supporting the organization's strategy, operations, regulatory, legal, risk and environmental requirements."

Institute of Medicine (IOM) An independent, nonprofit, nongovernmental organization that works to provide unbiased and authoritative advice to decision makers and the public.

Insurance plan The medical insurance contract under which a patient is covered; the extent to which services are covered. Also referred to as "the plan."

Insurance verification   The process of contacting the insurance carrier and receiving validation of coverage for that patient, deductible status, and co-pay amount.

Interface   The ability of one computer system or component to accept or send data to another system without loss of integrity or meaning.

International Classification of Diseases, 10th revision, Clinical Modification/Procedure Coding System (ICD-10-CM/PCS)   The classification system used to convert narrative diagnoses and procedures into numeric codes. Effective October 1, 2015, replaced ICD-9-CM.

Internet   A series of networks that allow instant access to information from around the world.

Interoperability   Many different functions can take place and information can be shared between computer systems, or within applications of the same computer system, which is not possible with a manual or paper record system.

Intranet   A secure environment or private internal network that is available only to a select group (e.g., the staff within an organization).

l

Library   In computer software, a listing or choice of entities, for instance, employers, insurance plans, ICD-10-CM codes, or CPT codes.

Live   The point at which computer software or systems are put into real-time use within a practice or hospital.

Local area network (LAN)   Links computers and related devices that are physically close to one another such as within a building.

m

Malware   Malware is short for malicious software and includes deviant software such as worms, viruses, and Trojan horses, all of which attack computer programs.

Managed care plan   Insurance plan that promotes quality, cost-effective healthcare through monitoring of patients, preventive care, and performance.

Master file   Dataset that provides structure and is the building block for parts of chart notes within an EHR.

Master Patient Index (MPI)/Patient List   A permanent listing of all patients who have received care in a hospital (inpatient or outpatient). In physicians' offices often referred to as a Master Patient List or Patient List. May also be known as a Master Person List or Master Person Index.

Meaningful Use   Part of the requirements of the Health Information Technology for Economic and Clinical Health (HITECH) Act which is meant to increase the use of an electronic health record through monetary incentives provided the EHR is used in a meaningful way to improve patient care. At the time of publication, the Meaningful Use regulations are undergoing revision.

Medical necessity   The fact that there is a medical reason to perform a procedure or service. Documentation exists in the patient's record to show there are sufficient signs, symptoms, or history to warrant the services provided.

Medical record number   A unique number assigned to each patient seen by a facility or office.

Medicare Access and CHIP Reauthorization Act (MACRA)   Ends the Sustainable Growth Rate formula that had been used to determine payments to providers for healthcare services billed to Medicare beneficiaries. Also known as the Doc Fix Act.

Menu objectives   Additional functions that allow for greater use of EHR functionality.

Merit-based Incentive Payment System (MIPS)   A reimbursement system that replaces the Sustainable Growth Rate formula previously used by Medicare Part B to a value-based system. The value-based system is called the Quality Payment Program.

Merit-based Incentive Program (MIPS)   A new Medicare provider payment program based on quality of care, resource use, clinical practice improvement, and meaningful use of certified EHR technology.

Minimum necessary information   As required by the Health Insurance Portability and Accountability Act (HIPAA), releasing the minimum information to satisfy the reason the information is needed or the minimum necessary to perform a job function.

n

National Health Information Network (NHIN)   A set of standards, services, and policies that enable the secure exchange of health information over the Internet.

National Practitioner Data Bank (NPDB)   Required by law, a database of malpractice payouts, revocation of privileges, licensure denial or suspension, denial of medical staff privileges, and similar actions.

National Provider Identifier (NPI)   A unique, 10-digit identifier, issued by the Centers for Medicare and Medicaid Services (CMS), that must be used on insurance claims to identify the care provider and/or group practice that rendered care to the patient.

Notice of Privacy Practices   A requirement of the Health Insurance Portability and Accountability Act (HIPAA) that patients are made aware (in writing) of their rights under HIPAA including the fact that the patient has the right to view/receive a copy of his/her own record, the fact that amendment to the documentation may be requested, the ways in which their health information will be used and released to outside entities, and the procedure to file a complaint with the Department of Health and Human Services.

o

Office of the National Coordinator for Health Information Technology (ONC)   The principal federal entity charged with coordination, implementation, and use of health information technology and the electronic exchange of health information.

Optical character recognition (OCR)   Technology that converts a document into a format that is computer readable—that is, into an electronic file.

p

Password   A unique code, known only to the user, that is used to gain access to computer applications.

Past medical history (PMH)   Previous medical condition(s) for which the patient has been treated.

Patient portal   A method of accessing portions of one's own health information from the care provider's or hospital's electronic health record.

Patient-Centered Medical Home (PCMH)   A model that was developed to care for patients with chronic conditions by the American Academy of Family Practitioners, to encourage and facilitate a patient's (and family's) involvement in his or her own care.

Personal digital assistant (PDA)   A mobile device that is small enough to fit in one's hand, yet allows access to local area networks (LANs), wide area networks (WANs), and the Internet; may also have telephone capability.

Personal health record (PHR)   A record, kept by the patient, that contains a person's health history, immunization status, current and past medications, allergies, and instructions given by a care provider; it often includes patient education materials as well.

Physical exam (PE)   An examination of the patient's body for signs of disease.

Physician Quality Reporting Initiative (PQRI)   A voluntary pay-for-performance incentive program. Participating care providers submit data on any of the 100 designated quality measures and receive monetary incentives for doing so.

Picture Archiving and Communication System (PACS)   Computerized system for enhanced viewing and sharing of images such as x-rays, scans, ultrasounds, and mammograms.

Point of care (POC)   Documentation, dictation, ordering of tests and procedures that occur at the same time the patient is being seen.

Practice management (PM)   Software used in physicians' offices to gather data on every patient and perform administrative functions from the time an appointment is made through the time the bill for each visit is paid.

Privacy   The right to be left alone; the right to expect that one's personal space is respected while undergoing healthcare.

Problem list   A listing kept in the patient's health record of all of his/her current (active) and resolved medical conditions.

Protected health information (PHI)   Any piece of information that identifies a patient, including a patient's name, date of birth, address, email, telephone number, employer, relatives' names, Social Security number, medical record number, account numbers tied to the patient, fingerprints, photographs, and characteristics about the patient that would automatically disclose his or her identity. PHI also includes any clinical information about an identified patient.

q

Quality Reporting Document Architecture (QRDA)   Based on HL7's approved Clinical Documentation Architecture (CDA), QRDA is a data standard used for reporting quality measure data and that is EHR compatible across different health IT systems.

Query   Searching a database for patients who meet certain criteria.

r

Regional extension center (REC)   An organization that assists healthcare providers with the selection and implementation of electronic health record systems.

Regional Health Information Organization (RHIO)   Healthcare organizations in a geographic area that exchange health information with the goal of improving patient care, reducing duplication, and reducing unnecessary costs.

Registry   A listing that is filed in chronological order based on when something occurred. Examples include a birth registry, a death registry, a cancer registry, and a trauma registry.

Remittance advice (RA)   A detailed accounting of the claims for which payment is being made by an insurance company. The remittance advice accompanies the payment from the insurance company.

Resolution   The quality of a scanned image as it will appear in the record. The higher the resolution, the crisper the image.

Review of systems (ROS)   A body-system-by-body-system inventory of any symptoms the patient is having or has had based on a series of questions asked by the care provider.

Routing Slip   A document (paper or electronic) that is used in medical offices to capture the diagnoses and services or procedures performed and from which the CMS-1500 billing form is completed. Also known as a Superbill or encounter form.

s

Scanner   A piece of equipment that digitizes documents into a format that is readable by a computer.

Scribe   An assistant who enters data either in writing or electronically into the health record as the care provider verbally dictates recent findings.

Smartphone   Telephone that allows Internet browsing, audio, video, and camera functionality.

SOAP   An acronym for the documentation used in a care provider's office to record the patient's symptoms, signs, assessment (diagnosis), and plan of care.

Social history (SH)   Lifestyle or social habits of the patient. Examples include smoking history or current use, use of alcoholic beverages and frequency, patient's profession, etc.

Social media   Interactive communication sites via the Internet. Examples are Facebook, YouTube, Instagram, Snapchat, and Twitter.

Speech recognition technology   Software that recognizes the words being said by the person dictating and converts the speech to text.

Structured data   Data that fit a particular model or format, which can be tracked and may be part of a database. Examples include ICD-10-CM/PCS codes, CPT codes, a patient's temperature, or a patient's age.

Subscriber   The primary person covered by an insurance plan.

Summary report   A statistical report that includes totals rather than data for individual patients. Examples include a report of total patients seen during a particular time by gender; a report of the total number of patients seen in the office with E&M code 99214.

Superbill   A document (paper or electronic) that is used in medical offices to capture the diagnoses and services or procedures performed and from which the CMS-1500 billing form is completed. Also known as a routing slip or encounter form.

Surgical history   Previous surgical procedure(s) the patient has undergone, the approximate date(s), name of surgeon, reason for procedure(s), and complications, if any.

t

Tablet computer   Computer that is larger than a PDA or smartphone yet smaller than a laptop computer; allows access to local area networks (LANs), wide area networks (WANs), and the Internet.

Telehealth   Associated with preventive care, telehealth is the use of audiovisual equipment through which the patient and the care provider or healthcare professional can connect remotely.

Telemedicine   The use of technology to remotely monitor a patient's vital signs and perform tests such as an EKG, or forward radiologic images.

Templates   Preformatted documents built into practice management and electronic health record systems.

Transactions   Posting of charges and the payment of claims in the practice management system to update patients' accounts.

u

UB-04   The form used to submit insurance claims for hospital patients.

Unstructured data   Data in the form of words or audio files that cannot be tracked. Examples include emails, written narratives, and audio files from speech recognition technology.

User rights   The limitations of one's access to the functionality of the software as defined by one's job description or position within the organization.

v

Variable   In relation to a statistical report, the factor that varies from one patient to the next. Examples include age, ZIP code, and diagnoses.

Virtual private network (VPN)   Software that encrypts (codes) the data being sent as well as interprets the data being received.

Vital signs   Measurements taken (temperature, heart rate, respiratory rate, blood pressure, height and weight, and sometimes body mass index) to determine the status of basic body system functions.

Voice recognition technology   Software that recognizes the words being said by the person dictating and converts speech to text; differs from speech recognition because voice recognition "learns" the voice of the dictator and is therefore more accurate.

w

Wi-Fi   Data exchange via high radio frequency.

Wide area network (WAN)   Connects computer networks together that are not physically close.